T0177561

ETHICAL CONSIDERATIONS AT THE INTERSECTION OF PSYCHIATRY AND RELIGION

Ethical Considerations at the Intersection of Psychiatry and Religion

Edited by John R. Peteet, M.D.
ASSOCIATE PROFESSOR OF PSYCHIATRY
HARVARD MEDICAL SCHOOL

Mary Lynn Dell, M.D., D.Min.
DIRECTOR OF PSYCHOSOMATIC MEDICINE
PROFESSOR OF CLINICAL PSYCHIATRY AND PEDIATRICS
NATIONWIDE CHILDREN'S HOSPITAL
THE OHIO STATE UNIVERSITY

Wai Lun Alan Fung, M.D., Sc.D., FRCPC
CHAIR OF RESEARCH ETHICS BOARD
NORTH YORK GENERAL HOSPITAL
ASSISTANT PROFESSOR OF PSYCHIATRY
UNIVERSITY OF TORONTO FACULTY OF MEDICINE

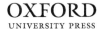

OXFORD
UNIVERSITY PRESS

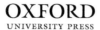

OXFORD
UNIVERSITY PRESS

Oxford University Press is a department of the University of Oxford. It furthers
the University's objective of excellence in research, scholarship, and education
by publishing worldwide. Oxford is a registered trade mark of Oxford University
Press in the UK and certain other countries.

Published in the United States of America by Oxford University Press
198 Madison Avenue, New York, NY 10016, United States of America.

© Oxford University Press 2018

All rights reserved. No part of this publication may be reproduced, stored in
a retrieval system, or transmitted, in any form or by any means, without the
prior permission in writing of Oxford University Press, or as expressly permitted
by law, by license, or under terms agreed with the appropriate reproduction
rights organization. Inquiries concerning reproduction outside the scope of the
above should be sent to the Rights Department, Oxford University Press, at the
address above.

You must not circulate this work in any other form
and you must impose this same condition on any acquirer.

CIP data is on file at the Library of Congress
978–0–19–068196–8

1 3 5 7 9 8 6 4 2

Printed by Sheridan Books, Inc., United States of America

In honor and appreciation of the late James W. Fowler, MDiv, PhD, whose knowledge and vision of practical theology, ethics and mental health have inspired clinicians, ethicists and theologians in their strivings for interdisciplinary dialogue and scholarship.

Contents

Acknowledgments

We are deeply grateful for the thoughtful contributions of chapter authors, the skilled encouragement of Oxford University Press staff, and the generosity and understanding of our families, without whom this work would not have been possible. In particular, Alan Fung would like to express his sincerest appreciation to his parents, Thomas and Joannie; his wife, Rhoda; and his son, Andrew - for their unceasing love and support throughout the preparation of this book.

Contributors

Shad S. Ali, M.D.
Child and Adolescent Psychiatry Fellow
Department of Psychiatry
University of Colorado School of Medicine

Tony B. Benning, M.D.
Clinical Instructor in Psychiatry
University of British Columbia
Vancouver, British Columbia

Nathan Carlin, Ph.D.
Christopher C. H. Cook, M.B., B.S., M.D.,
    M.A., Ph.D.
Professor of Spirituality
Theology & Health
Durham University, UK

Quirino Cordeiro, M.D., Ph.D.
Professor and chair of the Department of
    Psychiatry
Faculdade de Ciências Médicas da Santa
    Casa de São Paulo (FCMSCSP)
São Paulo SP, Brazil

Mary Lynn Dell, M.D., D.Min.
Professor of Clinical Psychiatry and Pediatrics
The Ohio State University
Director, Psychosomatic Medicine
Nationwide Children's Hospital
Priest Associate, St. Mark's Episcopal Church
Columbus, Ohio

Wai Lun Alan Fung, M.D., Sc.D., FRCPC
Chair of Research Ethics Board
North York General Hospital
Assistant Professor of Psychiatry
University of Toronto Faculty of Medicine
Toronto, Ontario, Canada

William Gaventa, M.Div.
Director, Summer Institute on Theology and
    Disability
Director, Collaborative on Faith and
    Disability
Waco, Texas

Eilish Gilvarry, M.B., M.Ch., B.A.O.
Honorary Professor of Addiction Psychiatry
Newcastle University, UK

Gerrit Glas, M.D., M.A., Ph.D.
Dooyeweerd Chair
Department of Philosophy
Vrije Universiteit Amsterdam
The Netherlands
Director of Residency Training, Dimence
    Groep, Zwolle, The Netherlands

Glenn Goss, D.S.W.
Open Doors International

James L. Griffith, M.D.
Leon M. Yochelson Professor and Chairman
Department of Psychiatry and Human Behavior
The George Washington University School of
    Medicine and Health Sciences
Washington, D.C.

Daniel H. Grossoehme, M.Div., D.Min.
Associate Professor of Pediatrics
Division of Pulmonary Medicine
University of Cincinnati Academic
    Health Center
Staff Chaplain III
Department of Pastoral Care
Cincinnati Children's Hospital
    Medical Center
Assisting Priest, St. Thomas Episcopal
    Church, Terrace Park, Ohio

Andrea Hearn, B.Sc. (hons), Ph.D., M.B., B.S.
Consultant Psychiatrist
Northumberland, Tyne & Wear NHS
    Foundation Trust, UK

Marta Herschkopf, M.D., M.St.
Beth Israel Deaconess Medical Center
Center for Bioethics
Harvard Medical School
Boston, Massachusetts

Allan M. Josephson, M.D.
Professor and Chief
Division of Child and Adolescent Psychiatry
    and Psychology
Department of Pediatrics
University of Louisville School of Medicine
Louisville, Kentucky

Samuel E. Karff, D.H.L. Chair
Associate Professor
Director of the Medical Humanities and
    Ethics Certificate Program
The University of Texas Health Science
    Center at Houston
McGovern Medical School
The McGovern Center for Humanities
    and Ethics
Houston, Texas

Nancy C. Kehoe, RSCJ, Ph.D.
Assistant Clinical Professor of Psychology,
    Part Time
Harvard Medical School
Boston, Massachusetts

Carol L. Kessler, M.D., M.Div.
Community Child and Adolescent Psychiatrist
Astor Services for Children
Bronx, New York
Ordained Pastor in the Evangelical Lutheran
    Church of America

Harold G. Koenig, M.D., M.H.Sc.
Professor of Psychiatry & Behavioral Sciences
    Associate Professor of Medicine
Director
Center for Spirituality, Theology, and Health
Duke University Medical Center
Durham, North Carolina

James W. Lomax, M.D.
Professor of Psychiatry
Baylor College of Medicine
Houston, Texas

Gina Magyar-Russell, Ph.D.
Fellow
Department of Psychiatry and Behavioral
    Sciences
Johns Hopkins Bloomberg School of
    Public Health
Baltimore, Maryland

Morgan M. Medlock, M.D., M.Div.
Commonwealth Fund Mongan Fellow in
    Minority Health Policy
Harvard Medical School
Boston, Massachusetts

Alexander Moreira-Almeida, M.D., Ph.D.
Associate Professor of Psychiatry
School of Medicine
Federal University of Juiz de Fora (UFJF)
Brazil
Director of the Research Center in
    Spirituality and Health (NUPES) at UFJF
Brazil

Michael A. Norko, M.D., M.A.R.
Associate Professor of Psychiatry
Yale University School of Medicine
Director of Forensic Services, Connecticut
Department of Mental Health and Addiction
  Services
New Haven, Connecticut

Abraham M. Nussbaum, M.D., M.T.S.
Chief Education Officer, Denver Health
Associate Professor
Department of Psychiatry
University of Colorado School of Medicine

John R. Peteet, M.D.
Associate Professor of Psychiatry
Harvard Medical School
Boston, Massachusetts

Don C. Postema, Ph.D.
Program Director for Medical Bioethics,
  HealthPartners
Minneapolis, Minnesota
Ethicist-in-Residence, Gillette Children's
  Specialty Healthcare, St. Paul, Minnesota
Professor of Philosophy Emeritus, College of
  Arts and Sciences
Bethel University, St. Paul, Minnesota

David H. Rosmarin, Ph.D., ABPP
McLean Hospital
Harvard Medical School
Boston, Massachusetts

Walid Sarhan, M.B., B.S., FRCPsych
Consultant Psychiatrist
Aman, Jordan

Len Sperry, M.D., Ph.D.
Professor of Mental Health Counseling and
  Director of Clinical Training
Florida Atlantic University
Boca Raton, FL

Samuel B. Thielman, M.D., Ph.D.
Adjunct Assoc. Professor of Psychiatry
Department of Psychiatry and Behavioral
  Sciences
Duke University School of Medicine
Durham, North Carolina

ONE

Introduction

John R. Peteet, M.D., Mary Lynn Dell, M.D., D.Min.,
and Wai Lun Alan Fung, M.D., Sc.D., FRCPC

PSYCHIATRY AND RELIGION/SPIRITUALITY SHARE A CONCERN FOR HUMAN flourishing, individual beliefs and values, and social context. Yet tensions between science and religion, and especially between psychiatry and the behavioral sciences and religion, have historically hindered constructive dialogue, creating uncertainty about how to approach ethical questions emerging at the interface between them. Many questions arise: What is the clinician's role in treating patients with unhealthy forms of religion? How should a therapist approach a patient's existential, moral, or spiritual distress? What are the ethical implications of taking into account a patient's religious beliefs as they bear on decisions about treatment, parenting, or end-of-life care?

Psychiatric ethics have traditionally focused on the implications of generally accepted principles and professional virtues, including respect for the patient's culture and values. Both the *Resource Document on Psychiatrists' Religious and Spiritual Commitments* published by the American Psychiatric Association (APA) and the *Position Statement on Spirituality and Religion in Psychiatry* published by the World Psychiatric Association (WPA) emphasize the need to understand the place of religion/spirituality as a source of these values. Conversely, religious ethics often emphasize caring for the ill and impaired. However, few resources are available for understanding the ways in which religion/spirituality informs the relevant values of patients and their clinicians, how clinicians should address conflicting values, or what principles should guide the interaction between clinicians' own professional and personal commitments. Discussions within the APA's Caucus on Spirituality, Religion, and Psychiatry of this conceptual and practical lack led to this project.

Our aim in this volume is to help readers think more clearly about these issues as they are encountered by psychiatrists and other mental health professionals, religious professionals working in mental health settings, bioethicists, healthcare ethics committee members, and trainees in all of these disciplines. Rather than philosophical arguments or practice guidelines, the contributors offer a conceptual framework for understanding the role of religion/spirituality in ethical decision making and pragmatic guidance for approaching challenging cases. Authors in Part One explore several dimensions of the ethical challenges presented by religious/spiritual in psychiatric practice, and those in Part Two describe ways of approaching these in different treatment contexts. Wherever appropriate, we have asked psychiatric and religious professionals to collaborate.

In Chapter Two, John Peteet addresses psychiatry's lack of a clearly articulated set of values with which to approach the complexities of clinical work within a pluralistic context. He suggests that four core values—prevention and treatment of disease, patient centeredness, relief of suffering, and enhancement of functioning—can be traced to psychiatry's roots in humanistic medicine. When each is counterbalanced by the others from the perspective of the clinician's and the patient's worldviews, they offer a value-based approach to understanding the patient's disorder, chief concern, and prerequisites for flourishing. This approach, reflected in the Jonsen Four Topics Model for ethical reasoning (Jonsen, Siegler, & Winslade, 2015), frames and illuminates the relevance of religious and spiritual commitments in clinical work.

In Chapter Three, Mary Lynn Dell and Daniel Grossoehme discuss the relationship between religion/spirituality and psychiatric ethics, beginning with a review of religious ethics and religious bioethics from the perspectives of several major world faith traditions. Elements of Jewish, Christian (Catholic and Protestant), Islamic, Hindu, and Buddhist religious ethics are considered, with particular attention to how ethical teachings of these traditions interact with common elements of psychiatric ethics. Our hope is that this chapter will be helpful as readers become more aware of when and where theological perspectives have particular relevance in psychiatric practice.

In Chapter Four, Allan Josephson explores religious/spiritual and ethical aspects of psychiatric diagnosis. He argues that because diagnosis involves knowing the patient "through and through," it of necessity includes knowledge of the patient's religious/spiritual or secular worldview and related commitments. After considering how these present challenges in the care of patients struggling with issues of meaning, moral distress, and authority/autonomy, he discusses ethical challenges for diagnosis presented by a pluralistic psychiatric culture, including overdiagnosis and a loss of perspective on the whole patient.

In Chapter Five, James Griffith and Gina Magyar-Russell acknowledge that personal spirituality sets a standard for relational and ethical living but consider three major ways in which religion can be unhealthy and potentially harmful: when "sociobiological" religion obscures personal spirituality, when religion becomes a venue for mental illness, and when individuals experience spiritual struggle.

In Chapter Six, Len Sperry considers how clinicians should approach the various spiritual and religious concerns that adult patients present in everyday psychiatric practice. These include those noted in the V code, Religious or Spiritual Problem, in the *Diagnostic and Statistical Manual of Mental Disorders, Fifth Edition* (DSM-5) (APA, 2013). The author presents a taxonomy of these concerns that is useful in making treatment decisions and an ethical framework for responding to them. He emphasizes the patient's informed consent and the competency of the psychiatrist in addressing religion and spiritual issues, which has implications for professionals' scope of practice.

In Chapter Seven, Nancy Kehoe examines the unique ethical dilemmas faced by religious professionals in dealing with mental health and illness. Some of these are rooted in a lack of understanding of mental illness and its impact on the community; others have to do with the multiple relationships with members of the congregation and lack of objectivity when conflicting concerns emerge. Still others relate to the inevitable boundary crossings and risk of boundary violations, decisions regarding confidentiality, and the situation of being the sole religious leader in the community with unclear guidelines for oversight or accountability.

In Chapter Eight, Don Postema considers the role of religion/spirituality in the work of ethics committees. He reviews the history of ethics committees and consultation, notes the re-emergence of the religious and spiritual in medicine and healthcare, and uses a challenging case to illustrate the need to integrate moral, religious/spiritual, and psychiatric perspectives.

In Chapter Nine, James Lomax and Nathan Carlin discuss the clinical implications of a mental health professional's personal religion/spirituality by focusing on the example of fundamentalism and the importance of understanding and managing one's countertransference reactions to the patients whom it has shaped.

Chapter authors in Part Two identify and address ethical challenges involving religion/spirituality in various areas of psychiatric practice: outpatient (Morgan Medlock and David Rosmarin), inpatient (Shad Ali and Abraham Nussbaum), geriatric psychiatry (John Peteet), community psychiatry (Tony Benning), consultation liaison (Marta Herschkopf and John Peteet), forensic psychiatry (Michael Norko), child and adolescent psychiatry (Carol Kessler and Mary Lynn Dell), addiction psychiatry (Chris Cook, Eilish Gilvarry, and Andrea Hearn), emergency and disaster psychiatry (Sam Thielman and Glen Goss), disability psychiatry (Bill Gaventa and Mary Lynn Dell), international psychiatry (Walid Sarhan and Alan Fung), psychiatric research (Alexander Moreira-Almeida, Quirino Cordeiro, and Harold Koenig), and psychiatric education (Gerrit Glas).

Given the lack of universally accepted definitions of religion and spirituality, we use the following working definitions in this book: *Spirituality* refers to one's relationship to something larger that gives life meaning, and *religion* refers to a tradition of spiritual beliefs and practices. The two are not identical but often travel together; we recognize this by using the term *religion/spirituality* wherever appropriate. The term *ethics* is also subject to various definitions; we use it simply to mean inquiry into what is good and right.

JONSEN, SIEGLER, AND WINSLADE'S FOUR TOPICS MODEL: A HELPFUL PARADIGM FOR ETHICAL ANALYSIS

Many of the chapters feature case examples that illustrate the relevance for decision making of medical indications, patient preferences, quality of life, contextual factors, and religion/spirituality in relation to culture. Several contributors use the Jonsen Four Topics (or Four Quadrant) Model in their discussion. The editors have employed this model as a helpful tool for almost three decades to provide a consistent framework for the systematic analysis of ethical dilemmas that have arisen in clinical work—primarily in consultation liaison psychiatry, as well as in work with ethics committees, in general clinical ethics consultations, and in educational sessions with trainees learning and working at many levels in numerous medical disciplines.

The originators of the Four Topics method, Albert R. Jonsen, Mark Siegler, and William J. Winslade, developed this four-part model to bring order and consistency to the way in which ethicists and clinicians consider ethical quandaries. This method is especially helpful when the emotions of patients, family members, and medical care providers risk coloring the understanding of the facts and the true nature of the ethical issues at hand. By working through and identifying the information requested in each section, all individuals involved in a particular dilemma are more likely than not to be assured that what matters most to them is included in ethical analysis and decision making. Although it was not originally intended and is not predominantly used by clinicians concerned with ethical issues at the intersection of psychiatry, ethics, and religion/spirituality, we have found the Four Topics Model to be very applicable to mental health and ethics quandaries because of its broad conceptualization of personhood.

The first topic or quadrant is Medical Indications. This section focuses on the medical problems at hand and the accompanying diagnostic, therapeutic, and prognostic considerations. Although it is not always the most important contributor to understanding and addressing the ethical quandary, this body of medical/psychiatric information must be understood as well as possible to provide the best conceptual understanding for matters included in the other three sections.

The second topic or quadrant involves Patient Preferences. What does the patient decide or want to do in the current circumstances? If the patient is not able to speak for himself or herself at the time of the consultation or when the ethical quandary arises, has anyone else been authorized to speak for and make decisions on behalf of the patient?

The third topic or quadrant refers to Quality of Life. How does the particular disorder or illness and its treatments affect patients' quality of life and their ability to earn a living, to engage with family and friends as they find meaningful, and to participate in and enjoy what has mattered to them in their lives before, during, and after treatment?

The fourth topic or quadrant considers Contextual Features, the nonmedical but nevertheless significant elements that influence the kinds of decisions patients make for themselves in healthcare settings, as well as how the "system" interacts with patients and their loved ones. This is the quadrant that ensures that finances, legal concerns, social concerns, and other institutional matters relevant to ethical analysis and decision making are not forgotten. It is in this fourth quadrant, Contextual Features, that Jonsen, Siegler, and Winslade placed the reminder for ethicists and clinicians dealing with ethical dilemmas to inquire about religious and spiritual factors that may be influencing clinical decisions.

The Four Topics Chart

Medical Indications	Preferences of Patients
The Principles of Beneficence and Nonmaleficence 1. What is the patient's medical problem? Is the problem acute? chronic? critical? reversible? emergent? terminal? 2. What are the goals of treatment? 3. In what circumstances are medical treatments not indicated? 4. What are the probabilities of success of various treatment options? 5. In sum, how can this patient be benefited by medical and nursing care, and how can harm be avoided?	The Principles of Respect for Autonomy 1. Has the patient been informed of benefits and risks of diagnostic and treatment recommendations, understood this information, and given consent? 2. Is the patient mentally capable and legally competent or is there evidence of incapacity? 3. If mentally capable, what preferences about treatment is the patient stating? 4. If incapacitated, has the patient expressed prior preferences? 5. Who is the appropriate surrogate to make decisions for an incapacitates patient? What standards should govern the surrogate's decision? 6. Is the patient unwilling or unable to cooperate with medical treatment? If so, why?

Quality of Life	Contextual Features
The Principles of Beneficence and Nonmaleficence and Respect for Autonomy 1. What are the prospects, with or without treatment, for a return to normal life and what physical, mental, and social deficits might the patient expereience even if treatment succeeds? 2. On what grounds can anyone judge that some quality of life would be undesirable for a patient who cannot make or express such a judgment? 3. Are there biases that might prejudice the provider's evaluation of the patient's quality of life? 4. What ethical issues arise concerning improving or enhancing a patient's quality of life? 5. Do quality-of-life assessments raise any questions that might contribute to a change of treatment plan, such as forgoing life-sustaining treatment? 6. Are there plans to provide pain relief and provide comfort after a decision has been made to forgo life-sustaining interventions? 7. IS medically assisted dying ethically or legally permissible? 8. What is legal and ethical status of suicide?	The Principles of Justice and Fairness 1. Are there professional, interprofessional, or business interests that might create conflicts of interest in the clinical treatment of patients? 2. Are there parties other than clinical and patient, such as family members, who have a legitimate interest in clinical decisions? 3. What are the limits imposed on patient confidentiality by the legitimate interests of third parties? 4. Are there financial factors that create conflicts of interest in clinical decisions? 5. Are there problems of allocation of resources that affect clinical decisions? 6. Are there religious factors that might influence clinical decisions? 7. What are the legal issues that might affect clinical decisions? 8. Are there considerations of clinical research and medical education that affect clinical decisions? 9. Are there considerations of public health and safety that influence clinical? 10. Does institutional affilation create conflicts of interest that might influence clinical decisions?

Jonsen AR, Siegler M, Winslade WJ. *Clincal Ethics: A Practical Approach to Ethical Decisions in Clinical Medicine.* 8th ed. New York, NY: McGraw-Hill; 2015.

RELIGION, SPIRITUALITY, AND CULTURE

It is noteworthy that religion/spirituality and culture share an intimate and complex relationship, with important implications for both mental health and ethics. Multiple cultures may practice the same religions, leading to challenges in distinguishing cultural from religious prohibitions (e.g., appropriate dress, accepting treatment from members of other faiths). Multiple religions can co-exist in one culture, and mental health practitioners may encounter problems stemming from their lack of familiarity with differences relative to values regarding health beliefs and practices, child rearing, sexuality, family, and death and dying.

To provide clinicians a framework for organizing cultural information relevant to diagnostic assessment and treatment planning, the Outline for Cultural Formulation (OCF) was introduced in the *Diagnostic and Statistical Manual of Mental Disorders, Fourth Edition, Text Revision* (DSM-IV-TR) (APA, 2000). In 2013, the DSM-5 updated the OCF and presented an approach to the assessment using the Cultural Formulation Interview (CFI), which has operationalized the process of data collection for the OCF. The revised OCF includes systematic assessment of the following domains: (1) cultural identity of the individual; (2) cultural conceptualization of distress; (3) psychosocial stressors and cultural features of vulnerability and resilience; (4) cultural features of the relationship between the individual and the clinician; and (5) overall cultural assessment (APA, 2013). The CFI contains 16 core questions (with both patient and informant versions) as well as 12 supplementary modules designed to expand on each domain of the core CFI for specific populations.

The core CFI is a 16-item semistructured interview that follows a person-centered approach to cultural assessment, focusing on the individual's experience and the social contexts of the clinical problem (APA, 2013). The questions cover four domains of assessment: (1) cultural definition of the problem (questions 1–3); (2) cultural perceptions of cause, context, and support (questions 4–10); (3) cultural factors affecting self-coping and past help seeking (questions 11–13); and (4) cultural factors affecting current help seeking (questions 14–16). Questions 6 through 12, 14, and 15 have been regarded as having specific relevance to spirituality/religion (APA, 2013).

In addition, supplementary module 5 of the CFI focuses on Spirituality, Religion, and Moral Traditions, and its 16 questions aim to clarify the influence of spirituality, religion, and other moral or philosophical traditions on the individual's problems and related stresses. These questions address (1) spiritual, religious, and moral identity; (2) role of spirituality, religion, and moral traditions; (3) relationship to the presenting problem; and (4) potential stresses or conflicts related to spirituality, religion, and moral traditions (APA, 2013). The core and supplementary modules of the CFI are available online from the Multicultural Mental Health Resource Centre website: https://www.multiculturalmentalhealth.ca/clinical-tools/cultural-formulation/.

We hope that the contributions in this book will broaden the perspective of readers on the multifaceted interface between mental health and religion/spirituality and stimulate thoughtful reflection and conversation about its important ethical dimension across multiple professional disciplines.

REFERENCES

American Psychiatric Association. (2000). *Diagnostic and statistical manual of mental disorders* (4th ed., text rev.). Washington, DC: Author.

American Psychiatric Association. (2013). *Diagnostic and statistical manual of mental disorders* (5th ed.). Washington, DC: Author.

Jonsen, A. R., Siegler, M., and Winslade, W. J. (2015). *Clinical ethics: A practical approach to ethical decisions in clinical medicine* (8th ed.). New York, NY: McGraw-Hill Education.

PART ONE

GENERAL CONSIDERATIONS

TWO

Values and Pluralism in Psychiatry

John R. Peteet, M.D.

ALTHOUGH MODERN PSYCHIATRY SHARES TERRITORY WITH BOTH SCIENCE and the humanities, it has tended to emphasize being evidence based rather than value based. One cost of this emphasis has been the unacknowledged adoption of value systems implicit in the culture (Hoff, 2005), such as biological or psychodynamic reductionism, pharmacological necessity, or Western individualism. Another cost has been a lack of consensus in dealing with the moral complexity of clinical work.

Several helpful attempts have been made to address the value dimension of psychiatry. Fulford (2004) and others have described the ways in which the process of psychiatric diagnosis is potentially value laden. Other psychiatrists in the United Kingdom have coined the term *value-based treatment* out of respect for the needs, wishes, and beliefs of the individual, the family, and the community. Their framework for understanding the policy implications of this approach has been adopted by The National Institute for Mental Health in England (Box 2.1). Psychiatric organizations such as the American Psychiatric Association and the Royal College of Psychiatrists in the United Kingdom have adopted codes of ethics calling for respecting patients' values and warning against abuses of basic principles such as confidentiality. Virtue ethicists such as Radden and Sadler (2010) have identified virtues intrinsic to being a good psychiatrist, and Waring (2016) has extended this perspective to include the ways in which psychiatrists foster the development of ethical and moral virtues in the process of treating conditions such as depression and demoralization. Elsewhere, I have suggested an approach to moral issues arising in treatment that is based on understanding moral functioning (Peteet, 2004). Finally, a number of authors have called attention to differing values expressed by various psychotherapeutic schools of thought (Bergin, Payne, & Richards, 1996), and held by therapists with various worldviews and religious/spiritual traditions (Josephson & Peteet, 2004).

However, a lack of articulated core therapeutic values has left clinicians with little guidance in making decisions across a range of clinical contexts. Consider a few examples:

1. A psychiatrist is asked to evaluate a patient requesting physician-assisted dying (PAD), in a jurisdiction where this is legal, and is unsure whether to participate.

Box 2.1. The National Institute for Mental Health in England (NIMHE) Values Framework—Policy Implications

Respect for diversity of values encompasses a number of specific policies and principles concerned with equality of citizenship. In particular, it is antidiscriminatory because discrimination in all its forms is intolerant of diversity. Respect for diversity within mental health is also

- *User centered*—it puts respect for the values of individual users at the center of policy and practice
- *Recovery oriented*—it recognizes that, building on the personal strengths and resiliencies of individual users and on their cultural and racial characteristics, there are many diverse routes to recovery
- *Multidisciplinary*—it requires that respect be reciprocal at a personal level (among service users, their family members, friends, communities, and providers), among different provider disciplines (such as nursing, psychology, psychiatry, medicine, social work), and among different organizations (including healthcare, social care, local authority housing, voluntary organizations, community groups, faith communities, and other social support services)
- *Dynamic*—it is open and responsive to change
- *Reflective*—it combines self-monitoring and self-management with positive self-regard
- *Balanced*—it emphasizes positive as well as negative values
- *Relational*—it puts positive working relationships supported by good communication skills at the heart of practice

---

2. A psychiatric resident sees a cancer patient with demoralization and diagnoses an adjustment reaction but is unsure whether or how to address the patient's existential distress.
3. A religious patient struggling with depression is uncertain whether to see a psychiatrist suggested by her primary care physician because she is concerned that the psychiatrist will focus more on her diagnosis and dysfunction than on her ability to grow.

Four core values—prevention and treatment of disease, patient centeredness, relief of suffering, and enhancement of functioning—can be traced to psychiatry's roots in medicine and humanism. In order for these values to make the process of diagnostic and therapeutic decision making more rational and transparent, clinicians need to appreciate the complementary ways in which they balance one another and how prioritizing them depends at least in part one's views of the world and of what constitutes human flourishing.

CORE THERAPEUTIC VALUES

Treatment and Prevention of Disease

The psychiatrist's role as a physician includes the treatment and prevention of disease, which is optimally evidence based. Because the diseases that psychiatrists treat can lead to harmful behavior, this value at times includes a directive role in ensuring safety. However, a commitment to treating disease leaves unclear whether psychiatrists should also attempt to treat conditions that are not considered disorders, such as the existential distress that is present in demoralization. If unchecked by attention to other core values, a disease orientation can lead to overemphasis on pathology and on narrow, technical solutions to complex, multidimensional problems such as depression (Peteet, 2010). The complaint of the author Parker Palmer (2000, p. 65) is not unique: "I had abortive meetings with two psychiatrists whose reliance on drugs and whose dismissive attitude toward the inner life would have made me angry enough to get well simply to spite them, if I had not been terminally depressed!"

Patient Centeredness

Patient centeredness is grounded in the fundamental ethical principle of respect for autonomy. It entails prioritizing the patient's good over that of the therapist or some other party. Respect for autonomy implies a commitment to the patient's self-actualization, freedom of action, and choice and extends to realization of the patient's goals. However, patients live in relationship to a larger context, and therapists also have a vision of health toward which they want to help patients move. Treatment shaped only by the patient's wishes can lead to overdependence on therapy or medication.

Relief of Suffering

The relief of distress and suffering is central to the calling of the physician to be compassionate, to care, and to comfort even when unable to cure. However, at times, some suffering may be required for the growth that comes from working through and taking responsibility (Waring, 2016). An unbalanced focus on relief of suffering can lead to collusion with the patient to limit functional goals and, in the extreme case of PAD for psychiatric indications, to the death of the patient.

Promoting Functioning

Finally, consistent with the World Health Organization's 2014 definition of mental health as "a state of well-being in which every individual realizes his or her own potential, can cope with the normal stresses of life, can work productively and fruitfully, and is able to make a contribution to her or his community," psychiatrists have a role in promoting positive health and functioning. This arguably includes adaptation, useful insights, skills, and growth, although a full definition of optimal functioning depends on one's view of human flourishing. An unbalanced emphasis on functional skills can lead to the indiscriminate prescription of strategies for coping (e.g., cognitive-behavioral therapy) for patients who are suffering too much to make use of them or have other priorities of their own, such as regaining a familiar sense of stability.

ETHICAL IMPLEMENTATION

Asking three key practical questions can help frame the clinician's approach to the value dimension of clinical work:

1. What is the diagnosis? In addition to the *Diagnostic and Statistical Manual of Mental Disorders, Fifth Edition* (DSM-5), the biopsychosocial model, George and Engel (1980)

and McHugh and Slavney's (1998) perspectival framework, developed at Johns Hopkins University to aid in more fully understanding the patient, are helpful ways to take into account the needs of the whole person within his or her context. Inexperienced clinicians can give the DSM diagnosis too much significance, allowing it to outweigh the need for attention to the dynamic formulation, or to existential issues such as demoralization or grief that may be an important part of a depression, or to family dysfunction that may be complicating the diagnosis of attention deficit disorder.

2. What is the patient's chief complaint? Unless they can appreciate the nature of the patient's distress and what is giving it priority now, clinicians may substitute their own agenda, such as completing a maximally billable assessment or offering the treatment with which they are most expert and familiar.

3. What does the patient need to flourish? At least as important as understanding the patient's diagnosis is assessing the strengths and resources, including the relationships, that have helped the patient grow and adapt. What has interfered with the patient's use of these resources to flourish?

Attention to core values can be useful in helping trainees consolidate their identities as more than DSM diagnosticians, teachers of skills, or facilitators of insights or practical dispositions. Avoiding mistakes requires listening and respecting the need to balance all four core values.

Consider the application of core values in the context of one's worldview in approaching the scenarios described previously:

1. PAD: If treatment of a disease is not at stake, considerations of relieving suffering and patient centeredness (in the sense of preference, although not in the sense of enhancing functional autonomy) need to be weighed against the potential for enhancing functioning through preserving life. Whether full human functioning takes into account and derives meaning from a higher context (an aspect of one's worldview) also influences what a clinician wants to do. Specifically, the patient's and the physician's spiritual and religious views inform their understanding of human flourishing.

2. Existential suffering: Clarifying what disease is present is important as a first step, but it takes one only so far in approaching a patient who is suffering from an intractable medical condition or illness. Patient centeredness takes one to the heart of that suffering, and enhancing functioning entails envisioning positive options for dealing with it. What these options are depends on one's view of the world.

3. A religious patient with depression: Because patients want, in addition to treatment of disease, help in dealing with the burden of illness and achieving health, how the clinician envisions these goals from the perspective of his or her worldview becomes an important consideration for the patient in choosing a therapist.

CORE VALUES WITHIN A PLURALISTIC CONTEXT

Core values can guide clinicians of differing theoretical orientations in addressing patients whose values differ from their own and who may need to understand what informs the direction of their psychiatrist's work with them. But how can these values be prioritized in making a difficult clinical decision? Principlism ethics offers a general framework for resolving tensions among competing values (i.e., to see whether a potential solution honors them), and virtue ethics helps to explain what is necessary for implementing them in therapy (Radden & Sadler, 2010; Waring, 2016). But weighing and choosing among values also depends on one's worldview. For example, the therapist of a patient who believes that people are created by God to worship Him and to sacrifice for one another may value individual autonomy less than spiritual maturity. If one is a materialist, scientific objectivity in deciding on a course of treatment for depression may have more weight than the goals of psychological, emotional, or spiritual growth.

As Poplin (2014) suggested, the most widely shared worldviews are radical materialism, secular humanism, pantheism, and monotheism, each differing from the rest in their core assumptions and clinical implications.

Radical materialists value scientific truth and the dramatic advances in medical knowledge and education seen since the publication of the Flexner Report on medical education in 1900 (Flexner, Pritchet, & Henry, 1910). For example, in advocating what he called the scientific worldview, Freud saw (1937) religiously based hopes as illusory and identified the goal of treatment as the substitution of ordinary unhappiness for neurotic suffering. Yet few scientists would limit admissible evidence to randomized clinical trials or view health as only the absence of disease. Most would acknowledge that reducing reality to what we can measure is not easily reconciled with how we actually live. As John Updike (1989) wrote, "[W]hen we try in good faith to believe in materialism . . . we are disavowing the very realm where we exist and where all things precious are kept—the realm of emotion and conscience, of memory and intention and sensation."

Secular humanists such as Michael Shermer (2015) and Stephen Pinker (2011) resisted such reductionism and suggested that humane, or positive, values emerge from an evolutionary process of improvement in the human condition informed by reason. Secular humanists see individual freedom and tolerance as the essential conditions for human flourishing and contend that medicine should aim to eliminate not only disease but also suffering, defined as distress that threatens the integrity of the individual. Healing, in their view, involves promoting self-realization and self-mastery. This may be expressed by some in a preference for the option of PAD when suffering is deemed intolerable or for Albert Ellis's Rational Recovery (now known as SMART Recovery) rather than twelve-step programs with their emphasis on the need for a relationship with a higher power. But secular humanism leaves unanswered a number of questions about the philosophical basis and practical motivation for altruism. For example, what meaning can a paraplegic or a patient on dialysis find in their suffering and dependence? What if an appeal to one's rational self-interest is not enough to overcome addiction? What can motivate sacrificial compassionate care?

Many individuals see themselves as part of a larger, collective existence that transcends scientific understanding but would identify themselves as "spiritual but not religious" or respond "none" when asked to list a classification for themselves. Their view that there is an essential unity to all of reality (which can be termed *pantheistic*) supports a biopsychosocial-spiritual understanding of illness and a holistic understanding of healing that includes a harmonious relationship to an underlying reality that cannot be scientifically grasped. Integrative approaches such as mindfulness, which help individuals become more selfless and attuned to this larger context, have achieved major importance within medicine and psychiatry. Yet pantheism, with its spiritually informed view, leaves several questions unanswered. For example, how does it help the individual whose relationship to the transcendent is marked by shame and guilt? What in a contemplative stance can motivate altruism and help make needed moral distinctions?

Most *monotheists*, while sharing many of the values and insights of the first three world-views, see themselves as created by a good God but living in a broken world. For them, healing is found in a relationship with the Creator that moves them toward the ideal of a "peaceable kingdom." In their view, individuals have intrinsic value and dignity by virtue of their related-ness to God and others—a relatedness marked by love and the motivation to serve. Believers in a loving God see relational intimacy as central to the way that individuals heal. For example, Christians' experience of God's love prompts them to embrace radical forgiveness and hospi-tality toward those in most need, as exemplified in Mother Teresa's Missionaries of Charity and Victoria Sweet's God's Hotel (2012). Yet, as Charles Taylor pointed out in *A Secular Age*, accept-ance of authority is psychologically difficult for many in the West. Religious faith is also difficult for many who are confronted with the competing claims and the failures of institutional religion to live up to its professed ideals.

How can psychiatrists ethically engage this multiplicity of worldviews as they weigh and implement their core values? One important consideration is cultivating an awareness of one's own point of view; this is important to avoid "smuggling in" unacknowledged values. A second consideration is transparency or candor with patients about one's values (Curlin & Hall, 2005), including, at times, informed consent to work in a value-laden area. And a third is finding con-sensus on mutually valued goals toward which to work. The contributors to this volume discuss examples of this value-laden process in the presence of growing spiritual/religious pluralism.

REFERENCES

Bergin, A. E., Payne, R., & Richards, P. S. (1996). Values in psychotherapy. *Religion and the Clinical Practice of Psychology*, 297–325.

Curlin, F. A., & Hall, D. E. (2005). Strangers or friends: A proposal for a new spirituality-in-medicine ethic. *Journal of General Internal Medicine*, *20*, 370–374.

Flexner, A., Pritchet, H., & Henry, S. (1910). Medical education in the United States and Canada bulletin number four (The Flexner Report). *New York (NY): The Carnegie Foundation for the Advancement of Teaching*.

Freud, S. (1937). *Studies in Hysteria*. Authorized Translation with an Introduction by A. A. Brill. (Nervous and Mental Disease Monograph Series No. 61.) Nervous and Mental Disease Publishing, New York.

Fulford, K. W. M. (2004). Ten principles of values based medicine. In J. Radden (Ed.), *The philosophy of psychiatry: A companion* (pp. 205–234). New York, NY: Oxford University Press.

George, E., & Engel, L. (1980). The clinical application of the biopsychosocial model. *American Journal of Psychiatry*, *137*, 535–544.

Hoff, P. (2005). Recent advances in research on the history of psychiatry: Chances and limitations of the global perspective. In G. N. Christodoulou (Ed.), *Advances in psychiatry* (vol. 2, pp. 13–18). Paris, France: World Psychiatric Association.

Josephson, A. J., & Peteet, J. R. (Eds.). (2004). *Handbook of spirituality and world view in clinical practice*. Arlington, VA: American Psychiatric Association.

McHugh, P. R., & Slavney, P. R. (1998). *The perspectives of psychiatry* (2nd ed.). Baltimore, MD: Johns Hopkins University Press.

Palmer, P. J. (2000). *Let your life speak: Listening to the voice of vocation.* San Francisco, CA: John Wiley & Sons.

Peteet, J. R. (2004). *Doing the right thing: An approach to moral issues in mental health treatment.* Arlington, VA: American Psychiatric Association.

Peteet, J. R. (2010). *Depression and the soul: A guide to spiritually integrated treatment.* New York, NY: Routledge.

Pinker, S. (2011). *The Better Angels of Our Nature: Why Violence Has Declined.* New York: Viking Press.

Poplin, M. (2014). *Is reality secular? Testing the assumptions of four global world views.* Downers Grove, IL: InterVarsity Press.

Radden, J., & Sadler, J. (2010). *The virtuous psychiatrist: Character ethics in psychiatric practice.* New York, NY: Oxford University Press.

Shermer, M. (2015). *The Moral Arc: How Science Makes us Better People.* New York: Henry Holt.

Sweet, V. (2012). *God's Hotel: A Doctor, A Hospital and a Pilgrimage to the Heart of Medicine.* New York: Riverhead Books.

Taylor, C. (2007). *A secular age.* Cambridge, MA: Harvard University Press.

Updike, J. (1989). *Self-consciousness: Memoirs.* New York: Random House, p. 250.

Waring, D. R. (2016). *The healing virtues: Character ethics in psychotherapy.* Oxford, England: Oxford University Press.

World Health Organization. (2014, August). Mental health: A state of well-being. Retrieved from www.who.int/features/factfiles/mental_health/en/.

THREE

Theological Ethics Relevant to Mental Health and Psychiatry

AN OVERVIEW

*Daniel H. Grossoehme, M.Div., D.Min.,
and Mary Lynn Dell, M.D., D.Min.*

THE ROLE OF THEOLOGY IN BIOETHICS TOO OFTEN IS UNRECOGNIZED and underappreciated by psychiatrists and other mental health clinicians who lack a formal background or significant interest in religion and spirituality. The discipline of theological ethics enriches both the academic study of bioethics and the practical applications of ethics at the bedside and in daily discussions with patients, families, and clinicians.

Religion and spirituality may offer hope, comfort, resiliency, and ways to cope with the challenges of psychiatric illness. On the other hand, religious and spiritual beliefs and practices can be perplexing, a source of angst for individual patients and division among family members and friends. Even when psychiatrists inquire about religion and spirituality, they often do not venture beyond the patient's background and current commitment to those beliefs. Perhaps they lack the time and a certain amount of clinical courage to engage patients about how their understandings of problems, coping, and dealing with mental illness, treatment, and subsequent ethical concerns arise in psychiatric assessment and care. How does one's spirituality—past, present, or lack thereof—form and influence one's worldview and approach to ethical quandaries? Just as important, how does the clinician's religiosity, spirituality, or lack thereof affect his or her assessments and care of patients, and how does that professional identify and work through ethical issues with a spiritual overlay?

These questions are central to many chapters in this book. To best explore the intersection of psychiatry, ethics, and religion/spirituality, several basic terms beg definition. *Religion* refers to "beliefs, practices, and rituals related to the sacred . . . . Religion may be organized and practiced within a community, or it may be practiced alone and in private" (Koenig, King, & Carson, 2012, p. 37). *Spirituality* refers to one's connection to the sacred or transcendent, which is both inside and outside oneself and may or may not involve an organized world faith tradition (Koenig et al., 2012). Theologian Lisa Sowle Cahill defined *theology* as a "process of reflection on religious experience, in which the systematic coherence of religious narratives and symbols is clarified and their practical ramifications developed" (Cahill, 2012, p. 61). Although Beauchamp and Childress described several subtypes of ethics, their most basic definition of *ethics* is "a generic term covering several different ways of understanding and examining the moral life" (Beauchamp & Childress, 2013, p. 1). Finally, Cahill held that *theological ethics* "is the explication and defense of the personal morality and the social behavior required or idealized by a religious tradition" (Cahill, 2012, p. 61).

This chapter offers brief summaries of six major world faith traditions, including historical origins, demographic information, basic theological tenets, and key themes in the religions' ethics. Attitudes and beliefs about life, illness, suffering, medical care, end of life, and mental health care are discussed. The chapter is not intended to be an exhaustive review of major world faith traditions but a concise overview of common religions to illustrate an approach to understanding aspects of traditions of importance to patients and ethical decision making.

BUDDHISM

Buddhism includes numerous traditions and practices that are rooted in teachings attributed to Siddhartha Gautama, a man known as the Buddha; it began in present-day India between the 4th and 6th centuries B.C.E. These teachings are known as the Dharma. In 2010, there were approximately 488 million adherents worldwide, comprising 7% of the world population, with an estimated 3.8 million in the United States (Hackett & Grim, 2012).

Buddhist bioethics is influenced by a strong emphasis on truth telling, and this is especially incumbent upon clinicians (Ratanakul, 1988). Lying is never permissible, and withholding information, even if perceived by a clinician to be in a patient's best interest, is considered lying. Buddhist teachings focus on accepting reality and coping with life as it is. This is not possible without truth, including medical truth. A second important precept is the sanctity of life. Suffering is to be borne with patience (even while pursing medical means of ameliorating it); neither euthanasia nor suicide is permitted. Karma is another tenet of Buddhism. Suffering in the present is understood as a consequence of actions in a prior life, and such suffering will continue until the effects of the prior action have been exhausted (Ratanakul, 1988). Suicide is not a means of escaping this process; suffering interrupted by a suicide in the present life will be continued in the next. Another precept of Buddhist ethics is justice and equal treatment of all. The concept of justice is exceeded only by the value of compassion. To give up something for the benefit of others is central to the path to the attainment of highest human fulfillment. Buddhist bioethics are also influenced by a preference for motives rather than outcome (Ratanakul, 1988).

Buddhists define death to have occurred when a person lacks consciousness (vitality and heat). Death should be faced directly in order to pursue nirvana, the final release from the cycle of life and death (Mizuno & Slingsby, 2007). Nirvana is achieved by attempting to renounce mental states that afflict the mind, including anger and other emotions. Once those feelings are removed, their consequences are also eliminated (Mizuno & Slingsby, 2007). Buddhism places great value on the role of consciousness of thoughts and feelings. If the mind is the seat of mental troubles, it is also the seat of healing them. Clinicians can thus engage Buddhist patients in the work of understanding the cause of their problem and in the work of reframing its meaning or changing their thoughts (Scotton, 1998). The Buddhist teaching to identify feelings in order to eliminate their consequences may lead Buddhist patients to present extended lists of symptoms rather than a global assessment of their functioning. Related to this teaching is a sense of the impermanence of feelings, which leads to patience that may appear to be passivity. Some Buddhist patients may be willing to endure dysfunction while engaged in the work of healing rather than pursue interventions aimed primarily at symptom relief. Finally, the cognitive, emotional, and spiritual aspects of health are not distinct; consultations with a Buddhist teacher, who is the spiritual authority, may well occur even while the patient seeks traditional Western medical care (Scotton, 1998).

HINDUISM

Hinduism is an ancient religion with adherents worldwide. Its ethics are fundamentally deontological—based on duty rather than rights (Coward & Sidhu, 2000). The word *Hindus* has geographic roots, denoting the people who lived in the region through which the river Indus runs (Sarma, 2008). Although some have suggested that there is no "Hindu bioethics" (Sarma, 2008), there are nevertheless some common beliefs related to health. These include karma and rebirth, purity, and an emphasis on the communal rather than the individual (Coward & Sidhu, 2000). Time and life are not linear but have always existed. To say "life begins at . . ." is a Western construct that does not have a Hindu counterpart. At the moment of conception, a full person has been reborn, who carries within unconscious traces of experiences in previous lives. Each event in the present life is influenced by similar events in prior lives; one may follow the influence and repeat the behavior in the present life, or one may consciously resist the influence and act differently. In either case, the present experience leaves its own influence that will affect the person in subsequent lives.

The law of karma is influential. Suffering, including psychiatric suffering, is karmic in origin. Bad thoughts are punished through suffering until their influence is eradicated. Treatment may focus on identifying the thought which led to suffering and developing new thoughts that are good and will be rewarded. Also influential is a sense of interdependence and the interconnectedness of all living beings. Violence, including violence against one's self through suicide, is counter to this interdependence.

Hindu patients generally present for mental health issues by referral from someone in the community and typically only after seeking spiritual healing on their own (Juthani, 1998). They may have certain expectations of mental health professionals, including the idea of mental health professionals serving as advisors and teachers; the inclusion in treatment or consultation of members of the patient's family; and the prescription of medications for the relief of symptoms.

ISLAM

Islam means "to submit to God's will or law" (Rahman, 1987). The faith began with a revelation to Muhammad in the 6th century A.D. It arose in what is now Saudi Arabia, and adherents are found worldwide. The number of Muslims (those who follow Islam) is hard to quantify; there may be 2 to 5 million adherents in the United States (Rahman, 1987) and approximately 1.6 billion in the world (23% of the world population) (Lipke, 2016). The basic tenets of Islam are summarized in the Five Pillars of Islam (Hathout, 1995): the declaration that there is no god but God (Allah) and that Muhammad is His messenger; performing daily prayers; paying the alms-tax; observing the month-long annual fast of Ramadan; and making the Hajj (pilgrimage to Mecca) once in one's lifetime if one is able to do so.

Illness is understood to have three spiritual aspects: it is a trial from Allah; it is a means of expiating sins; and provided one has remained faithful, it is a sign of the promised afterlife (Rahman, 1987). Illness provides an opportunity for life examination, repentance, and change. Death through illness is understood to be a form of martyrdom (Rahman, 1987). Islamic scholars are divided on the issue of whether illness must be treated or treatment is optional. Islam understands only Allah to be certain and unchanging: medicine and its pursuit are uncertain (Rahman, 1987).

The sanctity of life is paramount (Hathout, 1995). The principle of the sanctity of life extends to prohibitions against ending a life to avoid illness or suffering (e.g., suicide). Rather, patience and endurance, even in the face of suffering, are valued. The sanctity of life leads to an understanding of death as total brain death (including the death of the brainstem) (Hathout, 1995). Life is given by Allah, and Allah alone determines when life ends: "It is not for a believing man or woman, if a matter has been decided by God and His messenger, to have a choice of their own. If anyone disobeys God and His messenger, he is indeed on a clearly wrong path" (Qu'ran 33:36). Between those transitions, lives of the body and of the mind are to be pursued (Hathout, 1995). Medicine is important to seek and use for one's self and also as a vocation by which to help others preserve life (Rahman, 1987).

JUDAISM

Judaism is one of the three major monotheistic religions, together with Christianity and Islam. Judaism has helped set the pace and development of modern medicine, perhaps driven by the Talmudic comment, "And whoever saves a life, it is considered as if he saved an entire world" (Yerushalmi Talmud 4:9). A history of persecution led the Jewish people to take on a responsibility for their people, leading to the construction of hospitals, research institutions, and institutes of higher learning (Feldman, 1986). The Torah is the primary sacred text, and writings by rabbis, whether ancient collected writings such as the Talmud or more recent individual writings, interpret the scriptures.

The Hebrew Scriptures teach that God created the world, pronounced it "good," and created humanity in God's own image. This has significant implications for the care of the body. Since anything God has created has good, the body must also be good (Novick, 1998). Bodies are gifts from God, and the body is to be accorded the care and respect it deserves as being made in God's image. The body is to be maintained in good health, just as one seeks to maintain one's soul in good health. "Body" is understood inclusively: the ethics apply to the physical, mental, and spiritual components of a whole person (Flam, 2003). The belief that the body is a gift from God implies boundaries around its use: God may set limits on how it is used (Dorff, 2003). Bodies are "on loan" to people for the duration of their lives (Dorff, 2003), and all bodies, regardless of ability or disability, are considered of equal worth. Bodies are morally neutral in Jewish ethics, although they have the potential to be good (Dorff, 2003).

Preserving the life of the body is a major tenet of Jewish bioethics (Feldman, 1986). One means of preserving life is practicing good hygiene; this also has a spiritual dimension because body cleanliness leads to spiritual cleanliness (Feldman, 1986). Jewish ethics are flexible, however, and prescriptions may have exceptions. If a religious observance, such as Sabbath keeping or another ritual, threatens a person's life, then the prescriptions of Torah are to be set aside to focus on preserving the person's life (Feldman, 1986). When the body is diseased or broken in any way, a religious response combines both intercessory prayer to restore well-being and human effort to restore health (Feldman, 1986). Prayer alone is insufficient; one should expend the effort to seek healing. At the same time, attending to the needs of someone who is ill or injured and visiting them is a religious duty and an act of kindness that exceeds one's moral obligations to another (Flam, 2003). The ethic of preserving life is not absolute in Jewish bioethics. It is permissible to stop praying for continued life, and one may pray for God to end one's life, although no action may be taken to end life (Feldman, 1986).

As already noted, religious observances are secondary to health care needs. This includes mental health needs also. Jewish bioethics do not differentiate between the importance of attending to physical health and that of attending to mental health. Psychotherapy is a means of participating in one's mental and spiritual healing (Feldman, 1986).

PROTESTANTISM

Protestant is a broad term that refers to those Christian churches which arose out of the Reformation in various countries in Europe during the 16th century and which sought to reform what were considered the excesses of the Church of Rome. In the United States, these include Episcopalian, Lutheran, United Methodist, Presbyterian, and Reformed churches and the denominations that grew out of them. In 2011, there were approximately 160 million Protestants in the United States, representing approximately 52% of the population (Hackett & Grim, 2011).

Protestant Christians believe that God has identified with humanity most fully in the person and ministry of Jesus Christ. Jesus's words and behavior are seen as exemplifying love and life in a world of brokenness and suffering and are the basis of Protestant bioethics. The reality of suffering means that improvement is possible: There is something to be gained by seeking relationship with God through Jesus and fellow believers. Humans are able to draw strength for surviving the horrors of life through their experience of God's love and from that love as found in each other (Vaux, 1984). Life is obtained through aligning one's self more fully with God (Smith, 1986). Protestant churches emphasize the ability of individuals to discern God's will and to use their minds—in conjunction with sacred scriptures—to make decisions. Physicians are accorded respect and authority, but power in decision making is to be shared (Smith, 1986). Clinical and research professionals, as well as clergy and other members of the faith group, share equality before God and act together for healing (Marty, 1986). Protestant traditions emphasize the role of free will and self-determination. This allows that people may choose evil or suffering and also that the ills they suffer may result from another person's choice for evil (Vaux, 1984). Suffering may be physical or mental; mental suffering, together with physical suffering, is seen as a sign of the brokenness of the created world (Marty, 1986).

Some Protestants equate physical well-being with spiritual well-being (Vaux, 1984). This has two aspects. First, spiritual remedies may be utilized for physical ills. Second, physical ills may be a sign of spiritual "dis-ease." Medical and spiritual care are an integrated whole (Marty, 1986). Well-being is a gift from God, and some Protestants believe that wellness can come about only if God acts to save one from illness or evil (Marty, 1986). Well-being is seen as evidence of divine blessings, which depend on a person's obedience and righteousness (Vaux, 1984). As such, well-being cannot be demanded from an external Being (although it can be sought through prayer and rituals).

Protestants view death as the end of something good (life); although it would be an error to deny the badness of death, they also affirm its positive aspects, such as making change possible (Smith, 1986). Life is not something to be pursued at all costs, nor is death to be hastened. Any form of medical care (physical or mental) that could be considered necessary to treat disease or brokenness may be used. A differentiation may be made between ordinary and extraordinary care. Routine methods to preserve life must be utilized; however, extraordinary means are optional (Smith, 1986). Advances in healthcare necessarily mean that what constitutes extraordinary care in the present may well be considered ordinary care in the future, and the ethic to utilize care must likewise change.

Protestant ethics tend to lean toward the deontological rather than the utilitarian, and they tend to include the principle of limited liability: People are not solely responsible for either the great or the bad things that happen to them (Smith, 1986). Protestants also distinguish between being the direct or the indirect cause of death. Directly causing death is ethically wrong. However, taking an action such as requesting or giving medication to reduce pain even though it may depress respiratory effort and hasten death is ethically permissible (Smith, 1986).

ROMAN CATHOLICISM

Roman Catholicism is a branch of the Christian church that since 1054 A.D. has its authority centered in the person of the Bishop of Rome, also known as the Pope. In 2011, there were approximately 74 million U.S. adherents, who comprised 24% of the population (Hackett & Grim, 2011).

Human life is a creation and gift from God, and its value is beyond human evaluation and authority. It is sacred (Markwell & Brown, 2001). Suffering in the present is seen as a mechanism of opportunity to deepen one's life. Serious illness presents an opportunity to conform to the example of Jesus, repenting of sin and seeking to remain in a state of grace. Death is the consummate grace and a means of sharing in the mystery of Christ's resurrection life. Although life is sacred, if medical treatment can be expected to only prolong death, it is permissible to refuse it. Medical decision making should always be made by the patient or by his or her designated surrogate. That right to self-determination is limited by four constructs, including preventing suicide and protecting innocent third parties (McCormick, 1987).

Individuals are ethically bound to preserve their health, including mental health. Some people who are Roman Catholic may feel a strong religious compulsion to engage in acute mental health treatment even if they do not meet criteria for inpatient admission (Markwell & Brown, 2001). Particular issues that may be encountered include guilt and developmental aspects. Sins include thoughts, feelings, and actions conceived with the desire to carry them out; they should be distinguished from spontaneous thoughts or fantasies that may arise and lack the full consent of the person to actually engage in a behavior (Kehoe, 1998). Guilt stemming from sinful thoughts or actions may also require a spiritual intervention. In the Roman Catholic tradition, this is the ritual of reconciliation, in which sins are confessed and a priest pronounces absolution—the reconnection of the penitent with the Absolute (God).

The Roman Catholic tradition has long placed an emphasis on education, sometimes with limited flexibility in how doctrine is presented. One may encounter adolescents or adults who are emotionally troubled by language or images presented to them as children, if their spiritual development has not paralleled their physical and cognitive development (Kehoe, 1998). Assistance with reframing may be beneficial.

OTHERS

It is not possible to describe the theological ethics of each world religion with any justice. Questions may arise for psychiatrists working with patients from historically Eastern, Oriental, or Asian religions regarding the use of complementary and alternative treatments for psychiatric disorders. Followers of the many Native American spiritual traditions may also wish to use complementary and alternative medicinal substances, some of which may be harmful according to practitioners of standard allopathic medicine. Other traditions, such as Jehovah's Witnesses, maintain beliefs and practices that vary less from usual psychiatric care than from non-psychiatric specialty care but for which psychiatrists may find themselves involved either as consultants or as members of ethics committees. For additional information on various major world faith traditions and theological ethics relevant to the practice of psychiatry, readers are referred to the resource list at the end of this chapter.

THEOLOGICAL ETHICS
AND ETHICAL ANALYSIS

Jonsen, Siegler, and Winslade's (2015) Four Topics Model is well suited for inclusion of religious and spiritual factors in ethical analysis and decision making (see Chapter 1). The most obvious question pertaining to religion and spirituality is in the area of Contextual Features: "Are there religious factors that might influence clinical decisions?" However, one's theology and sense of rightness and justice, as informed by one's spirituality, enter into the other Topics as well. Theological ethics influence Preferences of Patients regarding medical decision making, cooperation with recommended care, and surrogate decision makers.

Several of the questions in the Quality of Life quadrant are also pertinent to issues addressed by theological ethics, including the sanctity of life and what constitutes a "good enough" quality of life. (Jonsen et al., 2015). Certainly, patients' and psychiatrists' views on suicide are shaped in profound ways by individual theological interpretations, even if only indirectly by the ways in which major world faith teachings and ethics are interwoven into the cultures of society, including health care systems, and the moral formation of those who choose vocations in medical professions.

CONCLUSION

The numerous major world faith traditions and their variations are simultaneously diverse and divergent, infusing the disciplines of theological ethics and bioethics and the clinical practice of psychiatry and medicine with unending riches and new challenges for clinicians and scholars. Although knowledge of literature and scholarship in theological ethics is always helpful, theological and doctrinal differences—even controversies—exist, including within religious and faith groups. In these situations, clinicians must remember to consult with the patient, family members, and religious professionals to ensure as complete a picture as possible of not only the patient's theological and spiritual heritage and its typical attitudes toward medicine and psychiatry but also the patient's personal, internalized beliefs and understandings that most contribute to his or her stance on questions of an ethical nature arising during care.

Finally, the intentional consideration of theological ethics should remind psychiatrists and mental health clinicians of the deep roots of bioethics in religion and spirituality and the immeasurable contributions of theology to medicine's understanding of its role in comfort and healing. Such an appreciation should serve to increase and strengthen interdisciplinary collaboration, consultation, and respect among medical practitioners and the theologians and clergy who partner with them in the care of the ill and suffering.

RESOURCES ON THEOLOGICAL ETHICS

Abbott, D., & Gottschalk, S. W. (2002). *The Christian Science tradition: Religious beliefs and healthcare decisions.* Park Ridge, IL: The Park Ridge Center.

Ashley, B. W., Deblois, J., & O'Rourke, K. D. (2006). *Health care ethics: A Catholic theological analysis* (5th ed.). Washington, DC: Georgetown University Press.

Barilan, Y. M. (2014). *Jewish bioethics: Rabbinic law and theology and historical contexts.* New York, NY: Cambridge University Press.

Bodnaruk, Z. M., Wong, C. J., & Bhugra, D. (2004). Meeting the clinical challenge of care for Jehovah's Witnesses. *Transfusion Medicine Reviews, 18*(2), 105–116.

Hill, D. L. (2006). Sense of belonging as connectedness, American Indian worldview, and mental health. *Archives of Psychiatric Nursing, 20*(5), 210–216.

Initiative on Islam and Medicine, Program on Medicine and Religion. (2017). Chicago, IL: The University of Chicago. Retrieved from https://pmr.uchicago.edu/iim.

Kalra, G., Bhui, K. S., & Bhugra, D. (2012). Sikhism, spirituality, and psychiatry. *Asian Journal of Psychiatry, 5*(4), 339–343.

Lysaught, M. T., & Kotva, J. J. (2012). *On moral medicine: Theological perspectives in medical ethics* (3rd ed.). Grand Rapids, MI: William B. Eerdmans.

Mathewes, C. (2010). *Understanding religious ethics.* West Sussex, UK: Wiley-Blackwell.

Ramsey, P. (1950). *Basic Christian ethics.* Louisville, KY: Westminster/John Knox Press.

Sachedina, A. (2009). *Islamic biomedical ethics: Principles and application.* New York, NY: Cambridge University Press.

REFERENCES

Beauchamp, T. L., & Childress, J. F. (2013). *Principles of biomedical ethics*. New York, NY: Oxford University Press.

Cahill, L. S. (2012). Theologians and bioethics: Some history and a proposal. In M. E. Lysaught, J. J. Kotva, S. E. Lammers, & A. Verhey (Eds.), *On moral medicine: Theological perspectives in medical ethics* (3rd ed.). Grand Rapids, MI: William B. Eerdmans.

Coward, H., & Sidhu, T. (2000). Bioethics for clinicians: 19. Hinduism and Sikhism. *Canadian Medical Association Journal, 163*(9), 1167–1170.

Dorff, E. N. (2003). *Love your neighbor and yourself*. Philadelphia, PA: The Jewish Publication Society.

Feldman, D. M. (1986). *Health and medicine in the Jewish tradition*. Health/Medicine and the Faith Traditions Series. New York, NY: Crossroad.

Flam, N. (2003). Healing of body, healing of spirit. In H. E. Person (Ed.), *The mitzvah of healing: An anthology of Jewish texts, meditations, essays, persons, stories and rituals* (pp. 53–56). New York, NY: Women of Reform Judaism/UAHC Press.

Hackett, C., & Grim, B. J. (2011). *Global Christianity*. The Pew Forum on Religion & Public Life. Washington, DC: Pew Research Center.

Hackett, C., & Grim, B. J. (2012). *Global religious landscape*. The Pew Research Center. Retrieved from http://www.pewforum.org/files/2014/01/global-religion-full.pdf.

Hathout, H. (1995). *Reading the Muslim mind*. Plainfield, IN: American Trust Publications.

Jonsen, A. R., Siegler, M., & Winslade, W. J. (2015). *Clinical ethics: A practical approach to ethical decisions in clinical medicine* (8th ed.). New York, NY: McGraw-Hill Education.

Juthani, N. V. (1998). Understanding and treating Hindu patients. In H. G. Koenig (Ed.), *Handbook of religion and mental health* (pp. 272–278). San Diego, CA: Academic Press.

Kehoe, N. C. (1998). Religion and mental health from the Catholic perspective. In H. G. Koenig (Ed.), *Handbook of religion and mental health*. San Diego, CA: Academic Press.

Koenig, H. G., King, D. E., & Carson, V. B. (2012). *Handbook of religion and health* (2nd ed.). New York, NY: Oxford University Press.

Lipke, M. (2016). Muslims and Islam: Key findings in the U.S. and around the world. Retrieved from http://www.pewresearch.org/fact-tank/2016/07/22/muslims-and-islam-key-findings-in-the-u-s-and-around-the-world/.

Markwell, H. J., & Brown, B. F. (2001). Bioethics for clinicians: 27. Catholic bioethics. *Canadian Medical Association Journal, 165*(2), 189–192.

Marty, M. E. (1986) *Health and medicine in the Lutheran tradition*. Health/Medicine and the Faith Traditions Series. New York, NY: Crossroad.

McCormick, R. A. (1987). *Health and medicine in the Catholic tradition*. Health/Medicine and the Faith Traditions Series. New York, NY: Crossroad.

Mizuno, T., & Slingsby, B. T. (2007). Eye on religion: Considering the influence of Buddhist and Shinto thought on contemporary Japanese bioethics. *Southern Medical Journal, 100*(1), 115–117.

Novick, B. (1998). *Making Jewish decisions about the body* (2nd ed.). New York, NY: United Synagogue of Conservative Judaism.

Rahman, F. (1987). *Health and medicine in the Islamic tradition*. Health/Medicine and the Faith Traditions Series. New York, NY: Crossroad.

Ratanakul P. (1988). Bioethics in Thailand: The struggle for Buddhist solutions. *Journal of Medicine and Philosophy, 13*, 301–312.

Sarma, D. (2008). "Hindu" Bioethics? *The Journal of Law, Medicine & Ethics, 36*(1), 51–58.

Scotton, B. W. (1998). Treating Buddhist patients. In H. G. Koenig (Ed.), *Handbook of religion and mental health.* San Diego, CA: Academic Press.

Smith, D. H. (1986). *Health and medicine in the Anglican tradition.* Health/Medicine and the Faith Traditions Series. New York, NY: Crossroad.

Vaux, K. L. (1984). *Health and medicine in the Reformed tradition.* Health/Medicine and the Faith Traditions Series. New York, NY: Crossroad.

Ethical Issues Related to Religious Considerations in Psychiatric Diagnosis

Allan M. Josephson, M.D.

RELIGION, ETHICS, AND PSYCHIATRY ARE ALL CONCERNED WITH MEANING, purpose, intention, and consequence. In determining how we as humans should live, we draw on these separate disciplines throughout our lives. Many times the concerns of each are overlapping and require a joint approach. This chapter considers how a patient's journey in psychiatry begins—that is, with a diagnosis.

The word *diagnosis* comes from the Greek *gnosis*, meaning "knowledge," and *dia*, meaning "all through" (Combrick-Graham, 1990). "To know all through" is the high standard of diagnosis, and the term connotes much more than labeling or measuring (Kendler, 2016). According to the *Diagnostic and Statistical Manual of Mental Disorders, 5th edition,* or DSM-5 (American Psychiatric Association [APA], 2013), an individual with a diagnosable mental disorder must have disturbance in cognition, emotion regulation, and behavior that reflects dysfunction in psychological, biological, or developmental processes. The disorder must be associated with distress and/or disability or impairment in important life functions.

Spirituality refers to one's connection to something transcendent and larger than oneself, a connection that gives life meaning. It is beyond the material or physical. It is an umbrella concept under which the specific category of religion is subsumed. The tendency to believe that there is more to existence than the material, that life has a spiritual element, is codified in various religions through beliefs or tenets and related historical events that are often documented in written form (i.e., Scriptures). Spirituality provides an experience, whereas religion provides an explanation. The term *worldview* may have even more utility in that it embraces religious views but also a cognitive perspective that includes nonreligious, secular, and atheist views (Josephson & Peteet, 2004).

Pargament (2007) has discussed the increasingly common tendency of individuals to align with spirituality but distance themselves from religion. At its simplest, identifying oneself as a follower of a particular religion often implies a commitment or responsibility to a supreme being, whereas spirituality does not typically involve such a commitment. Similarly, a secular ethic requires no commitment to a religious vision but is proposed to rest on reason alone.

If diagnosis is knowing through and through, it would seem to include understanding the factors that comprise this knowing, which should encompass a range of psychological, biological, social, and spiritual factors.

RELATIONSHIPS AMONG RELIGION/ SPIRITUALITY AND ETHICS/MORALITY

How are ethics and religion related? Peteet (2004) commented that the word *moral* has been used in numerous ways, often interchangeably with *ethical*. By convention, *moral* refers to what is good, right, or ideal (i.e., how things ought or ought not to be), whereas *ethical* refers to the means of achieving moral ends, with ethical reasoning describing the process of deciding about those ends. As soon as one begins to use terms that refer to what is ultimately good or an ideal course of action, philosophical, religious, and spiritual questions emerge: Are there moral universals, and what might their content be? Does morality depend on external, objective, transcendent reality? What might be the characteristics of this transcendent reality? Consideration of these issues often leads to an exploration of the patient's and therapist's worldviews.

Morality deals with content—that is, the right and wrong of things. Ethics deals with the process of reasoning about right and wrong, making it easier for some to deal with ethics without dealing directly with morality. Many believe that morality is more closely connected with religion than ethics, which is taken to be a primary product of pure reason. There is little philosophical support for this position; some philosophers believe that ethics is concerned with doing the right thing just as much as morality is concerned with doing what is right. Both depend on basic moral intuitions that defy efforts to place them in a substrate of an even deeper, purer reason. They are underived first principles, if you will. Although the question is crucially important, it is beyond the scope of this chapter to ask from what source we get these foundational and common notions of right, wrong, and justice.

Some issues may seem more ethically related, even unethical. Examples include diagnosing a 2-year-old with bipolar disorder and medicating him; changing diagnoses or medications to garner more days of hospitalization coverage from an insurance company; making a diagnosis of attention-deficit hyperactivity disorder to facilitate use of drugs for academic performance enhancement. On the other hand, some issues might be seen as primarily moral, potentially influenced by religion. Examples are a major depressive episode after an existential life crisis and anxiety and depression related to the discovery of a partner's extramarital affair.

This chapter first reviews religious/spiritual considerations in making a psychiatric diagnosis, then moves to ethical aspects of contemporary psychiatry affecting psychiatric diagnosis, and finally describes how those ethical aspects relate to religious/spiritual considerations.

FORMULATION AS DIAGNOSIS: RELIGIOUS/SPIRITUAL CONTRIBUTIONS

Before we address religious considerations in psychiatric diagnosis, comments on the contemporary status of psychiatric diagnosis are indicated. The current authority for psychiatric diagnostic nomenclature, the DSM-5 (APA, 2013), is anchored in description, even if it is seen by some as merely a nonsystematic grouping or hodgepodge of labels. The descriptive DSM-5 criteria are best used to index (measure or assess) psychiatric syndromes, but they have come to be seen as comprehensive statements of what is known about a disorder (Kendler, 2016). For many, the DSM-5 entries imply that the various disorders are illnesses, biologically derived. Yet diagnosis is much more than mere labeling and description.

McHugh (2005) cogently described the DSM compendium as a collection of disorders with different etiologies, essences, or causal processes known to promote them. He categorized these disorders as follows (McHugh & Slavney, 1986):

- Diseases (e.g., autism, schizophrenia): something the patient **has**
- Developmental deviations/dimensions (e.g., temperament, intelligence, personality): something the patient **is**
- Behavior patterns (e.g., conduct disorder, bulimia, alcoholism): something the patient **does**
- Life stories (e.g., posttraumatic stress disorder).

The advantage of such a conceptualization is that it allows life experience to be much more centrally involved in diagnosis. Because religious and spiritual experience is central to life experience, this opens up a much more direct way of including these experiences in making a psychiatric diagnosis. It also enriches the picture of the patient as a person, becoming congruent with the wisdom of Hippocrates: "It is more important to know what sort of person has a disease than to know what sort of disease a person has." Of course, it is best practice to know both things, and McHugh's approach facilitates this. It also allows dimensional approaches to be utilized in making a diagnosis, enriching the DSM categorical perspective. Because diagnosis tends to dictate treatment approaches, this method may lead to a more balanced use of medication and psychotherapy.

This broad approach is also congruent with the use of the biopsychosocial formulation as a diagnostic tool. Why do some genetically vulnerable individuals develop disorders and others with similar genetic vulnerabilities do not? Why do some with certain psychosocial experiences develop disorders and others with similar experiences do not? These questions are better answered by a holistic view of the patient than by the reductionistic view that disorders are entirely biologically based (Insel, 2014). Such a holistic view must include religious and spiritual perspectives. Formulation involves understanding the patient through and through, including everything that affects the patient and leads to symptomatic expression: developmental psychopathology, context, family, and meaning (Josephson, 2013; Masten, 2014; Peteet, 2010; Wakefield, 2010).

The biopsychosocial formulation clarifies clinical diagnoses by elucidating risk factors and protective factors. For example, a spiritually oriented, dependent woman who is genetically vulnerable to depression is at increased risk for decompensation as her children emancipate and leave the home, particularly if her husband is unsupportive of her spiritual life. By including the spiritual, such formulations are enriched, and rightly connote a "biopsychosociospiritual" diagnosis (Josephson & Peteet, 2004). As another example, a wife's terminal medical illness may be more distressing to a husband who views God as loving and always supportive. Or a fundamentalist family may look to Scriptures that address discipline to justify their controlling, even abusive parenting. These latter two spiritual factors would be seen as risk factors in a psychopathological formulation. In addition to influencing diagnosis, such risk factors can use distorted theology or harmful religion to interfere with and destabilize psychotherapeutic treatment.

On the other hand, religion and spirituality can protect against the onset and evolution of mental disorders. By providing core beliefs or explanations about life, supporting physically healthy lifestyles, offering direct and enduring social support, fostering social competency in children, and encouraging family continuity, religion and spirituality function as protective factors (Josephson & Peteet, 2004).

In developing a psychiatric formulation, the following five areas illustrate the salience of religion and spirituality: moral distress; meaninglessness; conflicts with authority; adolescent conduct disorder; and personality disorder (categories of diagnosis). The relationship can be synergistic, as in the interpersonal fulfillment of a marital commitment supported by a religious worldview, or antagonistic, such as when a religious worldview is not supportive of an individual's decision for abortion. This latter example illustrates the way in which personal autonomy is highly valued by the secular individual, whereas the religious individual sees personal autonomy as subject to a higher power.

Moral Distress

In a previous era, guilt was often seen as arising from an intrapsychic, "neurotic" process requiring psychotherapeutic resolution. In the current era, moral distress is usually anchored in real-life events. The recognition of symptoms of posttraumatic stress disorder arising from morally reprehensible acts has identified guilt as a realistic internal response of an individual committing such acts (Thielman, 2011). The relationship of wrongdoing and guilt to psychiatric symptoms is supported by more than anecdote. Sheehan and Kroll (1990), in a remarkable report, described psychiatric patients' belief in both general health factors and sin as causes of illness. Approximately 25% of study patients believed their illness or problems could be the result of sinful acts; 10% believed that they had committed such acts leading up to their psychiatric problems; 20% did not feel they would get better unless they did penance; and 40% said that they believed that living a moral life helps prevent illness. These were not psychotic individuals.

Katherine Ann Power was a young college student and an antiwar militant. In 1970, she was part of a group of five individuals who robbed a bank near Boston, part of an effort to support a movement against the Vietnam War. One of the group shot and killed a police officer during the robbery, and under Massachusetts law, all five were chargeable with murder. Power went underground, living in Oregon under an alias for 23 years. She remained on the FBI's Ten Most Wanted list longer than any other woman in history. During this time, she experienced depressive symptoms and received psychotherapeutic and pharmacotherapeutic treatments. Yet complete resolution of her symptoms was not achieved, and in 1993, she turned herself in and pleaded guilty to manslaughter. She completed her prison sentence in 1999 (Landman, 2001).

In this case, moral distress was directly associated with psychiatric symptomatology that did not remit with formal psychiatric treatments. Power recognized the need to confess publically, do public penance, and make efforts at reconciliation with the family of her victim. Most cases of moral distress are not the result of a tragic death. Yet social and relational modes of remediation are commonly indicated in morally charged situations (e.g., divorce). Many times, these situations are influenced by spiritual or religious contexts.

Meaning

Psychiatrists have increasingly recognized the importance of meaning to mental health. (Blazer, 2005, 2011; Frankl, 1992; Yalom, 1980). Although existential crises have been linked to depression, few examples match the power of the clinical vignette reported by Harvard psychiatrist and anthropologist, Arthur Kleinman (1988).

Dr. Bill Smith, a patient, wrote in his diary after a clinical appointment with his psychiatrist:

> I don't think he heard me. I wanted him to listen to me not for the diagnosis but for my story. I know I am depressed but I wanted to hear him tell me what was wrong. Depression may be the disease but it is not the problem. The problem is my life. The center doesn't hold. Things are falling apart. My marriage. My relationship with my kids. My confidence in my research. My sense of purpose. My dreams. Is this depression? Maybe it caused the depression. Maybe depression makes it worse or seem worse. These problems also have their own legitimate reality. It is my life, no matter if I am depressed or not. And that is what I want to talk about, to complain about, to make sense of, to get help with, to put back together again. I want this depression treated all right. But there something more I want. I want to tell this story, my story. I want someone trained to hear me. I thought that was what psychiatrists do.

The vignette of this depressed patient does not refer to religious/spiritual issues. However, the existential distress demonstrated would compel any clinician to explore such issues in making a diagnosis.

Autonomy and Authority

Religion and spirituality focus on a higher power and/or the transcendent (Alcoholics Anonymous, 1952). This leads to a question for the religious individual: What is my relationship to this higher power, and what are its expectations of me? Conflicts over autonomy and authority commonly influence presentations in many of these patients.

Glenda, a 19-year-old Caucasian woman, was referred to me for psychiatric treatment after an extensive evaluation at a major national pain program. She had had unexplained abdominal pain for several years which had necessitated multiple medical consultations, including several exploratory surgeries, to determine the source of the pain. Her abdominal pain, accompanied by headaches, eventually had no medical explanation. She was referred for psychotherapy.

In the initial interview, she stated that she had gone to a parochial school and was, at the time of the interview, home schooled. She recounted, with anger and rage, how her parochial school peers had shunned her. Most of her anger, however, was directed toward the priest. She had gone to confession with her priest and expressed aggressive fantasies toward the girl she perceived as initiating her social ostracism. By her report, she was not met with acceptance by the priest, who told her "anger was not of God."

Glenda had been instructed by the clinicians in her pain program that "keeping her anger inside" was related to her psychosomatic symptoms. She had interpreted her priest's comment as indicating that the expression of anger was forbidden by God, even a sinful expression. This placed her in significant conflict: She had experienced the benefits of following the clinical directive to express affect, yet this autonomous feeling was associated with guilt at the implicit challenge to the priest's authority. She was already conflicted about expressing anger because she was just accommodating to this new experience. This conflict and the attendant anxiety were only exacerbated by the priest's admonitions, as she perceived them.

Faith and religion intersected in the ongoing therapy. From a diagnostic standpoint, the psychosomatic and psychophysiological symptoms would not have been uncovered without an understanding of the patient's religion and spirituality. The clinician's sensitivity to her religious experience and the ability to help her elaborate it deepened the psychiatric formulation and facilitated treatment. Her treatment was furthered by an appreciation of an overly close, enmeshed relationship with her family, which also engendered anger. In this case, the clinician's worldview and the patient's worldview shared common characteristics. Thus, it became important to consider the transference-countertransference relationship and monitor whether the patient viewed the therapist as another negative religious authority figure.

Adolescent Conduct Disorder

On the whole, commitment to one's religious/spiritual beliefs has been consistently associated with more cohesive, less conflicted family environments. Such environments have been linked with fewer child mental health problems, particularly conduct problems (Mabe, Dell, & Josephson, 2011). Studies have further supported the position that religious beliefs and practices, together with strength of religion in the family and the community, are inversely related to antisocial behavior among youth. There are exceptions, but the religious/spiritual family communicates a structure and an expectation of behavior.

This positive aspect of family life must be accompanied by a strong parental attachment and personal warmth. If these are not present, the structure of religion can merge into harshness and rigidity (Pearce, 2004).

A 14-year-old boy was referred for the evaluation of conduct problems. His parents had experienced relationship difficulties related to his father's substance abuse. The father was a very angry man who had "medicated" his anger for years. This anger seemed to have arisen in a conflicted relationship with his own father, a perfectionistic minister who had high spiritual and behavioral expectations. As he worked through these psychological and spiritual issues, he and his wife could not agree on appropriate limits for their son. They vacillated between harshness and lenience until the father eventually understood the spiritual conflicts of his own developmental years and their impact on his parenting. These spiritual conflicts led to an incomplete and inaccurate diagnostic formulation, seeing the son's behavior as more deviant than his relatively mild conduct problems indicated. From an ethical perspective, the father was not acting with beneficence or non-maleficence (see later discussion).

The diagnosis of adolescent conduct disorder must be associated with a thorough family evaluation, including consideration of the family's religious/spiritual worldview.

Personality Disorders

In marking religious and spiritual distinctions in diagnosis, there is often overlap among the religious, the spiritual, and the scientific. This is perhaps most clearly demonstrated in making the diagnosis of personality disorders, defined as enduring maladaptive patterns of inner experience and behavior that deviate markedly from the expectations of the individual's culture (Bendelow, 2010). Yet these enduring patterns of behavior can also be conceptualized in religious and spiritual terms. Religious and spiritual virtues such as temperance, prudence, fortitude, love, hope, and faith are associated with mental health and happiness (Cloninger, 2011). But there also are religious and spiritual terms that describe enduring maladaptive patterns of thoughts, feelings, and behavior. These terms include *vice* and *sin* and describe behaviors and attitudes that need to be "made right again."

For example, what is the difference between the grandiose focus on self to the exclusion of another's needs, diagnosed as narcissism, and the sin of pride, defined by Karl Menninger (1973) as "the willful disregard of the welfare of others for the satisfaction of self?" Such patterns of behavior clearly hurt other individuals. They both require remediation. In the former, the narcissistic mode of behaving arises in a family context in which an individual becomes entitled and defensively self-serving. In the latter, an individual knows the right and chooses the wrong. He makes a free choice of self over other. This difference may be too close to call in some situations, but all would agree that these patterns of behavior need alteration.

Ellen, the wife of a 48-year-old pastor, filed for a divorce. Her decision occurred in a spiritual community which through its traditions, beliefs, and practices did not support divorce. Ellen had tried for years to attain a more equal marriage. Her talented husband, Richard, was worshipped by parishioners, but he also required constant admiration in interpersonal relationships. This led to an affair, for which he was not remorseful. As Ellen sank further into depression, feeling that she was, in effect, a single parent of her two daughters, her psychotherapist encouraged her to "individuate" and leave the toxic marriage.

Psychological change includes the examination of one's mental life and alteration of the interactions that have given rise to cognitive constructs; often this occurs in the context of psychotherapy. In this case, Ellen grew through psychotherapy, which opened her up to the spiritual act of forgiving her husband. Psychological and spiritual change reinforced each other.

At the same time, Richard refused to take part in psychotherapy of any type. Spiritual change involves an examination of one's spiritual choices and their effects on others, with acknowledgement of error and asking for forgiveness, potentially leading to a spiritual reconciliation. This process began with Ellen but not with her husband, who believed such an act of contrition was inappropriate for a leader of his stature. Richard's resistance to change is familiar to clinicians working with the narcissistic patient but may also be fueled by the sin of pride. A clinician's diagnostic formulation can be enriched by considering spiritual components that may be contributing to the tenacity of resistance to change. Such a formulation prepares the way for intervening at the psychological level, the spiritual level, or both.

In sum, these five areas are not the only examples of how religious and spiritual factors intersect with psychiatric diagnostic formulations. Koenig, King, and Carson (2012) described, in an exhaustive review, the dramatic increase in the number of research studies in religion and health, with a strong emphasis on medical/psychiatric diagnosis. They boldly stated that the enormous increase in attention paid to this topic by various disciplines indicated the birth of an entirely new field of religion, spirituality, and health. Research in religion and mental health is no small part of this growth. Any attempt at diagnosis must thoroughly assess religious and spiritual variables to determine their relevance and role in the causes and effects of mental disorders.

Given the clear relationship of religion and spirituality to psychiatric diagnosis and formulation, we now move to ethical considerations in diagnosis.

ETHICAL ISSUES RELATED TO PSYCHIATRIC DIAGNOSIS

Ethics deals with what is right and what facilitates human flourishing. More specifically, the traditional core principles of bioethics are to foster autonomy, to do no harm (non-maleficence), to promote good in all actions (beneficence), and to promote justice (Orr, 2009). Virtue ethics is person based rather than action based: It looks at the virtue or moral character of the person carrying out the action rather than at the consequences of particular acts (Radden & Sadler, 2010).

In relating ethics to psychiatric diagnosis, this discussion emphasizes non-maleficence (do no harm) and beneficence (act in the best interests of the patient). The chairman of the DSM-IV task force, Allen Frances, wrote that "an accurate diagnosis can save a life; and an inaccurate diagnosis can wreck one" (Frances, 2013, p. 242). In the language of ethics, when we make accurate diagnoses we are promoting good (beneficence), and by avoiding inaccurate diagnoses we are doing no harm (non-maleficence).

In making a diagnosis, it is often the case that the truth hurts. Formulating the role of psychopathology in one's problems or the problems of another is a difficult experience and often can take place only with professional guidance (i.e., psychotherapy). As appealing as it might be, diagnosis cannot be mitigated because of concern about possible stigma associated with its application. Sensitively conferring an accurate diagnosis is the only ethical way to proceed. This process should improve the doctor–patient relationship through its basis in openness, honesty, and integrity.

The inclusion of religious and spiritual aspects of patients' life experience improves diagnostic accuracy through the delineation of sick religion from healthy religion. The therapeutic alliance with religious/spiritual patients is further strengthened by thoughtful consideration of their religious/spiritual experience. This is facilitated by clinician self-knowledge of her worldview as she sensitively explores issues influencing diagnosis (e.g., drug abuse, abortion, divorce, teen sexuality).

The Ethics of Diagnostic Inflation

Misdiagnosis, evidenced by diagnostic inflation, seems to have reached epidemic proportions (Whitaker, 2010). A number of critics have wondered whether the benefits of increased identification outweigh the harms of overdiagnosis and overmedication. During the last 20 years, childhood bipolar disorder has increased by a miraculous 40 fold, autism is up an astonishing 20 fold, attention deficit disorder has tripled, and adult bipolar disorder has doubled (Frances, 2013, p.104). The increase in childhood bipolar disorder was so embarrassing that the disorder had to be replaced in DSM-5 by the newly described Disruptive Mood Dysregulation Disorder, to temper the outrage over this particular misdiagnosis.

For many, diagnostic inflation is a major threat to psychiatry's credibility. For others, an increase in diagnoses means that previously undetected cases will now receive treatment. This debate will continue for the foreseeable future. It does seem clear that more disorders means more medications used to treat them (Safer, Rajakannan, Burcu, & Zito, 2015). Clearly, the pharmaceutical industry has pushed the clinical and scientific agenda in this direction (Cipriani et al., 2016; Cosgrove & Wheeler, 2013; Fournier et al., 2010). When psychiatry moves away from a holistic approach and looks only to biomedicine, it moves away from the patient, the family, and the patient's faith commitments and worldview. This all too frequently harms the patient and certainly is not in his or her best interests. Simply, this approach is all too often "not right."

The increased emphasis on description and labeling has changed the nature of clinical care and the practice of psychiatry (Plakun, 2015). Clinical care now places less emphasis on family life and developmental issues, often medicalizing straightforward problems. Perhaps the bipolar epidemic could have been prevented if patterns of interaction in families had been examined more closely. At the height of the epidemic, it was not uncommon for a rageful child to be hospitalized after a violent outburst and to receive the diagnosis of bipolar disorder. Not uncommonly, careful examination of the family revealed that the rages were triggered when the child "did not get his way." Diagnostic shifts that take the clinician's focus away from developmental and family issues have potentiated the difficulty in discerning spiritual, religious, and existential issues in developing a diagnostic formulation.

During a family therapy session, a 6-year-old boy irritably and angrily told his mother to "shut up." He did not appreciate her limit-setting efforts and directly communicated his distress. The astonished clinician asked of the mother and the father, "Isn't someone going to do anything here?" The mother responded, "He has attention deficit disorder." This misdiagnosis, absolving her son of personal responsibility, is not uncommon. The boy's entitlement arose from a special position in the family. His somewhat older parents' difficulty in limit setting had its roots in their belief that his birth was a gift, bestowed upon them after they had spent a number of years trying to conceive.

A 10-year-old boy was referred to a child psychiatrist for evaluation of the medication used to treat his presumed bipolar disorder. The young boy had thrown a Lego block at his school art teacher, injuring her by striking her in the forehead. The teacher had accidentally knocked to the floor a ceramic object the boy had, with some pride, just completed painting in her art class. When the object shattered as it hit the floor, the boy reflexively threw the nearest object at the teacher because "she did this on purpose." In reviewing the case, the psychiatrist determined that the young boy was in foster care because his father had abused him and his mother had abandoned him. As a consequence, he had developed a suspicious, overly sensitive, somewhat paranoid view of the world. No one had taken the time to elicit the boy's story and make sense of what had happened. Clearly, he was not suffering from a major mental illness, and he did not need medication, let alone having it increased.

Wakefield wrote that knowledge of normal human variation, context, and meaning are essential to judge disorder. Without consideration of these variables, there is a strong tendency to make false-positive diagnoses (Wakefield, 2010). Both of these boys illustrate the problem of diagnostic false-positives.

The Ethics of Misdiagnosis: Inappropriate Treatment

Perhaps the most salient issue in the ethics of diagnosis is the harm (maleficence) of misdiagnosis. Diagnosis appears to have been hijacked, with a thorough assessment giving way to mere labeling, and a developmental understanding of patients based on their life experience giving way to symptom checklists (McHugh & Slavney, 2015). Misdiagnoses violate the principles of beneficence and non-maleficence. These diagnoses often lead clinicians away from effective treatments toward potentially harmful treatments and practices (e.g., polypharmacy). The harms associated with polypharmacy and excessive dosing are self-evident. Many patients who know nothing of non-maleficence feel wronged by this practice.

A young woman, Jenny, was having memory difficulty and other neurological symptoms after discharge from years of residential treatment. During that treatment, she received multiple psychotropic medications for behavior problems, medications that she felt she could not refuse. When she later came to experience the long-term side effects of excessive medication, she shrieked, "It wasn't right! It wasn't right. They shouldn't have done that to me" (De Sa, 2014). In this case, misdiagnosis led to harmful, unnecessary psychiatric treatment. The patient's response, however, was not simply that she had received poor care but rather that she had been "wronged." She used an ethical term to describe her treatment.

By implying that medication can solve the problems of family relationships, for example, a patient is taken even further away from understanding the source of his problems, the clinical truth. He thus is not guided in an effective way to manage life and deal with his clinical problems. Religious and spiritual considerations bring back ethical practice by enriching context, which facilitates clinical understanding and minimizes potentially harmful treatments. For example, Jenny's harmful and unethical treatments may have been avoided by psychotherapeutic attention to her anxiety, which had existential sources—"Why did God give me parents who didn't want me?"

The Ethics of Misdiagnosis: Specific Religious/Spiritual Factors

In the last generation, mainstream psychiatry has increasingly turned away from serious consideration of the importance of relationships, meaning, context, social issues, and values (Horowitz & Wakefield, 2007, 2012). The push for psychiatry to be an applied neuroscience dealing only with mental illnesses and corresponding brain dysfunctions has marginalized life experience (Insel, 2014). This has correspondingly impacted religion and spirituality, which have everything to do with life experience.

When we speak of mental illness, we speak of a territory that is relational and value laden. It is a world that cannot be grasped with the same form of medical epistemology that has worked well in, for example, cardiology and endocrinology. What would it take for psychiatrists to have the courage to think differently about what an assessment should cover and about the nature of interventions proposed? Would not the chance for misdiagnosis decrease significantly if religious and spiritual factors were included in the review of a patient's life experience? Although misdiagnosis can happen throughout psychiatric practice without specific reference to religion or spirituality, there are some challenging diagnostic decisions to be made in a psychiatric formulation that is sensitive to religious/spiritual issues.

On the one hand, clinicians can mistake spiritual phenomena for psychiatric disorders or problems. Clinicians may diagnose patients as having personality disorders (e.g., narcissistic and antisocial) and youth as having conduct disorders, missing the volitional aspect of their behavioral choices. Spiritual despair and existential struggles with meaning are often mistaken for depression. More controversially, there have been reports of spiritual interventions being helpful in patients diagnosed as psychotic, raising the possibility of a possession state being causal (Irmak, 2014). The fact that some behavioral phenomena (e.g., eating disorders, addictive disorders) turn out to be spiritually linked is now well appreciated (Alcoholics Anonymous, 1952; Dell & Josephson, 2007). Apart from psychiatric diagnosis, significant behavioral change attributed to spiritual conversion has been described in the spiritual literature (Colson, 1979; Lewis, 1955).

On the other hand, clinicians and religious professionals can also misidentify psychiatric disorders as spiritual problems. Depending on the setting, hallucinations can be seen as a spiritual communication rather than a sign of mental illness. In some settings, the treatment of depression is associated with a spiritual view that one just needs to pray harder to lessen depression's power. Similarly, the intractability of a drug abuse pattern could be attributed to a spiritual weakness, or a persistent obsessive-compulsive pattern of behavior seen only in a religious context could be viewed as scrupulosity. A persistent pattern of promiscuity driven by an attachment disorder generated by neglect and abuse can be seen as primary sexual sin.

The Ethics of Cultural Influences

A DSM diagnosis is needed in many situations and is usually applied appropriately, but cultural forces have influenced how diagnoses are actually made and implemented. Frances noted that there is a difference between the DSM documents as written and oral traditions used in the application of DSM diagnoses. DSM descriptions are used and misused through the influences of physicians, other mental health workers, drug companies, advocacy groups, school systems, the courts, the Internet, and advertising on cable television (Frances, 2013, p. 139). These cultural forces that impact how diagnoses are made and used are clearly influenced by individual and collective worldviews.

Misdiagnosis for the financial gain of others is a particularly egregious unethical practice. Manipulating diagnoses to gain hospital admission or to extend hospital stays is one way in which clinicians attempt to assist patients in getting financial coverage for mental health care. Drug companies, in developing new products, are dependent on the diagnoses for which the products are developed (Cosgrove & Wheeler, 2013). Analyses of these issues again draws one into a consideration of ethics and its interrelationship with the diagnostic process.

THE CLINICIAN'S WORLDVIEW, RELIGION/SPIRITUALITY, AND ETHICS

The APA encourages clinicians to obtain information from their patients regarding their religious/spiritual commitments (APA, 2006). Doing so more fully informs a diagnostic formulation and facilitates all subsequent treatment efforts. These diagnostic considerations parallel the increasing discussion of the clinician's religious/spiritual commitments in psychotherapy (Peteet, 2013). Aware that their process of diagnosis is influenced by their own worldview, psychiatrists must be careful to avoid imposing their religious/spiritual (or anti-religious) views on the patient. This intentional effort in the diagnostic process is critical given that it is increasingly recognized that value neutrality in psychotherapy is a myth (Josephson & Peteet, 2004; Peteet, 2013).

The ethical positions held by clinicians are shaped, consciously or unconsciously, by their specific worldviews. The differing worldviews of clinicians lead to differing views of what constitutes human flourishing and, correspondingly, to different approaches to diagnosis and formulation. In our contemporary, pluralistic society, these worldviews undergird competing values, which are derived from either secular or spiritual/religious sources (Poplin, 2014).

As suggested, clinicians with a religious/spiritual worldview may diagnose or formulate cases differently from their secular colleagues. For example, personal autonomy is not the highest value for religious people, whereas it rates highly for the secular person. For the religious person, autonomy is relative, seen in the context of autonomy under God. In sum, it makes a significant difference if the clinician believes that he practices in an accidental world or in a world that was intended. With some variation, these two worldviews are the primary ones influencing contemporary practice.

Ethics and psychiatric diagnosis are intertwined. Contemporary society reflects a so-called culture war of competing worldviews. This conflict serves as the backdrop for ethical influences on psychiatric diagnosis. Any culturally influenced clinical diagnosis suggesting a change in behavior patterns that have been accepted for centuries requires careful analysis and scrutiny. This happens most commonly in contemporary psychiatry in the value-laden area of human sexuality. For example, declaring that gender dysphoria is a variant of normal development is a statement that must be scrutinized. All patients must be treated with dignity and respect—yet, in the service of intellectual integrity, psychiatry must scrutinize all ideas, while maintaining tolerance toward the individuals holding them. Again, the ethical good is served by clinical/diagnostic accuracy. No idea is above scrutiny; no person is beneath dignity (Nawaz, 2013).

SUMMARY

Diagnosis in psychiatry is about knowing the patient "through and through." This knowledge of necessity includes the patient's religious, spiritual, and worldview perspectives and commitments, the clinical relevance of which is especially obvious when dealing with moral distress, a loss of meaning, concerns about autonomy in relation to authority, and disordered behavior (e.g., personality disorders, conduct disorder). As the basis for effective treatment, diagnosis has important ethical implications. Harmful misdiagnosis can result from a truncated view of the person, from religious or pharmacological bias, or from cultural pressures to conform. This complexity requires clinicians to be aware of the influence of their own commitments. Both clinical observations and research efforts suggest that taking religion, spirituality, and worldview into account is good for the patient and can be done without doing harm.

REFERENCES

Alcoholics Anonymous. (1952). *Twelve steps and twelve traditions.* New York, NY: Alcoholics Anonymous World Services.

American Psychiatric Association. (2006, December). *Resource document on religious/spiritual commitments and psychiatric practice.* APA Official Action. Corresponding Committee on Religion, Spirituality, and Psychiatry.

American Psychiatric Association. (2013). *Diagnostic and Statistical Manual of Mental Disorders, 5th edition (DSM-5).* Arlington, VA: Author.

Bendelow, G. (2010). Ethical aspects of personality disorders. *Current Opinion in Psychiatry, 23,* 546–549.

Blazer, D. G. (2005). *The age of melancholy: Major depression and its social origins.* New York, NY: Routledge.

Blazer, D. G. (2011) Spirituality and depression: A background for the development of the DSM-V. In J. R. Peteet, F. G. Lu, & W. E. Narrow (Eds.), *Religious and spiritual issues in psychiatric diagnosis* (pp. 1–21). Arlington, VA: American Psychiatric Association.

Cipriani, A., Zhou, X., Del Giovane, C. D., Hetrick, S. E., Qin, B., Whittington, C., . . . Xie, P. (2016). Comparative efficacy and tolerability of antidepressants for major depressive disorder in children and adolescents: A network meta-analysis. *The Lancet, 388*(10047), 881–890.

Cloninger, C. R. (2011). Religious and spiritual issues in personality disorders. In J. R. Peteet, F. G. Lu, & W. E. Narrow (Eds.), *Religious and spiritual issues in psychiatric diagnosis: A research agenda for DSM-V* (pp. 151–164). Arlington, VA: American Psychiatric Association.

Colson, C. W. (1979). *Life sentence.* Lincoln, VA: Chosen Books.

Combrick-Graham, L. (1990). *Giant steps: Therapeutic innovations in child mental health.* New York, NY: Basic Books.

Cosgrove, L., & Wheeler, E. E. (2013). Drug firms, the diagnostic categories, and bias in clinical guidelines. *Journal of Law, Medicine & Ethics, 41*(3), 644–653.

De Sa, K. (2014). Drugging our kids. *Mercury News.* Retrieved from http://webspecial.mercurynews.com/druggedkids.

Dell, M. L., & Josephson, A. (2007). Religious and spiritual factors in childhood and adolescent eating disorders and obesity. *Southern Medical Journal, 100,* 628–632.

Fournier, J. C., DeRubeis, R. J., Hollon, S. D., Dimidjian, S, Amsterdam, J. D., Shelton, R. C., & Fawcett, J. (2010). Antidepressant drug effects and depression severity: A patient-level meta-analysis. *JAMA Psychiatry, 303*(1), 47–53.

Frances, A. (2013). *Saving normal.* New York, NY: HarperCollins Publisher.

Frankl, V. E. (1992). *Man's search for meaning.* Boston, MA: Beacon Press.

Horwitz, A. V., & Wakefield, J. C. (2007). *The loss of sadness: How psychiatry transformed normal sorrow into depressive disorder.* New York, NY: Oxford University Press.

Horwitz, A. V., & Wakefield, J. C. (2012). *All we have to fear: Psychiatry's transformation of natural anxieties into mental disorders.* New York, NY: Oxford University Press.

Insel, T. R. (2014). The NIMH Research Domain Criteria (RDoC) Project: Precision medicine for psychiatry. *American Journal of Psychiatry, 171,* 395–397.

Irmak, M. K. (2014). Schizophrenia or possession? *Journal of Religion and Health, 53*(3), 773–777.

Josephson, A. M. (2013). Family intervention as a developmental psychodynamic therapy. *Child and Adolescent Psychiatry Clinics of North America, 22*: 241–260.

Josephson, A. M., & Peteet, J. R. (2004). *Handbook of spirituality and worldview in clinical practice.* Arlington, VA: American Psychiatric Association.

Kendler, K. S. (2016). The phenomenology of major depression and the representativeness and nature of DSM criteria. *American Journal of Psychiatry, 173*(8), 771–780.

Kleinman, A. (1988). *Rethinking psychiatry: From cultural category to personal experience.* New York, NY: The Free Press.

Koenig, H. G., King, D. E., & Carson, V. B. (2012). *Handbook of religion and health* (2nd ed.). New York, NY: Oxford University Press.

Landman, J. (2001). The limits of reconciliation: The story of a perpetrator, Katherine Ann Power. *Social Justice Research, 14*(2): 171–188.

Lewis, C. S. (1955). *Surprised by joy.* London, England: Collins.

Mabe, P. A., Dell, M. L., & Josephson, A. M. (2011). Spiritual and religious perspectives on child and adolescent psychopathology. In J. R. Peteet, F. G. Lu, & W. E. Narrow (Eds.), *Religious and spiritual issues in psychiatric diagnosis: A research agenda for DSM-V* (pp. 123–142). Arlington, VA: American Psychiatric Association.

Masten, A. S. (2014). *Ordinary magic.* New York, NY: The Guilford Press.

McHugh, P. R. (2005). Striving for coherence: Psychiatry's efforts over classification. *Journal of the American Medical Association, 293*(20), 2526–2528.

McHugh, P. R., & Slavney, P. R. (1986). *The perspectives of psychiatry* (2nd ed.). Baltimore, MD: The Johns Hopkins University Press.

McHugh, P. R., & Slavney, P. R. (2015). Mental illness: Comprehensive evaluation or checklist? *New England Journal of Medicine, 366*(20), 1853–1855.

Menninger, K. (1973). *Whatever became of sin?* New York, NY: Hawthorn Books.

Nawaz, M. (2013). *Radical: My journey out of Islamist extremism.* Guilford, CT: Lyons Press.

Orr, R. D. (2009). *Medical ethics and the faith factor: A handbook for clergy and health-care professionals.* Grand Rapids, MI: William B. Eerdmans.

Pargament, K. I. (2007). *Spiritually integrated psychotherapy: Understanding and addressing the sacred.* New York, NY: The Guilford Press.

Pearce, L. (2004). Intergenerational religious dynamics and adolescent delinquency. *Social Forces, 82,* 1553–1572.

Peteet, J. R. (2004). *Doing the right thing: An approach to moral issues in mental health treatment.* Arlington, VA: American Psychiatric Publishing.

Peteet, J. R. (2010). *Depression and the soul: A guide to spiritually integrated treatment.* New York, NY: Routledge.

Peteet, J. R. (2013). What is the place of clinicians' religious or spiritual commitments in psychotherapy? A virtues-based perspective. *Journal of Religious Health, 43*(4), 1190–1198.

Plakun, E. M. (2015). Correcting psychiatry's false assumptions and implementing parity. *Psychiatric Times, 325,* 56–60.

Poplin, M. (2014). *Is reality secular? Testing the assumptions of four global worldviews.* Downers Grove, IL: InterVarsity Press.

Radden, J., & Sadler, J. Z. (2010). *The virtuous psychiatrist: Character ethics in psychiatric practice.* New York, NY: Oxford University Press.

Safer, D. J., Rajakannan, T., Burcu, M., & Zito, J. M. (2015). Trends in subthreshold psychiatric diagnoses for youth in community treatment. *JAMA Psychiatry, 72*(1), 75–83.

Sheehan, W., & Kroll, J. (1990). Psychiatric patients' belief in general health factors and sin as causes of illness. *American Journal of Psychiatry, 147*(1), 112–113.

Thielman, S. B. (2011) Religion and spirituality in the description of posttraumatic stress disorder. In J. R. Peteet, F. G. Lu, & W. E. Narrow (Eds.), *Religious and spiritual issues in psychiatric diagnosis: A research agenda for DSM-V* (pp. 105–113). Arlington, VA: American Psychiatric Association.

Wakefield, J. C. (2010). False positives in psychiatric diagnosis: Implications for human freedom. *Theoretical Medicine and Bioethics, 31,* 5–17.

Whitaker, R. (2010). *Anatomy of an epidemic: Magic bullets, psychiatric drugs, and the astonishing rise of mental illness in America.* New York, NY: Random House.

Yalom, I. D. (1980). *Existential Psychotherapy.* New York, NY: Basic Books.

FIVE

Unhealthy and Potentially Harmful Uses of Religion

James Griffith, M.D., and Gina Magyar-Russell, Ph.D.

WHY THERE IS A PROBLEM

Religious coping is perhaps the most commonly utilized source of resilience worldwide when facing of harsh adversity (de Jong, 2014, pp. 817–819; Kleinman, 2006, p. 14). Yet religious beliefs and practices also can produce self-harm, motivate violence toward others, and amplify suffering for people enduring illness or misfortune (Griffith, 2010; Pargament, Smith, Koenig, & Perez, 1998). Healthcare professionals need a framework for assessing and intervening that protects vulnerable individuals without violating expressions of religiousness. This framework should be grounded in a scientific understanding of human behavior while also respecting moral values provided by religious traditions.

Instances in which religion has produced harm can be identified for any religion. What is harmful seems not to be the type of religion but *how* any religion is implemented such that person-to-person relatedness is violated. Harmful uses of religion characteristically fail to extend empathy and compassion to others who suffer, even though identity with a religious group may be strong (Griffith, 2010). Social psychology and social neuroscience research have clarified how personal spirituality and sociobiological religious life are organized by different social cognition systems within the human brain (Griffith, 2010, pp. 36–55). Personal spirituality is primarily organized by person-to-person social cognition, whereas categorical social cognition primarily organizes the sociobiological religious life of religious groups. Religion that produces harm typically emerges when sociobiological religious life obscures the sensibilities of personal spirituality.

Archeological relics of religion that organized group life have been found from the early days of agriculture; religious belief provided a source for magical powers or an organizational structure for god-like rulers to govern a society. Personal spirituality appeared much later in the history of religion. Well-being of individual persons did not emerge as a central concern for religion until the Axial Age, between 800 B.C.E. and 700 C.E., when charismatic religious leaders emerged who helped transform religion from its archaic tribal orientations to focus on the moral self-awareness of individuals (Armstrong, 1993; Barnes, 2000). These religious leaders sought to discriminate institutionalized religious practices from an individual's personal religious experience, with the latter emphasizing beliefs, practices, and communal ways of living that alleviated suffering of individuals. They moved religion's field of interest away from the welfare of the group to the interior lives of individuals. The fruit of their labors was emergence of personal spirituality as a form of religion within which the lived experience of an individual person is given priority. In her book, *A History of God*, Karen Armstrong (1993, p. 391) characterized the religious transformations of this historical era as follows:

> Compassion was a characteristic of most of the ideologies that were created during the Axial Age. The compassionate ideal even impelled Buddhists to make a major change in their religious orientation when they introduced devotion (bhakti) to the Buddha and bodhisattvas. The prophets insisted that cult and worship were useless unless society as a whole adopted a more just and compassionate ethos. These insights were developed by Jesus, Paul, and the Rabbis, who all shared the same Jewish ideals and suggested major changes in Judaism to implement them. The Koran made the creation of a compassionate and just society the essence of the reformed religion of al-Lah. Compassion is a particularly difficult virtue. It demands that we go beyond the limitations of our egotism, insecurity and inherited prejudice.

Spiritualities associated with Taoism, Judaism, Christianity, Islam, Buddhism, and other traditions share remarkably similar themes. These themes have also been central to the work of more recent spiritual leaders, from Mahatma Gandhi to Mother Teresa and Martin Luther King, Jr. (Griffith, 2010, pp. 28–31; Griffith & Elliot, 2002, pp. 22–27). These fundamental themes include the following:

- Whole Person Relatedness—Spiritualities give primacy to whole person–to–whole person relatedness, which means opening oneself and responding fully to the Other as a person. Desire to learn about the Other's experience, despite acknowledged differences, is characteristic. Distinctions about social status, class, ethnicity, gender, and other such social categories are put aside. Such whole person–to–whole person relations have been characterized as I–Thou (Buber, 1958) or face-to-face relations (Levinas, 1961).
- Commitment to an Ethic of Compassion—Even inward-focused spiritualties, such as Buddhism, make an ethic of compassion a central theme. Any suffering person receives care, concern, and efforts to heal or protect, without regard to social category or status.
- Compassionate Care for Self—Compassion for others is also extended to oneself by most spiritualities. Compassionate care for self provides containment for personal woundedness, which interrupts cycles of revenge and retaliation.
- Emotional Postures of Resilience—Spiritualities typically generate coherency, hope, purpose, gratitude, joy, and other existential postures that confer resilience in the face of threat, uncertainty, and suffering.
- Encounters with the Sacred as Personal Experiences That Stimulate Reflection, Moral Reasoning, and Creativity—Within spirituality, encounters with the sacred lead to personal reflection rather than efforts to use the power of the sacred to control other individuals through magic, as in primitive religions, or to rule societies or fight enemies, as has often happened in classical religions.
- Prioritizing Well-Being of Individual Persons Over the Needs of Religious Groups—At its heart, spirituality is centered on the individual person, even when that leads to conflict with agendas of the religious group.

Personal spirituality sets a standard for relational and ethical living against which the moral worth of religious acts can be judged, both within the personal lives of individuals and at a societal level. The question then becomes not what type of religion produces harm but what types of religious rhetoric and acts diminish or erase the influence of personal spirituality in religious life.

RELIGION THAT VIOLATES PERSONAL SPIRITUALITY

There are three major classes of religious life that commonly impede the moral standards set by personal spirituality. These difficulties account for most of the harmful uses of religion that clinicians encounter in their practices.

- Sociobiological Religious Life That Obscures Personal Spirituality—Human sociobiology utilizes religious beliefs and practices to engineer strong, well-organized groups. However, empathy and compassion for individual persons did not evolve as part of the behavioral agenda of sociobiology. Religious life largely organized by sociobiological systems can produce secondary harm to people outside, and sometimes inside, the religious group (Griffith, 2010).
- Religion That Becomes a Conduit for Mental Illness—Religious experiences that are tolerable, or even growth-producing, for other individuals can be disorganizing for vulnerable individuals with mental illnesses. Lack of knowledge by religious leaders or religious groups about potentially harmful interactions between religious experiences and mental illnesses can place individuals with mental illnesses at risk (Griffith, Myers, & Compton, 2016).
- Spiritual Struggle—A religious person experiences spiritual struggle in conflicted meanings, motivations, and actions within his or her personal religious life; in interpersonal relationships; in relation to religious tradition; or in relation to God or other supernatural forces, including demonic forces.

Sociobiological Religious Life That Obscures Personal Spirituality

Ironically, religious acts of hatred or violence often are committed by people who do not suffer from chronic mental illness and whose religious traditions emphasize empathy and compassion. However, the religious lives of these people have been regimented by sociobiological behavioral systems that utilize religion to organize cohesive, tightly organized groups. Religion then becomes a marker of identity rather than a source of concern, empathy, and compassion for the Other. Sociobiological and social neuroscience research have provided the most coherent explanations for religious violence (Griffith, 2010) by groups ranging from anti-immigrant Christians to Muslim suicide bombers, Jewish settlers attacking Palestinians, and Buddhists attacking Myanmar's Rohingya. Because protagonists of religious violence are unlikely to seek help from a mental health professional, these problems rarely present in clinical settings. However, clinicians are asked to address cases bearing risks for suicide, domestic violence, child abuse, or treatment refusal in which sociobiological behaviors have silenced the sensibilities of spirituality within religious life.

According to evolutionary psychology, sociobiological religious life appeared with the evolution of the social brain. The earliest human beings prevailed over wild animals and other early hominids due to social cognition whose evolution enabled cohesive, well-organized groups of families, clans, and tribes. This social cognition was constituted by multiple sociobiological subsystems within the human brain that operated automatically, with little conscious awareness. These sociobiological behavioral systems now routinely organize group behaviors in every sector of life, including religious life (Griffith, 2010, pp. 15–35).

The sociobiological organization of religious life can be adaptive or maladaptive, as illustrated by the following examples:

- Attachment System—*"God is my good parent."* For many people, God serves as an important attachment relationship. As a secure attachment, the felt presence of one's personal God provides emotional stability and protection against loneliness. When a person–God relationship reflects insecure attachment, however, it carries a risk for generating anxiety, similar to insecure attachments between among humans.
- Peer Affiliation System—*"I feel secure as a member of my religious group."* Relationships among members of a religious group often are akin to those of teammates on an athletic team or sibling relationships within a family. However, the same processes can serve to hide the abuses of a pedophile priest when in-group loyalty overrides concern for harm to children.
- Kin Recognition System—*"My religious group is a family that looks out for its own."* It is common for a greater level of empathy, compassion, and intimacy to be available to members of one's religious group compared with those outside it. If this is taken to the extreme, out-group members may no longer be regarded as full human beings. This sets the stage for stigmatization, discrimination, and guilt-free aggression that is justified by religion.
- Social Hierarchy (Dominance/Submission) System—*"I accept my role within God's order and rule."* Religious groups commonly create organizations with hierarchy, roles, and responsibilities similar to those of secular groups. A visceral sense exists that people ought to adhere to whatever assigned roles they occupy within their groups. This attitude continues to provide a basis for the religious caste system within Hindu societies. In the United States, such Christian admonitions as "Slaves, obey your earthly masters in everything" (Colossians 3:22) once was used to justify slavery on religious grounds.
- Social Exchange (Reciprocal Altruism) System—*"God will ensure that life will be fair."* There often is an intuitively felt sense that doing good should be rewarded by good, and that doing bad should be rewarded by bad. It can be difficult for a religious person to experience misfortune without feeling that it somehow constitutes a punishment by God for wrongdoings.
- Social Identity—A compilation of all these sociobiological systems provides a visceral sense of identity: *"Who am I? To whom do I belong?"* Social identity operates in terms of both personal relations (e.g., family, team, work group) and relations with an impersonal collective (e.g., tribe, religious group, ethnicity, gender). Threats to social identity mobilize powerful emotions that are akin to threats to physical survival in their intensity. Religious identity thus can provide emotional energy for either care and protection of vulnerable persons that is healing or aggression toward those outside the religious group that is harmful.

The power of these sociobiological systems to organize group life can be seen in every church, synagogue, mosque, and temple. In a positive sense, they largely account for the effectiveness of religious groups in meeting goals and fulfilling missions. Such missions can advance moral commitments to heal, protect, and provide succor for ill, vulnerable, and suffering people that go far beyond the capabilities of any individual, as evidenced by such religious groups as Catholic Charities, the Bhai Tahirih Centers, and the Islamic Medical Society.

Church attendance and religious observance have been associated with an estimated 25% reduction in mortality, an effect on physical health that has been fully attributed to the protective effects of membership in a cohesive group rather than depth of spiritual experience (Powell, Shahabi, & Thoresen, 2003). However, sociobiological religious life has a downside. Sociobiology operates only to strengthen group effectiveness in pursuit of group aims. Within the human nervous system, sociobiological group cohesion as such does not generate empathy or compassion for individual persons (Griffith, 2010, pp. 36–55). This becomes a risk factor for harm when personal spirituality is absent from setting the values and agendas of religious groups.

Clinical assessment of sociobiological religious life means assessing the patient as a group member, not as an individual. This requires skills for discerning attachment styles, social hierarchy, peer affiliation, kin recognition, and social exchange processes insofar as they constitute a religious identity that can motivate behaviors harmful to self or others. It also requires assessment of the person's religious group: What does the group regard as its vital concerns; what are its "identity flags"; and how does it conduct surveillance of social space? Clinical assessment must discern when any of these normal motivations for joining a group instead hinders the whole person–to–whole person relatedness of spirituality. A clinical formulation makes intelligible how group processes have suppressed capacities for empathy, compassion, and relatedness to self and others as persons, not as categories.

A basic strategy for countering excessive sociobiological religiousness is to engage the person in dialogue that reawakens awareness of self as a whole person living in relationship with one's self, with one's God, and with other persons, apart from any family, gender, ethnic, or socioeconomic role expectations. Awareness of spontaneous moral impulses as responses to self, God, and other persons constitutes personal spirituality. Existential questions can prompt this awareness.[1]

Existential questions can help a person to articulate his or her personal spirituality. Existential questions focus on personal encounters with adversity (Griffith, 2010, pp. 81–95; Griffith, 2013; Griffith & Gaby, 2005). Primo Levi noted in his observations about those with him in the Nazi death camp at Auschwitz: "Every human being possesses a reserve of strength whose extent is unknown to him, be it large, small, or nonexistent, and only through extreme adversity can we evaluate it" (Levi, 1988, p. 60).

Existential questions ask how a person responds to adversity:

- *What has sustained you through hard times? From where do you draw strength?*
- *Where do you find peace?*
- *Who truly understands your situation?*
- *When you are afraid or in pain, how do you find comfort?*
- *For what are you deeply grateful?*
- *What is your clearest sense of the meaning of your life at this time?*
- *Why is it important that you are alive?*
- *To whom or what are you most devoted?*
- *To whom do you freely express love?*

---

1. Existential questions are akin to *implicit questions* in spiritually integrated psychotherapy (Pargament, 2007).

Existential questions also can be asked directly about a person's spiritual practices, religious community, relationship with God, or current religious struggles:

- *What does God know about your experience that other people don't understand?*
- *Do you sense that God sees a purpose in your suffering?*
- *What does God expect of your life in days to come?*
- *How do your beliefs help you prevail through this illness?*
- *How do your spiritual practices help sustain you during a time like this?*

For example, Lester M., a 17-year-old boy, was admitted to the hospital after a medication overdose. The psychiatric consultant learned that Lester was gay but had not revealed his sexual identity to his family. His father was a minister in a fundamentalist Christian church.

"The Bible says homosexuality is a sin," Lester said.
"Is that what your father believes? Do you believe that yourself?" the psychiatric consultant asked.
"He believes it . . . and I believe it. The Bible is the word of God," Lester responded.
"Do you ever feel God's presence— like, whether God feels closer at some times and at other times more distant? Or is it that God is mainly a belief, not someone whose presence you feel?" the consultant asked.

Lester said he tried not to think about God because that worsened his shame. He said that most of his participation in his church felt like a family ritual. However, there had been times when he was alone and God had felt near.

"At moments when God feels near, did you feel God judging you?" the consultant wondered.
"No, it just felt comforting." Lester said.
"Would God encourage you one way or the other when you feel like ending your life?" the consultant asked.
"He wouldn't want me to kill myself" Lester responded.
"Why, do you suppose? Why would God want you to live?," the consultant asked.

The discussion continued with further reflections about how Lester's life might matter to God and with whom he might continue these conversations after leaving the hospital.

In this brief encounter, Lester revealed how his religious life had been constricted by its sociobiology—an empty participation in church and family roles. The consultant sought moments in which Lester as a whole person had encountered his God in order to ask fundamental questions: *"Why does it matter that you live? If God wants you to live— why?"* These questions opened conversations that potentially could re-enliven Lester's personal spirituality. The practical challenge would be finding someone whom Lester viewed as trustworthy in regard to his religious faith and who could continue this conversation outside of the hospital.

As another example, the Phillips family was meeting with a psychiatrist in family therapy after the 14-year-old daughter, Cindy, ran away to an emergency shelter and alleged emotional abuse by her parents. A 48-hour family ordeal ended when Cindy and her parents agreed for her to be voluntarily admitted to an adolescent psychiatric inpatient unit for evaluation. The parents felt visibly shamed that they were obliged to accept psychiatrist care.

The psychiatric evaluation found Cindy to have little evidence to support a primary psychiatric illness. However, she had engaged in recent high-risk sexual behavior that appeared to be a provocative rejection of her religiously conservative parents' values. She had had casual sexual encounters on dates with two different boys, unprotected from either pregnancy or sexually transmitted diseases. Her mother had discovered the sexual encounters from a letter in Cindy's room. She had responded by taking away Cindy's cell phone, stopping her access to e-mail, and grounding her to home indefinitely with no dating privileges. Cindy went into a rage and fled the home.

The psychiatrist felt stymied when meeting with Cindy and her parents. Each effort to promote a dialogue between Mrs. Phillips and Cindy erupted into arguing and accusations. While alone with the psychiatrist, Mrs. Phillips stated that all children begin life as "little heathens" until they are redeemed in God's love. A parent's task is to domesticate the child until he or she is fit for the Kingdom of God. The standard was clear: God declared in the Bible that a sexual relationship should not occur until marriage. Mrs. Phillips felt an awful sense of failure that after 14 years under her parents' stewardship, Cindy was rejecting God's teachings.

In the family meeting, Mrs. Phillips was determined to institute tough love by holding Cindy accountable to a strict behavioral protocol until such time as she had re-earned her parents' trust. Cindy flared with each of her mother's comments, accusing her parents of "making me be bad" through unreasonable expectations.

The psychiatrist noted how prominent hierarchy, roles, responsibilities, boundaries, and social identity were in the Phillips family, and he anticipated that this was in keeping with their religious culture. Meeting alone with the parents, he asked: "Are there others in the community whose opinions matter? If you were to take a chance with giving Cindy more say in her rules, is there anyone outside the family who would care?" Mr. Phillips said that he and his wife had been church youth leaders and that this role had included helping other parents through difficult times with their children. He acknowledged that he and his wife had felt in a quandary as exemplars for other parents. God's instruction was to "bring up the children in the discipline and instruction of the Lord" (Ephesians 4:6). If they could not parent their own child effectively, how could they be entrusted with other children? Had they broken the trust of other parents whom they had counseled as church leaders?

The psychiatrist empathized with their dilemma—their parenting was so much in the spotlight of their church community that they felt little flexibility for parenting their child. He helped them engage the counsel of other trusted leaders in the church, both for emotional support and for advice in how to manage the dilemma of their leadership within the church.

Sociobiology facilitates formation of cohesive religious groups that protect their members and compete effectively with other groups. When sociobiological group processes become too dominant, personal spirituality can be suppressed in the lives of group members.

Religion That Becomes a Conduit for Mental Illness

Whereas sociobiology is one path by which the embodiment of religion can set the stage for harm, another path appears when a religious person's nervous system suffers dysfunction due to a mental illness. Psychiatric illness represents a failure of information processing in the brain that distorts how life events and situations are experienced (Griffith, 2010, pp. 181–196). In vulnerable individuals, even normal levels of stress can secondarily activate anxiety, mood, psychotic, or dissociative disorders.

Distinguishing symptoms of psychiatric disorders from the breadth of thoughts, emotions, and behaviors that a non-ill religious person expresses can be difficult. Hallucinations, delusional fears, dissociative trance states, panic attacks, and anxiety each can occur among otherwise normal people during intense religious experiences. Clinical assessment for distinguishing idiosyncratic but normal religious behavior from psychiatric illness must consider the DSM-5 criteria for diagnosing a Religious or Spiritual Problem (see Chapter 6).

For example, Mrs. Ballston, a middle-aged woman, was admitted to an inpatient psychiatry unit with recurrent depression for the third time in 12 months. Her family brought her back to the hospital after she became unable to care for herself and her children at home. She had been ruminating all day over television images of New Orleans children who were rendered homeless by Hurricane Katrina, blaming herself that she had done nothing to protect them. "I want to live by the Word of the Lord," she told the admitting psychiatry resident, "not by the words of psychiatrists." She was spending hours each day praying and reading her Bible. Mrs. Ballston was diagnosed with psychotic depression that remitted after electroconvulsive treatment and antidepressant medications, after which her guilty ruminations dissipated and her religious practices moderated.

As another example, Laticia M. was admitted to a psychiatry inpatient unit after her manager at work escorted her to the hospital emergency department. She had filed a complaint with the manager that a co-worker was seeking to harm her. She had sensed a message from God— "Mess with me and I will mess with you"—that she delivered to the co-worker she feared. She had begun aggressively giving orders to others in the office. For at least two nights she had not slept, frequently getting up from her bed and pacing. When asked by her psychiatrist whether she had always heard such direct communications from God, she said that they had begun only recently. Now this direct awareness of God's presence brought comfort and assurance of safety. She felt certain that that it was "God and me against the world." She could not think of any person whom she trusted. Ms. M. was diagnosed with a brief reactive psychosis that responded quickly to antipsychotic medications and a quiet environment. After treatment, she said that she could sense God's presence but not as an audible voice.

Risks can occur from normative religious practices that nevertheless destabilize mental illnesses for vulnerable individuals. Patients with schizophrenia and severe mood disorders cannot tolerate emotionally arousing religious experiences without thought disorganization and disturbances in social cognition. Patients with posttraumatic and dissociative disorders often become panic-ridden and disorganized in their thinking after exposure to emotionally evocative reminders of traumas, which can occur during religious counseling. Anxiety disorders can be activated by guilt- or fear-inducing religious images and narratives.

Collaboration between mental health and religious professionals is important. Religious leaders or ministries often are the first point of contact for emotionally distressed religious persons with mood, anxiety, psychotic, or posttraumatic disorders. Sometimes a person with a serious mental illness will accept aid only from a religious professional due to stigma or a risk of shunning by a religious group. It is important that religious leaders and religious groups have a factual grasp of mental illnesses and their treatment, including risks for inadvertent activation of a mental illness by routine experiences of religious worship (Griffith et al., 2016).

For example, George T., a 25-year-old college student, was recently recovered from a first episode of schizophrenia when he attended a religious revival at a charismatic Christian church. During fervent singing and praising God, he began running about in a disorganized manner and speaking unintelligibly. Friends brought him to the emergency room, where he was admitted with a diagnosis of brief psychotic episode. He recovered uneventfully with antipsychotic medications and an emotionally quiet environment. Reflecting afterward, he attributed his relapse of symptoms to "too much zeal for the Lord."

SPIRITUAL STRUGGLE: HEARTFELT CONFLICTS WHEN ENCOUNTERING THE SACRED

Suffering can emerge when encounters with the sacred are conflicted. Pargament, Murray-Swank, Magyar, and Ano (2004) defined *spiritual struggles* as "efforts to conserve or transform a spirituality that has been threatened or harmed" (p. 247) and *spiritually integrated psychotherapy* as a treatment approach designed to aid individuals suffering from spiritual struggles. Most religious traditions agree that pathways leading to the sacred are fraught with obstacles, wrong turns, and sometimes dead ends. In fact, struggles on the spiritual journey are commonplace and are accepted by many traditions as necessary for the development of mature faith (Fowler, 1981). Certainly, many efforts to resolve spiritual struggles ultimately lead to growth, transformation, and a faith life experienced as more authentic or more accessible in daily living. However, prolonged or unsuccessful efforts can lead to despair, hopelessness, and meaninglessness. It is this second type of spiritual struggle that is particularly challenging in the context of mental health treatment.

There are different forms of spiritual struggle (Pargament et al., 2004) and different ways of conceptualizing and treating religious and spiritual problems (Murray-Swank & Murray-Swank, 2013). Exline, Pargament, Grubbs, and Yali (2014) described two types of struggle involving tension between the individual and the supernatural: divine struggle and demonic struggle. Divine struggle involves "negative emotion or conflict centered on beliefs about a deity or a perceived relationship with a deity," whereas demonic struggle "involves concern that the devil or evil spirits are attacking an individual or causing negative events" (Exline et al., 2014, p. 209). Struggles with darkness or evil figures may be present in various faith traditions. Other struggles are *interpersonal* in nature, involving conflict or negative interactions and experiences with individuals or religious and spiritual institutions (Exline et al., 2014; Pargament et al., 2004). Finally, *intrapersonal* religious and spiritual struggles are conflicts within the self; they can include moral struggle, doubting, and struggle surrounding questions of ultimate meaning (Exline et al., 2014).

In psychotherapy, thorough assessment and integration of religious and spiritual lives of patients is not only critical for the therapeutic relationship but also tied to treatment outcomes (Koenig, King, & Carson, 2012). Hodge (2013) defined religious and spiritual assessment as "the process of gathering, analyzing, and synthesizing information about these two interrelated constructs into a framework that provides the basis for practice decisions" (p. 93). Thus, assessment of religiousness and spirituality has a distinct purpose for informing clinical decision making. In the case studies presented throughout this chapter, emphasis is placed on the importance of incorporating information gained via religious and spiritual assessment into the treatment approach. Many times, an individual's religious or spiritual struggles cut across these realms of conflict and therefore involve multiple modes of assessment and intervention. In these instances, ethical and efficacious treatment stems from the mental health professional's willingness to engage in a process of deeper understanding of the client's religious and spiritual experiences, worldview, and language (Deal & Magyar-Russell, 2015).

There are three distinctive strategies for religious and spiritual assessment: (1) implicit approaches[2] that take "a more covert approach that does not initiate the discussion of religious or spiritual issues and does not openly, directly, or systematically use spiritual resources" (Tan, 1996, p. 368); (2) explicit approaches that involve a direct and intentional focus on the role of religion and spirituality within the context of the client's life (Pargament, 2007); and (3) tacit approaches that require clinicians to first recognize and become critically conscious of their own theological assumptions and to recognize how their very presence (Townsend, 2011) affects the possibility of change and healing in the therapeutic relationship (Doehring, 2009). Ultimately, the tacit dimension requires a critical focus on the self in order to learn how to be present and encounter the mystery of the Other without projecting the clinician's own faith, religiousness, and spirituality on those seeking care (Deal & Magyar-Russell, 2015).

Each dimension or strategy brings a distinct interpretive framework to the assessment and treatment process. Although the importance of each dimension may vary by client, taking a comprehensive approach that is attuned to the complex layers of the religious and spiritual life helps ensure ethical and competent assessment and treatment.

The case study of Alma R. presents an example of different types of religious and spiritual struggle as well as the three different forms of religious and spiritual assessment and their implications for guiding treatment decision making.

Alma R., a 47-year-old woman, presented to her initial session of outpatient psychotherapy with long-standing symptoms of depression. She also reported being 15 years free from alcohol abuse with ongoing, active involvement in Alcoholics Anonymous (AA). She worked part-time as a telephone operator for a healthcare company. The clinician began the assessment process in an explicit manner, embedding religious and spiritual questions within other routine intake questions.

> CLINICIAN: "Do you belong to any organizations, including religious or spiritual?"
> ALMA: "I have an eclectic religious background, but I'm not going to a specific church at the moment."

Alma did not share in great detail about herself in response to this question, which she appeared to hear as overtly religious in nature. (She did not mention her involvement with other organizations such as AA or her art-making group.) Responses to explicitly religious and spiritual questions certainly can, and often do, open the door for religious and spiritual conversation; however, patients may not initially wish to share these most intimate aspects of the self until rapport is established or until a specific question or statement touches on an aspect of life connected to the sacred (Richards & Bergin, 2000; Rose, Westefeld, & Ansley, 2008).

When Alma was asked an implicitly religious and spiritual question, her response went much deeper into the nature of her religiousness and spirituality, as well as into other important aspects of her life that she viewed as intimately linked to her religious and spiritual life.

---

2. Use of an implicit strategy for religious and spiritual assessment bears close kinship with the use of existential questions discussed earlier (Griffith, 2013; Griffith & Gaby, 2005).

CLINICIAN: "How easy is it to forgive yourself and others for past hurts?"

ALMA: "On the surface I think forgiving seems easy, and I often think that I have forgiven. If I'm being honest, though, I'm not sure if I've ever forgiven anyone, including myself. I was raised in the Roman Catholic tradition, and I've heard lots of messages about how important forgiveness is, but you see, my dad hit us and berated us [Alma, her mother, and her sister], and so I left home at 17 before graduating from high school. I started going to church with friends that I lived with and began to identify with religious denominations that do not focus on condemnation and judgment. I have lots of African American friends, and I am inspired by their close-knit faith communities. Spirituality is very important to me, and I now view myself as Anglican with African association."

The clinician recognized the presence of both intrapersonal (difficulty forgiving self, anger at self) and interpersonal (dad, Catholic Church) religious/spiritual struggles and was also aware of a change in Alma's tone and the level of emotion in the room. She therefore asked open-ended follow-up questions, such as "Please share more about what is important to you in a faith community" and "Tell me about your experiences with forgiveness," to gain a more thorough understanding of Alma's religious and spiritual worldview and the language she used to express her spirituality.

On walking into her second psychotherapy session, Alma asked permission from her therapist to talk about her relationship with God.

ALMA: "I have an assignment from my AA sponsor that involves sitting down and talking with God. I am having difficulty carrying it out. I think it has everything to do with my relationship conflicts. Despite feeling an instant connection with God, I had a difficult experience with faith growing up."

The clinician noted that divine religious struggles were also present for Alma (harsh God image, insecure attachment to God) and listened with the ear of the father. She explained that she felt the same way toward God as she did toward her father—mistreated and angry—and that these feelings directly affected her poor self-image, especially when in the presence of men.

ALMA: "I have layers of conflict regarding my aging body and beliefs about myself that are represented in attention seeking, shame, vulnerability, and creating distraction to avoid closeness with others I perceive as being capable of seeing my true self. I often feel shallow, shameful, and distressed."

The tacit dimension involves the clinician's very presence, including his or her unspoken communication that there are possibilities for the patient to heal and grow in a constructive way, both psychologically and spiritually. It is therefore important for the clinician to contemplate the manner in which he or she uses the self to listen to, and communicate nonverbally with, the patient. For instance, the therapist might consider how being in relationship, meaning-making, motivation, and mystery are in part nonverbal processes that affect connections between human beings.

With Alma, the tacit dimension influenced treatment by allowing her the possibility to see some room for change in her view of God (see also Pargament's discussion of "small gods" [Pargament, 2007, pp. 277–279]). Alma's "default God" was judgmental, vengeful, volatile, and male. However, through the connection and person of the therapist, she was able to be open to, and identify, an image of God as possessing what she perceived as the feminine characteristics of grace, generosity, love, and wisdom. Out of her work in sessions, in AA, and via art-making, Alma found it helpful to notice when she was viewing the world and her relationships through the lens of her "default God" rather than the God she began to call "her real God."

The therapist continually encouraged Alma to bring into the therapy room situations and thoughts with which she was struggling outside of sessions and to engage in a re-evaluation process with the spiritual and positive frameworks she embraced in order to find areas of agreement and disagreement. This helped Alma to think through "default feelings" connected to her "default God," reframe these feelings, and then bring her feelings in line with her more rational thoughts and the positive attributes of her "real God."

Alma experienced occasional setbacks in her struggle to turn away from the thinking, feelings, and view of the world linked to her "default God." After several weeks of steady progress, Alma burst into session, sharing that she felt she needed spiritual intervention because of demonic spirits. As the clinician set the tone of calmly exploring this possibility with her, Alma shared that she felt her anger was out of control and beyond that of a straightforward anger problem,—so much so that it must have come from the devil (demonic struggle). The clinician and Alma spent time talking about her recent situation with a group of young men at work that led to these feelings and explored her anger triggers from the past. Alma quickly recognized the themes of being misunderstood and belittled in the situation. She stated that being able to see the link between her anger response and the situation that triggered the anger helped her to feel that her experience was still in the human realm and not supernatural. Alma agreed to continue to monitor her feelings and thoughts outside of sessions. The clinician's presence and the space of the therapy room allowed Alma to stop and recognize the attributes of her "real God" present in the situation and within herself.

RELIGION AND SPIRITUALITY AS RESOURCES IN TREATMENT

Emma D.'s story provides an example in which recovery occurred despite a confluence of spiritual struggle, sociobiological religion, and mental illness that had disabled the patient's life for years. Recovery required the integration of psychotherapy, psychopharmacology, pastoral counseling, and the patient's her own spiritual practices.

"It's just so cruel. This disease attacks the very things I love most: my faith, my God." Emma was a 66-year-old woman and a devout Catholic who attended Mass daily and participated regularly in church ministries. She had had recurring, yet distinct, episodes of obsessive compulsive disorder (OCD) over a 45-year period. Seven years before first seeking mental health treatment, she found herself experiencing blasphemous thoughts about the Virgin Mary ("cunt") and Jesus ("dick") when praying to Mary or Jesus or on seeing a statue or picture of either. In her anguish, she created rituals to remove these thoughts from her mind. For instance, she would repeat the word "Out!" to herself when experiencing an obsessive thought. Later she began to try to replace the intrusive thought as it came into consciousness (e.g., thinking the word "cup" or "love" to replace "cunt"). She stated that every day was a struggle and that she felt anxious, sad, and unable to find joy in her faith.

Sociobiological elements of her religious experience placed Emma at risk. Religious groups provide opportunities for merging the self with the group (peer affiliation), engaging in dominance/submission behaviors with religious leaders (social hierarchy), and suspiciousness towards nonbelievers (kin recognition). The uplift in morale experienced when joining a cohesive religious group was termed the "relief effect" by Marc Galanter in his studies of religious cults (Galanter, 1978, 1999). This wedding of self to group becomes problematic when it motivates specific behaviors that place a person with a vulnerability to mental illness at risk for relapse.

As with other individuals who suffer from OCD, Emma had a particular vulnerability to anxiety combined with ritualized behaviors for relieving the anxiety. Religious rituals ranging from confession of sins to foot washing to recitations of prayers can thus "catch" a patient with latent OCD. Emma worried endlessly that her intrusive thoughts were sinful or in violation of Catholic doctrine (scrupulosity). She repeatedly attended the sacrament of reconciliation (confession) to confess her sinfulness and to seek absolution. She worried about conversations she had had with others as well as regrets and guilt about experiences from the distant past. At one point, a priest who became impatient with her inadvertently exacerbated her symptoms: "One priest I didn't feel comfortable with. I felt like he didn't like it if I confessed having the obsessions more than once. He said 'It should be gone by now' when I re-confessed having obsessions. I felt like he didn't really understand how bad it [my OCD] was, and then I was worried that re-confessing my obsessions was sinful." Emma's vulnerability for her psychiatric illness, OCD, was not necessarily present in the theological content of her beliefs, practices, and rituals but was manifest in their expression. In other words, repetitive religious behaviors provided reinforcing moments of anxiety reduction from both her religious and nonreligious fears, thereby continuing the destructive cycle of her religious-oriented OCD.

Emma's distress was contextualized by memories of her mother's mental illness, which was likely schizophrenia. Emma's mother had been institutionalized numerous times during Emma's childhood because of religious delusions and hallucinations. As a consequence, Emma had lived in an orphanage with her siblings from 1 to 4 years of age. Obsessive doubts about her salvation and fears that she would "go crazy" like her mother also drove Emma's anxiety. Confession of sins, praying the rosary, and attending daily Mass were ritualized practices that temporarily relieved anxiety. Yet the anxiety returned more fiercely when Emma felt unable to engage in the rituals of her faith due to obsessions. She would then turn to ritualized compulsions to manage her anxiety in response to the obsessions. At the time Emma D. began outpatient psychotherapy (with GMR) she was guilt ridden, emotionally distraught, exhausted, and fearful that she would become as debilitated as her mother.

Religious and spiritual assessment for Emma could be conducted in an entirely explicit manner for most of her psychotherapy because of the prominence of the religious content of her obsessions and her corresponding spiritual struggles. Emma's spiritual struggles were largely intrapersonal in nature, including doubt and questioning her own sinfulness and morality. She also experienced demonic struggles. As she related, "At first I did feel like the Devil was attacking the most important thing in my life: my faith. I just didn't understand why this was happening to me. I never once blamed God. I did ask, what is causing me to have these thoughts? Why did I have to get them? Is my faith weak? Why is the Devil able to do this to me?" In a posttreatment interview, Emma stated that she still felt as though the Devil could "get a foothold" on her via her OCD symptoms and that she must constantly remain vigilant by performing her exposure treatment and staying strong in her faith in order to avoid the Devil's temptation to give in to her symptoms.

During the initial session, it was evident from Emma's self-report and intense emotion that her religious and spiritual life was integral to her presenting problem and also an indispensable resource in her treatment. Intervention began during the first session with psychoeducation about OCD and the recommended course of treatment. Externalizing the disorder by giving it a name and separating it from her sense of self provided a preliminary level of relief for Emma. Despite the religious content of both her psychopathology and that of her mother, there was relief in learning that it had a name and was treatable. Early in therapy, Emma elected to be evaluated for psychotropic medications and was prescribed sertraline (200 mg) and trazodone (100 mg).

Emma's treatment focused on in vivo exposure and response prevention in therapy sessions to help her approach these most distressing symptoms head on. Emma felt strongly that God had brought her and the clinician together for the purpose of helping her with symptom relief, specifically through the use of her faith. Reviewing the Doctrine in the *Catechism of the Catholic Church* (United States Catholic Conference, 1997) regarding the involuntary nature of psychological disorders (Article 8, IV, 1860), consulting with a Catholic priest, limiting her use of confession, and repeating exposure (with response prevention) to her obsessions via rituals such as prayer to saints and praying of the rosary were used in Emma's treatment. The tacit dimension was also an important factor in Emma's therapy because of the manner in which Catholic tradition and rituals were acknowledged nonverbally through the presence of the clinician.

Emma's description of her spiritual struggles and her role in combating those struggles provides a good example of the therapeutic exchange and interplay between faith and psychological health. As Emma observed, "Before treatment I didn't know how to use my faith to help with my symptoms; now I know how to work *with* God against my OCD by praying for strength to keep letting the obsessions in without trying to stop them with rituals or compulsions." Similarly, she commented that her faith had matured because of the OCD: "I now know that I need God even more, and He strengthens me, and I am constantly in touch with Him because I know I need to pray to be strong and to engage in my treatment. God is always there to help me."

Emma's devotion to her faith was indeed a resource in her treatment. However, her inflexible adherence to Catholic ritual at times contributed to ethical tension for the clinician. Early in treatment, Emma reported excessive use of confession and engaged in ritualized prayer (e.g., novenas) that possessed elements of the deferring form of religious coping (Pargament et al., 1998). In other words, Emma seemed to be asking God, saints, or her priest to take away her OCD rather than engaging in the hard work of treatment. The deferring form of religious coping, or spiritual bypass (i.e., the use of spirituality to avoid dealing with difficult issues [Welwood, 2000]), can be challenging to identify and should be managed sensitively. Although the use of the client's faith in treatment should generally be honored and supported, if beliefs or rituals seem to be used *instead of* treatment strategies, the clinician should address the concern in psychotherapy. After the clinician talked directly with Emma about her frequent use of confession and repetitive prayer, she demonstrated awareness of her excessive use of these coping strategies and also of their gradual loss of effectiveness with overuse. One aspect of Emma's treatment then became to use other religious resources (e.g., Bible study, church dinners, reading the Bible) in place of more ritualized religious expressions that, while supported in her faith tradition, served to "catch" Emma's propensity for ritual and keep her passively stuck in her symptoms rather than helping her more actively work through them.

A particularly powerful point in Emma's treatment, and in her religious life, occurred shortly after she began treatment. She and her husband had lunch with the priest at their parish, and Emma shared her OCD symptoms and diagnosis with him. She asked the priest whether she should stop administering the Eucharist at Mass. In her words, the parish priest said, "Keep at it!" She felt her pastor understood her and knew about OCD and its cruel symptoms. She felt reassured that her obsessions were not sinful based on the priest's authority in the Catholic Church and his encouragement for her to continue to minister to others despite her illness. Emma's experiences in her faith community helped her to persist in approaching her OCD symptoms in a therapeutic manner while continuing her ministry and making her feel accepted, included, and valued.

The religious and spiritual assessment process is dynamic in nature, evolving and changing over the course of therapy. For Emma, implicit spiritual assessment began after more than 6 months of treatment, after she had experienced significant symptom reduction and had begun to sense her personal spirituality again. At that point, she was able to engage with the implicit question, "When do you feel peace, or relief, from your OCD?" Emma responded by describing an experience she had had: "I was in Mass praying after communion, and a profound peace came over me. I felt so close to Jesus after a terrible week with my obsessions. It was miraculous! I went forth from Mass, and the thoughts were no longer there for at least a week." She went on to say, "Sometimes when I am in church, reading the Bible, or praying, I can really sense Jesus, really feel God's presence." This type of implicit question, followed by Emma's reflection on her experiences of personal spirituality, was not possible at the height of her symptom distress. Later in treatment, however, this implicitly spiritual question tapped into an important resource for Emma's ongoing treatment. The therapist and Emma began to focus on letting worry and obsessions enter her mind while simultaneously focusing on being present and getting in touch with God's presence in the moment. Emma found this strategy to be remarkably helpful for symptom relief and as a means of feeling closer to God.

It was also at this later point in treatment that Emma described how treatment had enabled her to use her faith as a vibrant resource rather than continually pleading to God to take her affliction away. In other words, she began to benefit from her personal spirituality and sense God's presence with her in her battle against OCD, rather than fearing God's judgment about her symptoms. She stated, "I discovered that we all have crosses to carry in life. When St. Paul prayed to God to take his burden away from him, God said, 'My grace is sufficient for thee,' and Paul said, 'I will bear it.' And so I will bear the burden of my OCD cross." Emma continued to bear this burden by collaboratively working with God. She prayed for the strength to engage in her exposure treatment and to let go of worry and doubt via cognitive restructuring and engaging in relationship with her faith community and family members.

In an interview with Emma after psychotherapy, she explained her situation like this:

> I still have obsessions about Mary and Jesus occasionally, but I know what I need to do [exposure and response prevention with present-centered focus on Divine presence]. I don't have them every day, just periodic bouts or episodes when they re-occur. I know how to fight OCD now, and I know I have this disease. That has done wonders. It's not my faith that's weak, it's not something I'm doing that is bad, it's my disease. But I still struggle. And I will continue to do my part: fight OCD and pray for the strength to do so.

CONCLUSION

The three types of religious acts discussed in this chapter each pose risks of harm due to potential violations of person-to-person relatedness, a moral standard that has been established by the various traditions of personal spirituality. This standard has been supported by social psychology and social neuroscience research that associates personal spirituality, but not group-based sociobiological religiousness, with the brain's social cognition for mentalization, empathy, and compassion.

Each of these three problems requires a different kind of solution. Sociobiological religion does harm when religious life is largely constituted by religious identity or loyalty to one's religious group, with the sensibilities of personal spirituality bearing little influence. This risk can be countered by opening authentic reflection about existential concerns in a manner that re-energizes personal spirituality. Discerning mental illness in the guise of religion requires learning basic principles for differential diagnosis and treatment of the mental illness. Recognizing risks that normative religious practices pose for vulnerable individuals means that religious leaders and groups should learn how psychotic, mood, anxiety, and posttraumatic disorders can be activated inadvertently by intense or prolonged religious experiences (Griffith et al., 2016). Religious persons caught in spiritual struggles often engage in psychotherapy or spiritual guidance that utilizes dialogue and reflection to resolve intrapsychic, interpersonal, or person-God conflicts. Throughout the course of treatment, clinical assessment should balance the patient's spiritual and religious life as a potential resource with its potential risk for harm.

REFERENCES

Armstrong, K. (1993). *A history of God*. New York, NY: Ballantine Books.

Barnes, M. H. (2000). *Stages of thought: The co-evolution of religious thought and science*. New York, NY: Oxford University Press.

Buber, M. (1958). *I and thou* (2nd ed.). New York, NY: MacMillan.

Deal, P. J., & Magyar-Russell, G. (2015). Religious and spiritual assessment. In E. A. Maynard & J. L. Snodgrass (Eds.), *Understanding pastoral counseling* (pp. 115–137). New York, NY: Springer.

De Jong, J. T. V. M. (2014). Challenges of creating synergy between global mental health and cultural psychiatry. *Transcultural Psychiatry*, 51, 806–828.

Doehring, C. (2009). Theological accountability: The hallmark of pastoral counseling. *Sacred Spaces: The e-Journal of the American Association of Pastoral Counselors*, 1, 4–34.

Exline, J. J., Pargament, K. I., Grubbs, J. B., & Yali, A. M. (2014). The Religious and Spiritual Struggles Scale: Development and initial validation. *Psychology of Religion and Spirituality*, 6(3), 208–222.

Fowler, J. W. (1981) *Stages of faith: The psychology of human development and the quest for meaning*. New York, NY: HarperCollins.

Galanter, M. (1978). The "relief effect": A sociobiological model for neurotic distress and large-group therapy. *Am J Psychiatry*, 135(5), 588–591.

Galanter, M. (1999). *Cults: Faith, healing, and coercion* (2nd ed.). New York, NY: Oxford University Press.

Griffith, J. (2010). *Religion that heals, religion that harms*. New York, NY: Guilford Press.

Griffith, J. L. (2013). Existential inquiry: Psychotherapy for crises of demoralization. *European Journal of Psychiatry*, 27, 42–47.

Griffith, J., & Elliot, M. (2002). *Encountering the sacred in psychotherapy*. New York, NY: Guilford Press.

Griffith, J. L., & Gaby, L. (2005). Brief psychotherapy at the bedside: Countering demoralization from medical illness. *Psychosomatics, 46*, 109–116.

Griffith, J., Myers, N., & Compton, M. (2016). How can community religious groups aid recovery for individuals with psychotic illnesses? *Community Mental Health Journal, 52*(7), 775–780.

Hodge, D. R. (2013). Assessing spirituality and religion in the context of counseling and psychotherapy. In K. I. Pargament, A. Mahoney, & E. P. Shafranske (Eds.), *APA handbook of psychology, religion, and spirituality* (vol. 2, pp. 93–123). Washington, DC: American Psychological Association.

Kleinman, A. (2006). *What really matters: Living a moral life amidst uncertainty and danger*. New York, NY: Oxford University Press.

Koenig, H. G., King, D., & Carson, V. B. (2012). *Handbook of religion and health* (2nd ed.). New York, NY: Oxford University Press.

Levi, P. (1988). *The drowned and the saved*. New York, NY: Vintage Books.

Levinas, E. (1961). *Totality and infinity* (A. Lingis, trans.). Pittsburgh, PA: Duquesne University Press.

Murray-Swank, A., & Murray-Swank, N. A. (2013). Spiritual and religious problems: Integrating theory and clinical practice. In K. I. Pargament, A. Mahoney, & E. P. Shafranske (Eds.), *APA Handbook of Psychology, Religion, and Spirituality* (vol. 2, pp. 421–437). Washington, DC: American Psychological Association.

Pargament, K. I. (2007). *Spiritually integrated psychotherapy: Understanding and addressing the sacred*. New York, NY: The Guilford Press.

Pargament, K. I., Murray-Swank, N., Magyar, G. M., & Ano, G. (2004). Spiritual struggle: A phenomenon of interest to the psychology of religion. In W. R. Miller & H. Delaney (Eds.), *Judeo-Christian perspective on psychology: Human nature, motivation, and change* (pp. 245–268). Washington, DC: APA Press.

Pargament, K. I., Smith, B. W., Koenig, H. G., & Perez, L. (1998). Patterns of positive and negative religious coping with major life stressors. *Journal for the Scientific Study of Religion, 37*, 710–724.

Powell, L. H., Shahabi, L., & Thoresen, C. E. (2003). Religion and spirituality: Linkages to physical health. *American Psychologist, 58*, 36–52.

Richards, P. S., & Bergin, A. E. (Eds.). (2000). *Handbook of psychotherapy and religious diversity*. Washington, DC: American Psychological Association.

Rose, E. M., Westefeld, J. S., & Ansley, T. N. (2008). Spiritual issues in counseling: Clients' beliefs and preferences. *Psychology of Religion and Spirituality, S*(1), 18–33.

Tan, S. Y. (1996). Religion in clinical practice: Implicit and explicit integration. In E. P. Shafranske (Ed.), *Religion and the clinical practice of psychology* (pp. 365–387). Washington, DC: American Psychological Association.

Townsend, L. (2011). A grounded theory description of pastoral counseling. *The Journal of Pastoral Care & Counseling, 65*(3), 1–16.

United States Catholic Conference. (1997). *Catechism of the Catholic Church* (English transl.). New York, NY: Doubleday.

Welwood, J. (2000). *Toward a psychology of awakening: Buddhism, psychotherapy and the path of personal and spiritual transformation*. Boston, MA: Shambhala Publications: 2000.

SIX

Spiritual and Religious Concerns Presenting in Psychiatric Treatment

Len Sperry, M.D., Ph.D.

AS PSYCHIATRISTS AND OTHER MENTAL HEALTH PROFESSIONALS BECOME more sensitive to the spiritual and religious concerns of patients, they need to know more about these concerns and how they can best respond to them. Although it is assumed that all mental health professionals will perform a thorough spiritual assessment and that this assessment will identify specific religious and spiritual concerns, it does not follow that every mental health professional will or should directly provide interventions targeting those identified concerns.

This chapter addresses various spiritual and religious concerns that adult patients present in everyday psychiatric practice. These include those noted under the V code, Religious or Spiritual Problem, in the *Diagnostic and Statistical Manual of Mental Disorders, Fifth Edition* (DSM-5). A taxonomy of these concerns that is useful in making treatment decisions is provided. Ethical considerations in responding to these concerns are discussed with an emphasis on the patient's informed consent and the competency of the psychiatrist in addressing religion and spiritual issues, which has implications for scope of practice. Because of the limits of scope of practice, most psychiatrists necessarily collaborate and/or make appropriate referral to other spiritual and religious providers for certain cases involving spiritual and religious concerns. Accordingly, a brief description of these providers of spiritual and religious services is included. Finally, two extended case examples illustrate this discussion.

RELIGIOUS AND SPIRITUAL CONCERNS OF PATIENTS

Although there is no consensus on the definition of spirituality, there is increasing agreement about what constitutes a spiritual problem or concern and what constitutes a religious concern. Generally speaking, a religious or spiritual problem is a "problem involving religious or spiritual beliefs, experience, or practices as indicated by an individual's distress or impairment in functioning" (Murray-Swank & Murray-Swank, 2012, p. 423).

Some contend that there is value in defining religious and spiritual problems separately. For example, religious problems have been defined as those that involve an individual's conflicts over beliefs, rituals, practices, and experiences related to a religious belief system or community. Spiritual problems, on the other hand, are those that involve distress associated with an individual's personal relationship to a higher power or transcendent force that may not be related to a religious belief system or community (Lukoff, Lu, & Yang, 2011). This section includes the DSM-5 specification of religious and spiritual concerns as well as a number of other characterizations of such concerns. It summarizes the discussion in a taxonomy.

Religious or Spiritual Problem in DSM-5

DSM-5 provides a V code for Religious or Spiritual Problem (V62.89). "This category can be used when the focus of clinical attention is a religious or spiritual problem. Examples include distressing experiences that involve loss or questioning of faith, problems associated with conversion to a new faith, or questioning of spiritual values that may not necessarily be related to an organized church or religious institution" (American Psychiatric Association, 2013).

The wording of this code was based on research reviewed prior to 1991 (Lukoff, Lu, & Turner, 1992). The wording has not been updated since DSM-IV (1994) even though the research and professional literature has greatly expanded. Recommendations for changes in the DSM-5 V code have been made based on updated research and on separate typologies for religious problems and spiritual problems (Lukoff et al., 2011). Even though DSM-5 does not incorporate these recommended changes, the suggested changes can be particularly useful to psychiatrists and other mental health professionals who deal with patients presenting with spiritual and religious concerns.

RELIGIOUS PROBLEMS

This typology includes loss or questioning of faith; changes in membership, practices, and beliefs (including conversion); new religious movements and cults; and life-threatening and terminal illnesses (Lukoff et al., 2011). Life-threatening and terminal illnesses are not implied in V62.89.

SPIRITUAL PROBLEMS

This typology includes the so-called spiritual emergencies such as mystical experiences; near-death experiences; psychic experiences; alien abduction experiences; meditation and spiritual practices-related experiences; and possession experiences. A detailed description of each of these types was provided by Lukoff et al. (2011).

Whereas DSM-5 emphasizes that religious/spiritual problems result in significant distress or impairment, there has been an effort to differentiate the impact of spiritual distress from the impact of spiritual impairment. Accordingly, "religious and spiritual struggles" can be distinguished from "clinically significant religious impairment."

RELIGIOUS AND SPIRITUAL STRUGGLES

Religious and spiritual struggles are struggles that involve spiritual or religious beliefs, practices, or experiences that are causing or perpetuating distress. They are indicators of religious/spiritual disorientation, tension, or strain. The distress may involve the divine (e.g., anger at or feeling alienated from God), the intrapersonal (e.g., inability to forgive oneself for a transgression), or the interpersonal (sexual abuse or feeling of betrayal by a priest or minister) (Pargament, 2007).

CLINICALLY SIGNIFICANT RELIGIOUS IMPAIRMENT

Clinically significant religious impairment is defined as a "reduced ability to perform religious/ spiritual activities, strive for religious/spiritual goals, or experience religious/spiritual states because of a psychological disorder" (Hathaway, Scott, & Garver, 2004, p. 97).

SPIRITUAL INJURY

Although spiritual injury is somewhat similar to the distress involving the divine in religious struggles, it appears to be sufficiently unique to merit a separate category of concerns. These concerns are included in the Spiritual Injury Scale, which is part of a computerized spiritual assessment instrument (Berg, 1994). Indicators of spiritual injury include feelings of guilt, grief, shame, rage, or unfair treatment by God or life and other injustices related to an individual's religious world view (Berg, 1998).

TAXONOMY OF RELIGIOUS, SPIRITUAL, AND CLINICAL CONCERNS

Box 6.1 provides a taxonomy of religious and spiritual concerns along with various clinical concerns that are common among psychiatric patients. The next section describes which categories of concerns are most likely to be addressed by the various providers of religious and spiritual services (i.e., pastoral care and chaplaincy, pastoral counseling, spiritual care, spiritual direction, and spiritually oriented psychotherapy).

SPIRITUAL AND RELIGIOUS TREATMENTS

Although psychiatrists are expected to perform a spiritual history that identifies specific spiritual and religious concerns, this does not mean that they are responsible for directly addressing the identified concerns. Many if not most psychiatrists refer or collaborate with other professionals to provide such treatments or services. This section provides a capsule summary of these services.

Box 6.1. Taxonomy of Religious, Spiritual, Life, and Clinical Concerns

I. CONCERNS DIRECTLY INVOLVING RELIGIOSITY

- Loss or questioning of faith*
- Problems associated with conversion to a new faith*
- Changes in membership, practices, and beliefs (including conversion)
- New religious movements and cults
- Life-threatening and terminal illness
- Religious and Spiritual Struggles (including sexual abuse by clergy)

II. CONCERNS DIRECTLY INVOLVING SPIRITUALITY

- Mystical experiences
- Near-death experiences
- Psychic experiences
- Meditation and experiences related to spiritual practices
- Possession experiences
- Questioning of spiritual values not related to an organized church or religious institution*
- Spiritual injury

III. CONCERNS INVOLVING THE MEANING OF LIFE

- Finding one's purpose in life
- Discernment regarding major life decisions
- Issues involving self-development (i.e., growth in virtue)

IV. CONCERNS INVOLVING MORALITY AND ETHICS

- Moral/ethical issues regarding self
- Moral/ethical issues regarding relationships
- Moral/ethical issues regarding work or social institutions

V. CONCERNS INVOLVING PROBLEMS OF LIVING

- Losses and bereavement
- Relational conflicts
- Imbalances in life-work demands
- Failed expectations
- Mild to moderate symptoms or impairment

VI. CONCERNS INVOLVING CLINICAL CONDITIONS

- Personality-disordered behaviors
- Alcoholism and addictions
- Sequelae of early life trauma
- Moderate to severe psychiatric symptoms or impairment

---

*V62.89 Religious or Spiritual Problem of DSM-5.

Pastoral Care

Pastoral care is care provided by chaplains and community-based clergy. It refers to pastoral or religious communication that helps and nurtures individuals and interpersonal relationships as part of the work of chaplains and clergy in the community (Sperry, 2013). For centuries, clergy have provided pastoral care to believers and others interested in religious or spiritual change and to those facing personal problems and crises. Some have also provided pastoral care to individuals with mental illness.

Formal training in pastoral care is commonly referred to as Clinical Pastoral Education (CPE). CPE is the primary method of teaching pastoral care to chaplains, community clergy, and other hospital and hospice care providers. Typically, a minimum number of CPE units (credits) are required for ordination in many denominations. Additional training is required to become a certified chaplain.

CPE training emphasizes listening and responding to individuals experiencing change, confusion, or distress with health and non-health concerns. Some basic counseling skills may be taught, but in a briefer and less therapeutically complex manner than in pastoral counseling or psychotherapy. Pastoral care could therefore be considered a form of precounseling that takes place outside a formal counseling context (Montgomery, 2010).

Pastoral Counseling

Like pastoral care provided by clergy, pastoral counseling is rooted in clinical pastoral education and chaplaincy. Unlike those providing pastoral care, pastoral counselors have specialized professional training and certification or licensure (Stone, 1999). The primary emphasis of pastoral counseling is to assist individuals in coping with physical, emotional, or moral stressors or with a crisis of meaning. A basic assumption of pastoral counseling is that addressing spiritual or religious needs is essential in effectively dealing with personal problems and crises, particularly for believers.

Whereas in the past, the terms *pastoral care* and *pastoral counseling* were often used synonymously, today they are differentiated. Distinct from pastoral care, pastoral counseling is a more structured and complex form of pastoral communication involving an articulated request for help that occurs within a formal counseling context. Furthermore, specific arrangements for formal sessions, times, and fees are mutually negotiated in pastoral counseling, as in traditional psychotherapy. Pastoral counseling requires graduate training, endorsement by a religious body, and certification.

Pastoral counseling is well suited to address religious and spiritual crises and concerns. It is a unique form of counseling that uses religious and spiritual resources as well as psychological understanding for healing and growth. Besides spiritual growth, its goals include problem resolution and restoration of psychological health.

The assessment in pastoral counseling typically includes the individual's awareness of God; acceptance of God's grace; repentance and responsibility; and the nature of the client's involvement in her or his faith community (Benner, 2003). Treatment interventions usually include active listening and other problem-solving or solution-focused counseling methods. It can also include advice on religious or spiritual matters (e.g., forgiveness) and on employing the resources of the client's faith community. Most psychiatrists do not appear to identify pastoral counseling as an area of competency. Pastoral counselors are likely to refer individuals with more complex presentations for psychotherapy or other psychiatric treatment (Sperry, 2013).

Spiritual Care

Spiritual care is psychiatric care or spiritually sensitive care that is provided by non-chaplain health care professionals (Koenig, 2013). Spiritual care addresses the person's relationship to the transcendent and the spiritual needs resulting from that relationship. It is considered the basic level of functioning for psychiatrists who do not have specialized training and experience in other religious and spiritual modalities and interventions (Koenig, 2013). Spiritual care involves four functions: taking a spiritual history, identifying spiritual needs, ensuring that those needs are addressed by someone, and providing mental health care in a spiritual way. Specifically, this means "providing care with respect for the patient as a unique individual; it means inquiring about how the patient wishes to be cared for; it means providing care in a kind and gentle manner; it means providing care in a competent manner; and it means taking extra time with patients who really need it" (Koenig, 2013, p. 75).

Basic to spiritual care is taking a thorough spiritual history as an essential part of the psychiatric evaluation. The spiritual assessment should include inquiry about "any past negative experiences with religion, including disappointments due to unanswered prayers, major losses, stressful events, or conflicts with clergy or other members of the congregation. Religious beliefs and activities (public and private) should be explored . . . . Unlike in medical patients where any indication that the patient is not religious would stop further inquiries, the [mental health] specialist may need to gently probe further to obtain a better understanding of the patient's prior negative experiences with religion. Situations that may have turned patients off to religion (such as sexual abuse by a religious authority or a traumatic event that altered a patient's religious worldview) could be contributing to the current psychiatric problems" (Koenig, 2013, p. 221). Besides identifying the patient's spiritual and religious concerns, a thorough spiritual assessment also identifies the patient's spiritual beliefs, practices, and involvement in a religious community.

Spiritual Direction

Spiritual direction is also referred to as spiritual guidance, spiritual friendship, and spiritual companionship; although it is primarily associated with the Catholic tradition, it is also practiced in other Christian denominations, including Episcopal, Lutheran, and Methodist, as well as in Judaism and in Buddhism (Bhikku, 2003; Edwards, 2001). The primary emphasis in spiritual direction is to facilitate spiritual growth, and the secondary emphasis is psychological change. Spiritual direction focuses on the maintenance and development of spiritual health and well-being. It assumes that an individual is already whole but has not yet fully embraced this truth. Therefore, spiritual direction is not for everyone, because it presumes a moderate degree of psychological health and well-being, the relative absence of psychopathology, and moderate to high psychological functioning (Sperry, 2002).

Interventions in spiritual direction include instruction in prayer and the prescription of rituals and other spiritual practices. A focus on developing and monitoring the directee's prayer life, including meditation or contemplation, is central to spiritual direction. When indicated, spiritual directors may refer directees with certain psychological problems for concurrent psychotherapy or suspend spiritual direction until the course of therapy is completed (Sperry, 2013).

Formal training typically includes a master's degree in spirituality and formal training and supervision. Some psychiatrists, such as Gerald May, M.D., have focused their practice on spiritual direction (May, 1992).

Spiritually Oriented Psychotherapy

Spiritually oriented psychotherapy differs from pastoral counseling and spiritual direction in that it is based on psychological theory and research (Pargament, 2007). It is practiced by licensed health professionals, including psychiatrists, psychologists, social workers, and mental health counselors with specialized training and experience. Its primary emphasis is psychological change; its secondary emphasis is religious and spiritual change or growth.

Spiritually oriented psychotherapy focuses primarily on three religious and spiritual issues that surface in the context of psychotherapy: those in which spirituality offers a key resource for coping with serious problems; traumatic situations that may lead to spiritual struggles, such as a crisis of faith or meaning in life; and the quest for increased well-being and spiritual growth (Sperry, 2012b; Sperry & Shafranske, 2005). Although a focus on spiritual growth may seem more consistent with traditional spiritual direction, patients today are increasingly seeking out mental health professionals rather than ministers and other spiritual guides to foster their spiritual growth and development. Individuals seeking explicitly spiritually oriented psychotherapy range from relatively healthy spiritual seekers to disordered clients presenting with symptomatic distress and/or impairment in one or more areas of life functioning (Sperry, 2012a).

The goals of treatment vary according to patient presentation and need. They may include help with spiritual struggles, spiritual emergencies, spiritual growth, increased psychological well-being, self-fulfillment, or individuation or the reduction of symptomatic distress and restoration of baseline functioning (Sperry, 2012a). Various psychotherapeutic and psychospiritual interventions are used, depending on patient need and indication. These can include spiritual practices such as prayer and meditation and, when indicated, collaboration with or referral to a clergy member or chaplain. Medication and hospitalization may also be used (Sperry, 2013).

ETHICAL CONSIDERATIONS

Various ethical considerations arise in the provision of religious and spiritually sensitive treatment. These considerations can be considerably complex for those providing spiritually oriented psychotherapy and pastoral counseling, less complex for psychiatrists who provide only spiritual care as defined in this chapter. Nevertheless, there are four core ethical considerations that impact the practice of all health and religious professionals: confidentiality, informed consent—particularly value imposition, conflict of interests, and competency—particularly scope of practice (Sperry, 2007). Issues most common in the provision of spiritual care are informed consent and competence or scope of practice.

Informed Consent

Ethical practice requires that a patient's consent be given freely without coercion and without value imposition. Because spiritual care is value based, it is necessary to distinguish value imposition from value exposure. Value exposure involves the disclosure of the provider's values when appropriate and without an agenda, whereas value imposition involves disclosure with an agenda. Typically, value imposition occurs when providers impose their values or religious beliefs on clients or use them to persuade a client to accept a course of treatment or an intervention. It is unethical because it undermines the patient's right to decide about the specifics of treatment (Sperry, 2007). Value imposition can be less a concern for individuals seeking spiritual direction or pastoral counseling because they have opted for spiritually oriented treatment. However, it can be a concern when spiritual or religious issues are not the primary reason for seeking treatment.

Numerous complaints have been filed by patients or their guardians to state licensing boards or professional organizations about spiritually oriented treatments being provided that were not sought or wanted. Case law contains a number of examples of health professionals who have been fired, sanctioned, or convicted for providing unwanted spiritual treatment to patients (Bullis, 1996). Accordingly, a mental health provider would do well to elicit patients' expectations for treatment and to engage in mutual treatment decision making so that adequate informed consent is achieved.

Competence and Scope of Practice

Competence is "the capacity of practitioners to provide a minimum quality of service within their scope of practice" (Sperry, 2008, p. 20). Scope of practice is defined as the "extent and limits of professional activities by an individual who is licensed or certified and that is considered acceptable professional practice as defined by the profession or by statute. It also refers to a recognized area of proficiency, competence, or skills gained through appropriate education and experience" (Sperry, 2008, p. 89). Scope of practice is an ethical consideration that has legal ramifications, and it is one of the most complex and challenging considerations for those providing treatment that is spiritually sensitive. Such practice assumes that a provider has sufficient formal training, supervision, and experience in a specialized area to practice ethically, legally, and competently. Relatively few mental health training programs currently offer formal training in a specially areas such as spiritually oriented psychotherapy, pastoral counseling, or spiritual direction. Therefore, graduates of such programs must seek additional specialized training and experience to extend their scope of practice in such specialty areas.

The practice of spiritual care as described in this chapter (Koenig, 2013) appears to be within the scope of practice of most psychiatrists and other mental health professionals with little, if any, additional formal training required. In contrast, specialized formal training and experience are needed to practice spiritually oriented psychotherapy.

As noted earlier, the four functions of spiritual care are taking a spiritual history, identifying spiritual needs, ensuring that those needs are addressed by someone, and providing mental health care in a spiritual way. Neither the Joint Commission nor Medicare and Medicaid appears to require specialized training for these functions. For example, the Joint Commission requires a spiritual assessment for patients receiving psychosocial treatment for substance abuse and emotional and behavioral disorders, and eligibility for Medicare or Medicaid payment to health professionals requires both identification of and respect for patients' spiritual beliefs (Koenig, 2013).

MATCHING RELIGIOUS, SPIRITUAL, AND CLINICAL CONCERNS TO SERVICE PROVIDERS

Individuals commonly bring various concerns to their providers, be they psychiatrists, psychologists and others psychotherapists, pastoral counselors, spiritual directors, chaplains, or community clergy. It is not uncommon for these concerns to spread across the various categories in the taxonomy of religious, pastoral, spiritual, life, and clinical problems and concerns (see Box 6.1). It is not unreasonable to expect patients to present with concerns that span many of these six categories. Using scope of practice as a criterion for an appropriate "fit" between concerns and provider, the following observations are offered.

Category I concerns are primarily the province of pastoral care and pastoral counseling. However, life-threatening and terminal illness may also be addressed by physicians and psychiatrists. When it comes to religious and spiritual struggles, spiritually oriented psychotherapy may be indicated. If sexual abuse by clergy is involved, specialized trauma-based therapy and pastoral care may be necessary.

Category II concerns are primarily the province of a form of spiritually oriented psychotherapy called *transpersonal psychotherapy* (Cortright, 1997). It is usually indicated for these spiritual emergencies, which are more common in geographic regions where meditation and New Age practices are common.

Category III concerns are primarily the province of spiritual direction. They were the mainstay of pastoral care and counseling in the era before pastoral counseling became psychotherapeutically focused. Recently, pastoral counseling appears to be reclaiming this category of concerns.

Category IV concerns are primarily the province of spiritual directors, who in the past were often priest-confessors. They would routinely deal with an individual's moral or ethical issues. More recently, pastoral counselors work with individuals who may be confused about moral choices or who have violated established Christian norms. These individuals may be offered moral guidance, or they may be guided through a process of forgiveness and restoration to the community.

Category V concerns are primarily the province of pastoral counseling (i.e., the so-called problems of daily living). This category has been considered the bread and butter of psychotherapy practice, including spiritually oriented psychotherapy.

Category VI concerns are the primarily the province of psychiatry and also of psychotherapy. That does not mean that a spiritual director would avoid these symptoms or concerns. Rather than attempting to process them psychotherapeutically, the spiritual director might ask, "Where is God for you in this situation?" to assist clients to reflect on the spiritual dimension of their symptoms or concerns.

What about spiritual care practiced by psychiatrists? To the extent that spiritual and religious concerns are identified in the spiritual assessment and life and clinical problems are identified in the psychiatric evaluation, the psychiatrist practicing spiritual care could reasonably address concerns in all categories, probably with the exception of Category IV. However, collaboration and referral may be indicated for concerns in Categories I through III.

CASE ILLUSTRATIONS

Case 1

A 36-year-old, married, Catholic woman presented for outpatient treatment to a psychiatrist requesting help in dealing with a depression and guilt feelings. An initial psychiatric evaluation was performed, which reportedly did not include a spiritual assessment, and a provisional diagnosis of a mood disorder was made. After four therapy sessions, the client became increasingly symptomatic, and the diagnosis was changed to Dissociative Identity Disorder and Major Depressive Disorder. She was given an antidepressant; later, when she began to decompensate, an antipsychotic was added. Two months later, she became increasingly distressed and was admitted to the psychiatric unit of a local Catholic hospital where the psychiatrist was the medical director.

During the hospitalization, a chaplain completed a spiritual assessment, but there is no indication that it was incorporated into the psychiatrist's case conceptualization. However, as the patient became more regressed and described nightmares, the psychiatrist talked with her about using a spiritual intervention in which she would "be exorcized of the demons" that were distressing her. Presumably, the psychiatrists's diagnosis now included Religious or Spiritual Problem (V62.89).

Although the idea of being possessed was confusing and frightening to the client, she reluctantly agreed to the plan. The next day, the psychiatrist proceeded to follow the Roman Catholic rite of exorcism. During it, the patient became frightened and repeated asked him to stop, to which he reportedly replied that it was only the devil inside her telling him to stop. After the spiritual intervention, the patient appeared to be somewhat less distressed but was still quite depressed. She was discharged and soon dropped out of treatment. Subsequently, she sued the psychiatrist for malpractice, alleging that he was negligent in her treatment, particularly in performing the exorcism.

In court testimony, two expert witnesses questioned the diagnosis of Dissociative Identity Disorder and posited that the patient likely suffered from depression, insomnia, and Borderline Personality Disorder. Much testimony centered on the spiritual intervention as the chosen treatment. Although there is no consensus on the treatment of choice for Dissociative Identity Disorder, expert witnesses questioned the use of exorcism and the manner in which it was performed. In related testimony, the psychiatrist's knowledge of and experience with proper diagnosis and treatment of possession states were demonstrated to be inadequate. For example, under cross-examination, he admitted that his only formal training with this intervention was a "weekend workshop and reading a book about demons." He also admitted that on the day of the intervention he stopped at K-Mart and bought a fire extinguisher "in case she spontaneously combusted."

It appears that the psychiatrist's use of the spiritual intervention was based on an inaccurate recognition of "demonic activity," which in this case was more likely an exacerbation of the patient's borderline personality. In addition, he failed to demonstrate clinical sensitivity in several respects, particularly by his failure to heed the patient's repeated requests that he stop the rite. With regard to clinical interventions, although it appears that a reasonable therapeutic alliance was established between doctor and patient at the beginning of treatment, it had eroded considerably during the hospitalization.

In terms of ethical considerations, full informed consent for the exorcism was not achieved. The patient testified that the psychiatrist never warned her of any risks involved in the spiritual intervention and that she felt taunted as the psychiatrist "screamed at the devil to leave my body." This suggests that value imposition occurred. The question of whether the exorcism was within the scope of practice as well as the psychiatrist's competency to perform it were brought up during the trial. As already noted, his only experience was very limited. He also stated that he had performed the deliverance to "gain experience and see how it worked." This statement suggests a conflict of interests.

Overall, it did not appear that the patient's spiritual needs were appropriately and sufficiently addressed. There was no indication that the psychiatrist knew or was aware of the patient's spiritual history and considerations because he did not take a spiritual assessment nor utilize information from the chaplain's assessment. In addition, it did not appear that the psychiatrist considered organizational ethical issues (Sperry, 2007) that could have positively or negatively affected the appropriateness and sufficiency of treatment. The first issue was that the bishop of the diocese required that an extensive neuropsychiatric and pastoral investigation be performed and submitted to him before he would approve any request for exorcism, and that an exorcism could be performed only by a priest assigned by the bishop. The second issue was that because the hospital had no specific policy and procedures concerning exorcism, any staff member wanting to perform a nonconventional treatment had to make a formal request to the hospital's ethics committee and executive committee for approval. This, of course, was not done. Most psychiatrists do not appear to identify exorcism as an area of competency. Not surprisingly, the psychiatrist lost his privileges at the hospital as well as his position as inpatient director. Even if a lawsuit for malpractice had not been brought against this healthcare professional, the case clearly demonstrates failures in competence and spiritual sensitivity. As unimaginable as it might seem, this is a very real case (*Cool v. Olson*, 1994).

Case 2

A 24-year-old, unmarried, Caucasian woman was referred from her primary care physician to a male psychiatrist after reporting that she had begun to experience anxiety, nightmares, and headaches after watching a television documentary on sexual abuse. The initial session with the psychiatrist consisted of a psychiatric evaluation that included a thorough spiritual assessment. The following diagnoses were made: Major Depressive Disorder, Unspecified Trauma- and Stressor-Related Disorder, and Dependent Personality Disorder. After a medication evaluation, therapy with an antidepressant was begun. The spiritual assessment revealed that the patient had been raised within the Catholic faith and attended Catholic grade school and high school. Because her parents were deeply involved with their parish community and religious services and practices, the patient, their only child, had also consistently and compliantly practiced her faith, at least until she left home for college. When she no longer had her parents monitoring her religious activities, she "lost her faith" and stopped all religious practices. It was only in therapy that it became clear to her why she had relinquished the practice of her faith.

The spiritual assessment also disclosed that the client had been sexually abused by a parish priest for approximately 4 months when she was 12 years old. The abuse stopped when the priest was abruptly transferred because of a complaint of sexual misconduct by another family in the parish. The patient was afraid that her parents would not believe she was also abused, so she never told them or anyone else until the disclosure to the psychiatrist. In terms of religious and spiritual concerns, religious concerns were prominent. These included religious and spiritual struggles of the interpersonal type related to the sexual abuse, feelings of betrayal by the priest, and loss of faith.

Because the psychiatrist did not have specialized training in trauma work, after discussion with the patient, he made a referral to a female Christian psychologist with an expertise in clergy sexual trauma. The plan was for the patient to work with the psychologist weekly to focus on trauma and to meet with the psychiatrist monthly for medication and supportive psychotherapy. After 16 months of trauma-based therapy, both the psychiatrist and the patient evaluated her progress and agreed that her trauma symptoms had remitted and her overall well-being had increased. Accordingly, they agreed that she would terminate the trauma-based therapy and continue with the psychiatrist on a bimonthly basis. The client also felt that she was ready to accept the psychiatrist's invitation to meet with a compassionate priest to discuss her "faith journey," as she referred to it. After a few discussions with the priest, she joined one of her female friends in a parish activity and soon became active again.

Clinically, it appears that the patient was accorded both appropriate and effective psychiatric treatment including spiritual care. That the patient had come to trust her psychiatrist in a matter of a few months is a testament to the deep level of his caring and concern. It is noteworthy that the trauma specialist commented that the patient's overall treatment appeared to have been accelerated by her relationship with the psychiatrist.

In terms of ethical sensitivity, the psychiatrist demonstrated sensitivity and respect for the patient's religious values. In addition, her privacy and confidentiality were well preserved. The referral to the trauma specialist reflected the psychiatrist's respect for scope of practice considerations. With the patient' permission, the psychiatrist conferred with the psychologist over the course of the trauma therapy. It appears that full informed consent was secured for all treatments, including the psychiatrist's consultation with the psychologist. No evidence of conflict of interest or lack of competence on his part was evidenced.

Overall, it appears that the patient's religious and spiritual concerns were appropriately and sufficiency addressed by the spiritual care the psychiatrist provided. Clearly, the psychiatrist was knowledgeable about religious and spiritual matters, and based on his psychiatric evaluation and spiritual assessment of the patient, he was able to plan and implement an integrative treatment plan that addressed her two main religious concerns as well as her psychiatric symptoms.

Case Commentaries

A distinctive feature of Case 1 is that the psychiatrist concluded that his patient's primary spiritual concern was a possession state, a Category II concern. Even though this concern was not elicited from a spiritual assessment—because the psychiatrist did not perform one—he implemented a spiritual intervention that did not result in a reduction of symptoms but rather caused an increase in symptoms and set the stage for premature termination and a malpractice suit. Not only was his formulation of demonic possession not shared by the patient, it was not shared by the expert witnesses in their court testimony. Instead, they concluded that the patient's presentation was more likely due to an exacerbation of her Borderline Personality Disorder (Category VI). There is little indication that the psychiatrist practiced spiritual care. In addition to the diagnostic failure and verdict of malpractice, the psychiatrist's behavior would be considered grossly unethical and spiritually insensitive. Finally, this case is really about incompetence and poor judgment in assessment, diagnosis, case conceptualization, and the choice and implementation of a particular spiritual intervention. It is not simply about possession and exorcism. In short, this case exemplifies how *not* to deal with spiritual, religious, and clinical issues in psychiatric practice.

In contrast, Case 2 exemplifies how to deal appropriately and effectively with spiritual and religious concerns in psychiatric practice. In contrast to Case 1, treatment decisions were based on an accurate psychiatric evaluation and a thorough spiritual assessment. From this evaluation and assessment, religious, spiritual, and clinical concerns were identified, and treatment decisions were made about the psychiatrist's role and involvement in spiritual care, medication evaluation and monitoring, and supportive therapy. Treatment decisions also included referral and collaboration with the trauma specialist and parish priest. Accordingly, the patient was provided appropriate and effective treatment, her psychological well-being was promoted, and her spiritual concerns were addressed. The result was that the clinical and spiritual outcomes were achieved in an ethical and spiritually sensitive manner.

CONCLUDING COMMENT

Not all psychiatrists who are sensitive to clinical, ethical, and religious/spiritual considerations have sufficient specialized training to provide spiritually oriented psychotherapy or other specialized spiritual and pastoral treatments. However, all psychiatrists are expected to provide spiritual care as described in this chapter (Koenig, 2013), and this includes performing a spiritual history. As described in the text and illustrated in the case examples, psychiatrists are faced with a number of ethical considerations in assessing and responding to the spiritual and religious concerns of all their patients, particularly those involving informed consent and competency as they relate to scope of practice.

REFERENCES

American Psychiatric Association. (2013). *Diagnostic and statistical manual of mental disorders, fifth edition*. Alexandria, VA: American Psychiatric Association.

Benner, D. (2003). *Strategic pastoral counseling: A short-term structured model* (2nd ed.). Grand Rapids, MI: Baker Academic.

Berg, G. (1994). The use of the computer as a tool for assessment and research in pastoral care. *Journal of Health Care Chaplaincy, 6*(1), 11–25.

Berg, G. (1998). A statement on clinical assessment for pastoral care. *Chaplaincy Today, 14*(2), 42–50.

Bhikku, T. (2003). Making a cup of tea: Some aspects of spiritual direction within a living Buddhist tradition. In N. Vest (Ed.). *Tending the holy: Spiritual direction across traditions* (pp. 3–18). New York, NY: Morehouse Publishing.

Bullis, R. (1996). *Spirituality in social work practice*. Philadelphia, PA: Taylor & Francis.

Cool v. Olson. (1994). Circuit Court, Outagamie County, Wisconsin, No. 94CV707.

Cortright, B. (1997). *Psychotherapy and spirit: Theory and practice in transpersonal psychotherapy*, Albany, NY: State University of New York Press.

Edwards, T. (2001). *Spiritual director, spiritual companion: Guide to tending the soul.* New York, NY: Paulist Press.

Hathaway, W., Scott S., & Garver, S. (2004). Assessing religious/spiritual functioning: A neglected domain n clinical practice. *Professional Psychology, Research and Practice, 35L*, 97–104.

Koenig, H. (2013). *Spirituality in patient care: Why, how, when, and what* (3rd ed.). West Conshohocken, PA: Templeton Press.

Lukoff, D., Lu, F., & Turner, R. (1992). Toward a more culturally sensitive DSM-IV psychoreligious and psychospiritual problems. *Journal of Nervous and Mental Disease, 180*, 673–682.

Lukoff, D., Lu, F., & Yang, P. (2011). DSM-IV religious and spiritual problems. In J. Peteet, F. Lu, & W. Narrow (Eds). *Religious and spiritual issues in psychiatric diagnosis: A research agenda for DSM-V* (pp. 171–198). Arlington, VA: American Psychiatric Association.

May, G. (1992). *Care of mind, care of spirit: A psychiatrist explores spiritual direction.* San Francisco, CA: Harper San Francisco.

Montgomery, D. (2010). *Pastoral counseling and coaching.* Monticello, CA: Compass Works.

Murray-Swank, A., & Murray-Swank, N. (2012). Spirituals and religious problems: Integrating theory and clinical practice. In K. Pargament (Ed.), *APA handbook of psychology, religion and spirituality* (vol. II, pp. 421–437). Washington, DC: American Psychological Association.

Pargament, K. (2007). *Spiritually integrated psychotherapy: Understanding and addressing the sacred.* New York, NY: Guilford.

Sperry, L. (2002). *Transforming self and community: Revisioning pastoral counseling and spiritual direction.* Collegeville, MN: Liturgical Press.

Sperry, L. (2007). *The ethical and professional practice of counseling and psychotherapy.* Boston, MA: Allyn & Bacon.

Sperry, L. (2008). *The dictionary of ethical and legal terms and issues: Essential guide for mental health professionals.* New York, NY: Routledge.

Sperry, L. (2012a). *Spirituality in clinical practice: Theory and practice of spiritually oriented psychotherapy* (2nd ed.). New York, NY: Routledge.

Sperry, L. (2012b). Spiritually-integrated psychotherapy: Philosophical and clinical considerations in fostering spiritual growth. In L. Miller (Ed.), *The Oxford handbook of psychology of spirituality* (pp. 223–233). New York, NY: Oxford University Press.

Sperry, L. (2013). Distinctive approaches to religion and spirituality: Pastoral counseling, spiritual direction, and spiritually integrated psychotherapy. In K. Pargament (Ed.), *APA Handbook of psychology, religion and spirituality* (vol. II, pp. 223–238). Washington, DC: American Psychological Association.

Sperry, L., & Shafranske, E. (Eds). (2005). *Spiritually oriented psychotherapy.* Washington, DC: American Psychological Association.

Stone, H. (1999). Pastoral counseling and the changing times. *Journal of Pastoral Care, 53*, 47–56.

SEVEN

The Role of Religious Professionals in Ethical Decision Making in Mental Health

Nancy C. Kehoe, RSCJ, Ph.D.

THE TERM *RELIGIOUS PROFESSIONAL* REFERS TO MEN AND WOMEN WHO are recognized by a faith tradition as leaders/teachers within the tradition. Examples include elders, pastors, imams, rabbis, ministers, gurus, priests, nuns, and spiritual guides. Their required education and training vary widely but focus on the doctrines of the faith tradition, understanding the oral and written traditions of the community, liturgical leadership of services, and the fostering of personal spiritual growth. In practice and in their respective ministries, religious professionals encounter many issues, including ethical dilemmas related to mental health, but their preparation to deal with these issues varies greatly. The unique ethical dilemmas that faith leaders face is the focus of this chapter.

Within some traditions, a trained and appointed leader is the person responsible for the local congregation, while in others that responsibility is borne by the wider community. In the Roman Catholic Church and the Episcopal Church, a bishop is responsible for the diocese and assigns the minister to a particular congregation. In other faith traditions, such as Baptist, Muslim, and Jewish communities, the congregation hires the minister, imam, or rabbi, who is accountable to a board of trustees or a vestry instead of a superior religious authority. This is relevant because, when ethical violations arise, counsel is often sought from a higher authority. In Muslim, Jewish, or Baptist communities, there may be no clear authority to whom the affected party can appeal.

Anyone in the community doing ministry in some capacity is bound by the same ethical codes as an ordained leader. Examples include pastoral counselors, spiritual directors, leaders of youth groups, and directors of adult education. Chaplains are ordained or designated leaders within their faith tradition who may serve in schools, hospitals, correctional facilities, or the armed services.

Like mental health professions, religious organizations have their own sets of ethical guidelines. Although these vary across religious denominations, they share common features that resemble the universal concerns found in the codes of ethics for disciplines such as medicine, psychiatry, psychology, and social work. Some of these universal concerns are respect for the individual, avoidance of discriminatory practices, respect for boundaries including physical contact, maintenance of competence and record keeping, conflicts of interest, relationships with colleagues, dual relationships (e.g., a minister who is a close friend of a family in the congregation), and the reporting of ethical violations.

The *Principles of Medical Ethics* of the American Psychiatric Association states, "A psychiatrist shall not gratify his or her own needs by exploiting the patient. The psychiatrist shall be ever vigilant about the impact that his or her conduct has upon the boundaries of the doctor–patient relationship and thus upon the well-being of the patient. These requirements become particularly important because of the essentially private, highly personal and sometimes intensely emotional nature of the relationship established with the patient" (American Psychiatric Association, 2010, p. 3).

The American Psychological Association's *Ethical Principles of Psychologists and Code of Conduct* states, "In applying the Ethics Code to their professional work, psychologists may consider other materials and guidelines that have been adopted or endorsed by scientific and professional psychological organizations and the dictates of their own conscience, as well as consult with others within the field" (American Psychological Association, 2003).

Uniquely and constructively, the *Code of Ethics* of the National Association of Social Workers names the value and the underlying principle that supports it: "Ethical decision making is a process. There are many instances in social work where simple answers are not available to resolve complex ethical issues. Social workers should take into consideration all the values, principles, and standards in this *Code* that are relevant to any situation in which ethical judgment is warranted. Social workers' decisions and actions should be consistent with the spirit as well as the letter of this *Code*" (National Association of Social Workers, 2008).

The guidelines for mental health professionals call for performance evaluations and the requirement of ongoing education as a necessity for maintaining their professional licenses to practice. Remarkably, except for pastoral counselors, no such requirement is cited for religious professionals.

A religious professional or faith leader is serving in the name of God, Allah, or Yahweh and is responsible for the spiritual health and development of the faith community as a whole as well as the individuals within it. Among the ethical guidelines reviewed for this chapter, only the codes for Jewish rabbis and for North American Baptist ministers stated a need to maintain a balance between one's family commitments and religious duties. Whereas the ethical guidelines for religious professionals call for the person to be responsible for his or her spiritual formation and physical, emotional, and mental health, there currently exists no explicit process for accountability.

GUIDELINES FOR RELIGIOUS PROFESSIONALS IN VARIOUS FAITH TRADITIONS

The following quotations are illustrative of some the guidelines for religious professionals.

Responsibilities of Professional and Volunteer Imams

"The standards act as a resource for imams and other staff as they struggle with ethical issues and dilemmas in the context of their daily practice. The same standards also enable the imam and staff to be accountable to Allah, themselves and to the community . . . . The imam must accept his office as an *amanah* (trust) from God and the people he serves. An imam's approach to his job should be professional, ethical and accountable . . . . Each person has the right to respect and dignity as a human being and to counseling services . . . . Each person has the right to privacy and thereby the right to expect the Imam to comply with all laws, policies and ethical standards pertaining to confidentiality" (Siddiqui, 2014).

The Ethical Code for Upaya Zen Center

Different centers have similar though not identical ways of expressing the ethical guidelines for those engaged in a Buddhist practice. For all Buddhists, the Eight-Fold Path and the Five Precepts are the guides for life. In the guidelines enunciated by the Upaya Zen Center, the leaders are those "who are given the responsibilities of leadership and teaching within our sangha." The leaders "acknowledge that we are first of all continuing students of the Great Way. We also acknowledge there are power differentials in our relationships and how with leadership our words and actions carry even greater weight than might be the case in other circumstances. As such we agree to bind ourselves consciously to a code of conduct that nurtures our community as well as our own continuing practice" (Upaya Zen Center, 2013).

Code of Ethics for Rabbis

"As rabbis, we are expected to abide by the highest moral values of our Jewish tradition: personal conscience and professional integrity, honorable social relationships, and the virtues of family life. As teachers and role models, we are called upon to exemplify the ideals we proclaim. Should we fail, we need to do *teshuvah* [repentance], ask forgiveness, avoid repetition, and make restitution whenever possible" (Central Conference of American Rabbis, 2015).

The Catholic Tradition

Each Roman Catholic diocese has its own ethical guidelines, which vary slightly. One is referenced here.

"The ethical Church leader is one who embraces the principles of ecclesial commitment, integrity, respect for others, personal responsibility for one's health, ongoing formation and competence."

"They [the priests] are to be aware of warning signs of potential problems in regard to their own health and in their personal and professional lives and are to strive for greater self-awareness in order to recognize the unique dynamics at work in pastoral relationships" (Catholic Diocese of Richmond, 2016, p. 3).

Code of Ethics of North American Baptists

"As a minister of Jesus Christ, called by God to proclaim the Gospel, and gifted by the Spirit, I dedicate myself to conduct my ministry in accord with the *Statement of Beliefs* of the North American Baptist Conference and the church to which I am called . . . . I will constantly prepare myself in body, mind and spirit for the task to which God has called me . . . . I will seek to build up the church without discrediting other churches or ministries." The minister signs the document stating that he/she "is in full and complete agreement with the North American Baptist *Statement of Beliefs* and *Code of Ministerial Ethics*" (North American Baptist Conference, 2015). This is the only code reviewed that required a signature.

Assemblies of God

"A valid code of ethics for ministers must contain a key internal ingredient—integrity. Many professions have a code of ethics that contributes to the ethical environment by providing professionals a general understanding of what is expected. They are nonetheless missing this essential element.

In its biblical uses, integrity is wholeness and completeness. To be whole is to make all areas of life consistent with internal values, commitments, and allegiances. Regardless of the meticulous details of a code, a list of rules cannot produce wholeness in an individual. Codes supply basic rules for external action but cannot forge the steel of one's internal character . . . . A code of ethics mutually agreed upon by clergy and congregation gives reasonable assurance to both when they plan how the structure will be built" (Reasons, 2015).

RELIGIOUS PROFESSIONALS AND MENTAL HEALTH ISSUES

To review, the following were some of the concerns highlighted in the codes of ethics of religious professionals that were reviewed: being "professional, ethical and accountable"; acknowledging that "we are first of all continuing students of the Great Way"; knowing that, "should we fail, we need to do *teshuvah*"; and defining the ethical church leader as "one who embraces . . . responsibility for one's health, ongoing formation and competence."

Whereas faith leaders encounter various ethical dilemmas, such as the reception of gifts, the use of discretionary funds, and dual relationships that are unavoidable, the guidelines emphasize the importance of competence and ongoing spiritual formation. What is startling is the absence of any guidelines that recognize necessary levels of competence to deal with mental health issues, save for those stated in the Canadian code of ethics for imams (Siddiqui, 2015). Given the recent promulgation of many of these guidelines and the awareness that religious professionals regularly encounter mental health issues, this is an important omission. The following discussion focuses on what has been written about this intersection and some dilemmas that involve issues related to mental health or mental illness.

REVIEW OF THE LITERATURE

A paucity of research exists on the ethical dilemmas that faith leaders encounter in relation to mental health issues. According to Keenan (2006), author of "Toward an Ecclesial Professional Ethics" in *Church Ethics and Its Organizational Context*, this absence may be due to the fact that

> Clerical cultures, episcopal cultures, and the cultures of religious life do not regularly promote for their own members an awareness of the goods and benefits that are engaged by the practice of critical ethical thinking in routine decision-making. That is, unlike many other professions, religious leaders rarely turn to ethical norms to consider what constitutes right conduct in their field of leadership and service. I do not mean by this that religious leaders or their decisions are unethical. Rather, I mean that when religious, clergy, and bishops exercise routine decision-making, they turn to a multitude of considerations, but articulated ethical norms, their specific values and goods, the virtues, and the type of critical thinking that estimates the long-standing social claims these values, goods, and virtues have on use are not explicitly, professionally engaged. In a word, ethical norms and critical ethical reasoning, which frequently aid other professionals in their considerations, play a much less explicit role in ecclesial leadership practices. (p. 83).

Numerous articles address the fact that it is the clergy person to whom members of the congregation turn in time of stress (Nieuwsma et al., 2014; Wang, Bergland, & Kessler, 2003; Weaver, Revilla, & Koenig, 2002), while also recognizing that the clergy lack sufficient training to deal with serious mental illness (Noort, Braam, Gool, & Beekman, 2012). Seminary training frequently includes a requirement that those in training take at least one semester in Clinical Pastoral Education, a training program most often conducted in hospitals and correctional facilities, to teach clergy pastoral care, but this is inadequate to enable ministers to identify and deal with serious mental health issues (Moran et al., 2005; Nauert, 2014). The local church is called upon to provide either a mental health ministry or counseling activities and referrals and/or to be the source for health education (Chatters, 2000; Chatters, Levin, & Ellison, 1998; Clinebell, 1972, Moran et al., 2005; Wang et al., 2003; Weaver et al., 2002; Young, 1989). This is a lot to expect when requisite training is not provided.

Within African American faith communities, more attention is often paid to providing health services. This may be because trust in religious professionals is greater than trust in mental health professionals, many of whom are of other ethnic backgrounds. Although stigma is widespread, there seems to be within the African American community a greater fear of reaching out to mental health professionals and a greater belief in the power of spiritual supports, such as prayer (Neighbors, Musick, & Williams, 1998; Taylor, Ellison, Chatters, Levin, & Lincoln, 2000; Young, Griffith, & Williams, 2003).

For many in the Muslim community, it is important to work with a counselor who understands one's religious orientation; hence, the role of the imam as counselor is frequently sought (Abu-Ras & Laird, 2010; Kehoe, 2014; Padela, Killawi, Heisler, Demonner, & Fetters, 2010; Wahiba & Lance, 2011). Most Muslims seek informal help from imams on a variety of issues, including mental distress. Imams nationwide, report that their congregants come to them for a full range of emotional problems, marital and family problems, and psychological and social concerns (Ali et al., 2005), and 100% of imams reported an increase in help-seeking follow-ing the 9/11 attack (Ali et al., 2005). Muslims have a broad range of beliefs about the cause of mental illness, but by virtue of religious belief, they attribute the ultimate cause of everything, including disease, to God (Wahiba & Lance, 2011). In order to promote a greater understanding between the Muslim community and the mental health community, Dr. Farha Abbais, an Assistant Professor of Psychiatry at Michigan State University, has since 2001 led an annual conference for mental health professionals and religious leaders in the Muslim community to network and discuss ways to address mental health issues.

Although boundary issues, confidentiality, and ethical dilemmas are discussed as they relate to the dual roles that faith leaders often play, very little of the literature reviewed included any specific remarks on mental illness (Bleiberg & Skufca, 2005; Justice & Garland, 2010; Kitchener, 1988; Miller & Atkinson, 1988; Parent, 2004; Smith & Smith, 2001). The issue of dual roles is one that other professionals also encounter. (Aravind, Krishnaram, & Thasneem, 2012; Gutheil & Gabbard, 1993). Faith leaders whose primary responsibility is for the spiritual life and care of the community have administrative, teaching, and possibly counseling relationships with individuals or families. Counseling relationships present particular complexity; their development may become problematic because the faith leader is likely to encounter the congregants in social, civic, and community settings. Even though many faith leaders develop these kinds of dual relationships, they nonetheless require an awareness of the potential difficulty inherent in boundary crossings and an ability to solve issues that are likely to arise.

One article (Stanton, 2015) made reference to small communities, such as those in rural areas, where the faith leader or the only doctor may be the one that individuals turn to for mental health issues despite their lack of training. In such areas, mental health resources are frequently limited or absent.

In this chapter on religious professionals, ethical dilemmas, and mental health, we must not ignore the sexual abuse crisis within faith communities. However, because much has already been written on this topic, we will not expand upon it here except to raise the issue as it relates to accountability. Many religious professionals are operating on their own with little or no ethical oversight or accountability as is often provided in other professions. With no ethical oversight, as is often provided in other professional roles, accountability is never addressed.

As Karen Allen (2012) wrote in "What Is an Ethical Dilemma?":

> There are three conditions that must be present for a situation to be considered an ethical dilemma. The first condition occurs in situations when an individual, called the "agent," must make a decision about which course of action is best. Situations that are uncomfortable but that don't require a choice are not ethical dilemmas . . . . The second condition for an ethical dilemma is that there must be different courses of action to choose from. Third, in an ethical dilemma, no matter what course of action is taken, some ethical principle is compromised. In other words, there is no perfect solution.

Because of the nature of their roles involving a multiplicity of varied demands, faith leaders potentially face numerous situations that involve ethical dilemmas. Although we cannot address all of the ethical dilemmas that might confront religious professionals within the limits of this chapter, we will mention some that relate to the setting, training, and the dual roles of counselor and faith leader.

SETTING

Religious professionals work in a variety of settings, including communities and institutions. A community may or may not have a clearly defined geographical boundary. It may be in an urban or a rural area with some other faith communities proximate or distant. These differences may affect the availability of colleagues, a support system, and mental health resources. Boundaries are more fluid within a geographically defined community. A religious professional may be a chaplain in a hospital setting, in a correctional facility, in an academic setting, or with the armed services. In these institutional situations, boundaries and roles may be more easily defined.

A minister, called to be a representative of God, Allah, or Yahweh to his or her congregation and to the community as a whole, may encounter a conflict between the good of the individual congregant or congregation and that of the community (e.g., taking a stand on a political issue based on conscience that is opposed by congregants). A faith leader who lives in a small community where there are insufficient mental health resources may be asked to address mental health needs and issues that far exceed his or her competency.

TRAINING AND RESOURCES

As noted earlier, the education and training of religious professionals is theological and spiritual and typically has not included formation in relation to issues of mental health and mental illness, yet congregants with such issues frequently turn first to their faith leader. Depending on the setting, faith leaders may have few mental health resources to whom they can refer. They may, through a mistaken notion of being all things to all people, think that they can help anyone who consults them. Sometimes there is a certain hubris or arrogance in assessing what one can or cannot do. Some ethical guidelines state that ministers are responsible for their own physical, mental, emotional, and spiritual well-being, but lines of accountability or supervision are not clearly stated. Although a minister is called to live a life of selfless service, his or her personal and family needs may be in conflict with the need to respond to the community. Ministers often serve a community alone, and in the absence of any requirement regarding accountability or supervision, they may not recognize personal problems that interfere with performance. With increasing demands on their time, they may give insufficient reflection to their various involvements with individuals, resulting in boundary crossings and boundary violations.

For example, in many religious traditions, prayers are said publicly for members of the community who are ill. It may create an ethical dilemma for a minister to pray for someone who is suffering with mental illness without identifying the illness. Or, a family may feel that their confidentiality has been compromised by praying for the person in public. A faith leader's position of upholding certain theological beliefs within the faith tradition may also conflict with his or her pastoral response to an individual (e.g., by providing a pastoral response to someone who is gay when the faith community condemns homosexuality).

DUAL ROLES

Dual roles are inevitable for religious professionals because they serve within the context of a larger community; this is true as well for chaplains serving in hospitals, in correctional facilities, or in the armed services. For the religious professional, ethical dilemmas can arise in situations such as the following: when the faith leader is also a therapist or mental health professional; when the faith leader does counseling for a congregant and is not a trained mental health professional; when the faith leader is privy to information regarding a congregant's mental illness or that of a family member; when in a small geographic area the faith leader becomes aware of a mental health issue in a social setting; and when the faith leader has a personal and social relationship with members of the congregation that affects his or her objectivity about a mental health issue. Although a congregant might recognize that religious professionals are responsible for maintaining confidentiality, he or she may still be concerned that what is shared in a counseling setting could inadvertently be communicated and therefore may withhold vital information.

CASE STUDIES

The following cases illustrate some ethical dilemmas. All identifying information has been changed to protect those involved.

Case 1

During the summer, Sheila, a woman in her late thirties, began attending services at a Christian church. Over time, she offered to do volunteer work for the congregation in preparation for its Christmas craft fair. After the holidays, she joined the Bible study group in the congregation—a group of women who had been meeting for many years and were good friends with the minister. The young woman had shared with the minister that she was living with bipolar disorder, seeing a psychiatrist, and taking medication.

In the Bible study group, Sheila shared that her father was an atheist who found it difficult to understand why she was now attending a Christian church. Several weeks later, when she vehemently questioned what one of the older women in the group said about God, the latter retorted that since Sheila was an atheist, of course she wouldn't understand how God acts. Enraged, Sheila responded with an angry outburst and stormed out of the meeting. The next day, some of the members of the group met with the minister and told him what had occurred. He contacted Sheila and told her that she could no longer do volunteer work nor attend the Bible study group and that her attendance at services needed to be restricted.

Multiple aspects of this case can be explored to shed light on different issues involved. Sheila had shared her diagnosis with the minister. He had the duty to respect her confidentiality and not share this information with the Bible study group. However, he also had a responsibility to discuss with the members of the group the precipitant of this outburst. This presented him with a true dilemma. Before limiting her involvement (acting solely on behalf of the group), he could have sat down with Sheila to ask whether he might share with the group her struggles with certain issues. He also might have advised her to take some time before returning to the group and asked whether she would be willing to share with them how the response had triggered something in her. In order for the minister to tell the group about her diagnosis, he would first need to obtain permission from Sheila.

This minister's action revealed that he does not understand mental illness. This is, unfortunately, common in faith leaders because their training in this regard has often been inadequate.

If he had had some understanding of what it means to live with bipolar disorder, he might have had conversations with Sheila and discussed with her the unacceptable nature of some behaviors while also communicating his understanding that her reaction was triggered by an inappropriate remark. Rather than summarily restricting her involvement in the church, he might have sought consultation to identify a satisfactory way to handle the situation. Ethical guidelines call for consultation when the professional is dealing with areas in which he or she may lack adequate competence.

The minister acted solely on behalf of the group, perhaps affected by his dual relationship with the member of the group who called Sheila an atheist. The family of the person who reacted to Sheila was a big donor to the church, and this also might have affected the minister's hesitancy in challenging the group member.

There are a number of different courses of action that the minister could have taken in response to Sheila's case. Before acting, the minister could have consulted a mental health professional. He also could have spoken to the group and assured them that he was going to address the issue but that they also needed to reflect on their response to Sheila. Were Sheila to give permission for her diagnosis to be shared with the group, this could have presented an invaluable opportunity to educate members of the congregation about mental illness, but the minister would have needed some other, knowledgeable person to do this. As in this instance, faith leaders are often taken off guard or caught at inopportune moments and may act precipitously.

If the minister had stopped to reflect, he might have understood the complexities of the situation. Sheila, although living with a mental illness, needed to abide by the rules of conduct within the church. The minister's rash behavior and response to the situation in unreservedly supporting the group was detrimental to Sheila. He did not recognize that his relationship with the involved group member could have been affected by the fact that this member and her family were big donors to the church.

Case 2

A chaplain affiliated with a Humanistic spiritual tradition was seeing Anna, a 40-year-old woman who was on the hospital's medical floor being treated for cancer. Anna also suffered with bipolar disorder including some psychotic symptoms. Anna was rejecting chemotherapy because of the belief that God would heal her. The medical staff thought that Anna was incapable of making a rational decision because of her bipolar disorder and that her beliefs were being shaped by her mental illness. They knew that the chances for remission with chemotherapy were high, but they could not force a patient to accept chemotherapy treatment. The medical team was also unsure whether the chaplain could help convince the patient that God's healing and chemotherapy were not necessarily antithetical to each other, and how long that would take.

The ethical dilemmas for the chaplain included whether to proactively support the patient's religious beliefs, to advocate with the medical staff for more time to work with the patient, or to help the patient accept the idea that her faith in God's healing might also be compatible with chemotherapy. The chaplain believed that God can work through medical treatment. She wanted to respect Anna's religious beliefs while also maintaining awareness of how her psychotic symptoms could affect the way she thought about her faith: What was Anna's faith? What were the symptoms of her illness? What was her understanding of the treatment and possibly her fears in relation to the treatment? The chaplain wished to support the patient, to advocate for her on religious grounds, and to work with her on understanding how God heals, while also recognizing with the patient that in the past her delusions had been problematic. The medical staff was putting pressure on the chaplain to convince the patient that only chemotherapy could achieve healing and were dismissive of the faith dimension. They were concerned that refusal of the treatment plan would lengthen the hospital stay, which would not be covered by insurance.

In this case, the chaplain did understand mental illness, so she was able to talk with Anna about the reality of her illness and also, recognizing that her faith was important to her, explore with the patient just exactly what she did believe about how God works. The dilemma for the chaplain had more to do with working with the medical staff who were both skeptical of the faith dimension and impatient to begin the procedure, anticipating a lengthy process of education with the patient concerning God, medical interventions, and her mental illness. In a short time, the patient, with the support of the chaplain, did accept chemotherapy treatment.

Case 3

An imam in a small Midwestern city was asked by one of his congregants to see her for counseling. The woman and her husband were friends of the imam and his wife. The imam agreed to meet with the woman in order to understand some of her concerns. When they met, the woman shared with the imam that she had been suffering with serious depression for months and that it was affecting her marriage. Although the imam had taken some counseling courses as part of his training, he was not trained to deal with serious depression and recommended that she see a psychologist in the area. The woman said that she wanted to see the imam because he understood the relationship between depression and her religion; she believed that no secular psychologist understood Islam and the connection between a psychological illness and a person's relationship with God. She refused to see a secular therapist. The imam then faced an ethical dilemma. He had to choose between refusing to see the woman in recognition that he was not competent to deal with her depression, agreeing to see her in some supportive role while encouraging her to ask her primary care doctor for medication, seeing her on condition that he can consult with a therapist who understands serious depression, or suggesting that together they do three-way Skype sessions with a therapist whom he knows well in another city.

Case 4

A new Rabbi, Carole, was serving on an inpatient psychiatric unit and met with Joseph, a 27-year-old man suffering with serious depression who had made a suicide attempt. Joseph asked the chaplain to pray with him and asked that what was shared in the prayer not be put into his treatment notes. Being new on the psychiatric floor and new to hospital ministry, the Rabbi agreed, thinking that this came within the bounds of confidentiality between a chaplain and the person to whom she was ministering. After praying with the patient, she realized that by agreeing to the patient's request she was compromising the man's treatment by withholding information the staff needed to know.

The ethical dilemma the chaplain faced was whether or not to disclose the information. If she disclosed it without permission, there was a risk that the patient would feel betrayed and lose trust in her, and he might tell other patients on the unit that the chaplain could not be trusted. If she did not disclose it and something happened to the patient, she would be responsible. A resolution of the dilemma could be for the chaplain to convince the patient that it was in his best interest to share the information with the staff. Because of what was shared during the prayer, she could inform the patient that although she had agreed initially, she was obliged to reveal the information to the medical staff.

CONCLUSION

In ministering, religious professionals commonly encounter ethical dilemmas related to mental health and illness. Some of these dilemmas are rooted in a lack of understanding of mental illness and its impact on the community. Others have to do with the inevitable multiple relationships with members of the congregation and lack of objectivity when conflicting concerns emerge; inevitable boundary crossings and risk of boundary violations; decisions regarding confidentiality; and being the sole religious leader in the community with unclear guidelines for oversight or accountability. These are complex and demanding sets of issues that need constant attention.

REFERENCES

Abu-Ras, W., & Laird, L. (2010). How Muslim and Non-Muslim chaplains serve Muslim patients? Does the Interfaith chaplaincy model have room for Muslims' experiences? *Journal of Religion and Health, 50*(1), 46–61. doi:10.1007/s10943-010-9357-4

Allen, K. (2012, Spring). What is an ethical dilemma? *The New Social Worker.* Retrieved from http://www.socialworker.com/feature-articles/ethics-articles/What_Is_an_Ethical_Dilemma%3F/.

Ali, O. M., Milstein, G., & Marzuk, P. M. (2005). The Imam's role in meeting the counseling needs of Muslim communities in the United States. *Psychiatric Services, 56,* 202–205.

American Psychiatric Association. (2010). *Principles of medical ethics with annotations especially applicable to psychiatry.* Retrieved from http://www.psychiatry.org/psychiatrists/practice/ethics.

American Psychological Association. (2003). Introduction and applicability. In *Ethical principles of psychologists and code of conduct.* Retrieved from http://www.apa.org/ethics/code/index.aspx.

Aravind, V. K., Krishnaram, V. D., & Thasneem, Z. (2012). Boundary crossings and violations in clinical settings. *Indian Journal of Psychological Medicine, 34*(1), 21–24. doi:10.4103/0253-7176.96151

Bleiberg, J. R., & Skufca, L. (2005). Clergy dual relationships, boundaries, and attachment. *Pastoral Psychology, 54*(1), 3–22. doi:10.1007/s11089-005-6179-5

Catholic Diocese of Richmond [Virginia]. (2016). *The priests' handbook.* Retrieved from http://richmonddiocese.org/wp-content/uploads/2015/10/PriestHandbook2017-1.pdf.

Central Conference of American Rabbis. (2015). *CCAR ethics code.* Retrieved from https://www.ccarnet.org/rabbis-communities/professional-resources/.

Chatters, L. M. (2000). Religion and health: Public health research and practice. *Annual Reviews of Public Health, 21,* 335–367.

Chatters, L. M., Levin, J. S., & Ellison, C. G. (1998). Public health and health education in faith communities. *Health Education & Behavior, 25*(6), 689–699. doi:10.1177/109019819802500602

Clinebell, H. J. (1972). *The mental health ministry of the local church.* Nashville, TN: Abingdon Press.

Gutheil, T. G., & Gabbard, G. O. (1993). The concept of boundaries in clinical practice: Theoretical and risk-management dimensions. *American Journal of Psychiatry, 150*, 188–196.

Justice, J. A., & Garland, D. R. (2010). Dual relationships in congregational practice: Ethical guidelines for congregational social workers and pastors. *Social Work and Christianity, 37*(4), 437–445.

Keenan, J. F. (2006). Toward an ecclesial professional ethics. In J. Bartunek, M. A. Hinsdale, & J. F. Keenan (Eds.), *Church ethics and its organizational context* (pp. 83–96). New York, NY: Sheed and Ward.

Kehoe, N. (2014). Conversations on religion and mental illness [YouTube video]. Retrieved from http://projects.iq.harvard.edu/rshm/conversations-religion-and-mental-illness.

Kitchener, K. S. (1988). Dual relationships: What makes them so problematic? [Abstract]. *Journal of Counseling and Development, 67*, 217–221. doi:10.1002/(issn)1556-6676

Miller, H. M., & Atkinson, D. R. (1988). The clergyperson as counselor: An inherent conflict of interest. *Counseling and Values, 32*(2), 116–123. doi:10.1002/j.2161-007x.1988.tb00705.x

Moran, M., Flannelly, K. J., Weaver, A. J., Overvold, J. A., Hess, W., & Wilson, J. C. (2005). A study of pastoral care, referral, and consultation practices among clergy in four settings in the New York City Area. *Pastoral Psychology, 53*(3), 255–266. doi:10.1007/s11089-004-0556-3

National Association of Social Workers. (2008). *Code of ethics.* Retrieved from http://socialworkers.org/pubs/code/default.asp.

Nauert, R. (2014). Little seminary training to counsel mental illness. *Journal of Research on Christian Education,* https://psychcentral.com/news/2014/09/09/little-seminary-training-to-counsel-mental-illness/74651.html (accessed on 9/7/2017). Baylor University.

Neighbors, H. W., Musick, M. A., & Williams, D. R. (1998). The African American minister as a source of help for serious personal crises: Bridge or barrier to mental health care? *Health Education & Behavior, 25*(6), 759–777. doi:10.1177/109019819802500606

Nieuwsma, J. A., Fortune-Greeley, A. K., Jackson, G. L., Meador, K. G., Beckham, J. C., & Elbogen, E. B. (2014). Pastoral care use among post-9/11 veterans who screen positive for mental health problems. *Psychological Services, 11*(3), 300–308. doi:10.1037/a0037065

Noort, A., Braam, A., Gool, A. V., & Beekman, A. (2012). Recognition of psychopathology with religious content by clergy members: A case vignette study. *Mental Health, Religion & Culture, 15*(2), 205–215. doi:10.1080/13674676.2011.569705

North American Baptist Conference. (2015). *Code of ministerial ethics of the North American Baptist Conference.* Retrieved from https://nabconference.org/wp-content/uploads/2016/12/CODE-OF-MINISTERIAL-ETHICS.pdf.

Padela, A. I., Killawi, A., Heisler, M., Demonner, S., & Fetters, M. D. (2010). The role of Imams in American Muslim health: Perspectives of Muslim community leaders in southeast Michigan. *Journal of Religion and Health, 50*(2), 359–373. doi:10.1007/s10943-010-9428-6

Parent, M. S. (2004). Respecting boundaries: Preventing dual relationships. *Social Work Today, 4*(5), 27–29.

Reasons, J. A. (2015). A minister's code of ethics: A higher level of commitment and conduct. Assemblies of God, *Enrichment Journal.* Retrieved from Enrichmentjournal.ag.org/200404/200404_102_code.cfm.

Siddiqui, S. (2015). *A professional guide for Canadian imams.* (p. 6). Islamic Social Services Association. Retrieved from http://www.issacanadian.com/.

Smith, J. A., & Smith, A. H. (2001). Dual relationships and professional integrity: An ethical dilemma case of a family counselor as clergy. *The Family Journal, 9*(4), 438–443. doi:10.1177/1066480701094012

Stanton, A. (2015, Sept 3). Faith communities help provide mental health care. *IEI Newsletter.* Retrieved from https://iei.ncsu.edu/wp-content/uploads/2015/09/Sep2015Health.pdf.

Taylor, R. J., Ellison, C. G., Chatters, L. M., Levin, J. S., & Lincoln, K. D. (2000). Mental health services in faith communities: The role of clergy in black churches. *Social Work, 45*(1), 73–87. doi:10.1093/sw/45.1.73

Upaya Zen Center. (2013). *Ethics code for Upaya Zen Center.* Retrieved from https://www.upaya.org/about/ethics/.

Wahiba, Abu-Ras, & Lance, L. (2011). How Muslim and Non-Muslim chaplains serve Muslim patients? Does the Interfaith chaplaincy model have room for Muslims' experiences? *Journal of Religion and Health, 50*(1), 46–61.

Wang, P. S., Berglund, P. A., & Kessler, R. C. (2003). Patterns and correlates of contacting clergy for mental disorders in the United States. *Health Services Research, 38*(2), 647–673. doi:10.1111/1475-6773.00138

Weaver, A. J., Revilla, L. A., & Koenig, H. G. (2002). *Counseling families across the stages of life: A handbook for pastors and other helping professionals.* Nashville, TN: Abingdon Press.

Young, J. L., Griffith, E. E., & Williams, D. R. (2003). The integral role of pastoral counseling by African-American clergy in community mental health. *Psychiatric Services,54*(5), 688–692. doi:10.1176/appi.ps.54.5.688

Young, M. C. (1989). Professional and ethical issues for ministers who counsel. *Journal of Pastoral Care & Counseling, 43*(3), 269–275. doi:10.1177/002234098904300309

Ethics Committees and Consultation in Mental Health

Don C. Postema, Ph.D.

INTRODUCTION

The request for an ethics consultation comes from the consulting psychiatrist. The patient is refusing to eat, refusing dialysis, and not taking his medications. He is alternately withdrawn and combative. The psychiatrist has been asked to evaluate the patient's medical decision-making capacity and has requested an ethics consultation to determine whether compelled treatment and feeding would be ethically justified. Your review of the case opens up a complex mix of factors, one of which identifies the patient's "hyperreligious behaviors" as a problem to be assessed.

Mr. Abdullah is a 45-year-old, single, Somali man. His past medical history is notable for hypertension, diabetes, end-stage renal disease receiving hemodialysis, anemia, and depression. He is blind, reportedly because of his failure to manage his diabetes consistently. He has been in the United States for 20 years and was a math teacher. He attempted to start his own learning center, but was unsuccessful. More recently he has been living in a skilled nursing facility due to his inability to find stable housing and medical care on his own. When he refused to eat and take his medications as well as refusing dialysis, the nursing home nurse practitioner offered him hospice care because she believed he had chosen to die.

When you interview Mr. Abdullah, he appears to be a devout Muslim. Informed by the psychiatrist that without dialysis he would die, he responded that "Allah has told me that I cannot escape death in any case, whether from renal failure or something else." He thinks he can manage his diabetes by adhering to a strict diet and has "fixed beliefs about what he should or should not have for care." The psychiatrist noted that "his beliefs are inaccurate and out of step with good evidence-based practices." When challenged on his beliefs, Mr. Abdullah was "quite argumentative."

What can an ethics consultation add to the treatment of Mr. Abdullah and to the diagnosis and recommendations of the psychiatrist?

ETHICS COMMITTEES: ROLES AND HISTORY

An ethics consultation such as that requested for Mr. Abdullah is but one of the activities of a hospital-based ethics committee. An ethics consultation focuses on the ethical questions or issues identified in the care of a patient, resulting in recommendations for providers and patients that will help them rightly pursue their goals of care. In addition, an ethics consultation is often the occasion for stepping back from the immediate issues in order to construct the larger narratives within which those issues are to be addressed.

Education in ethics and ethics-related topics is a second role for an ethics committee, and education and consultation frequently overlap. There are many venues in which education may be offered; practice-related teaching is one of the most effective and most challenging. An immediate need related to patient care spawns a personal incentive to seek the wisdom of others. The immediacy may also mitigate the learning experience in that an answer as to what to do may obviate the need to know why this is the right and good thing to do. In the clinical context, ethics and medical education both face this challenge.

Ethics committees also initiate and review ethics-related policies. For example, the hospital may have a policy that details the nature of and parameters for informed decision making, including the conditions under which patient refusal of a recommended treatment should be honored. There are also policies detailing the limits of medical authority at its boundary with patient autonomy. Limited treatment policies, for example, carve out an area in which patients may choose options other than those recommended by medical professionals.

In addition to these three roles (consultation, education, and policy review), some ethics committees conduct research into ethics-related practices, such as the nature and frequency of ethics consultation requests and the degree to which they are found to be valuable in patient care. Overall, an ethics committee aims to increase the organizational awareness of the ethical dimension of healthcare practices, viewing it as salient to those practices. (For more on the work of ethics committees, see Post and Blustein, 2015).

The work of ethics committees is historically and theoretically situated in ways that enhance current understanding of the roles and values of ethics in healthcare. (The most frequently cited work on this history is Jonsen, 1998). Modern medical bioethics grew out of an era (mid-20th century) in which religious traditions and organizations were prominent in healthcare. Many hospitals trace their roots back to religious grounds, and some evidence these origins in their names (e.g., Methodist Hospital, The Jewish Hospital, St. Mary's Hospital). Bioethics as a distinct academic discipline emerged in the late 1950s from religious and theological concerns related to the growth of science and the medicalization of health. Two of the early leaders in bioethics were Dr. Joseph Fletcher (an Episcopalian who taught at Harvard Divinity School; see Morals and Medicine, 1954) and Dr. Paul Ramsey (a Methodist who taught at Princeton Theological Seminary; see The Patient as Person, 1970). They frequently disagreed on the major issues of the day even though they both were situated in the Christian tradition; sharing a common broad religious tradition is no guarantee of unanimity on any issue in medical bioethics.

Bioethics was "secularized" in subsequent years, and religious perspectives were often relegated to ancillary status. In part, this was driven by the academic birth of bioethics when philosophers, physicians, social scientists, and those in the humanities adopted the emerging field and created academic disciplines (i.e., medical ethics, bioethics, healthcare ethics, biomedical ethics, clinical ethics, and medical humanities). These academic disciplines presumed some degree of ethical autonomy from religious traditions and grounds, seeking rational justification for ethical principles and values or relying on broadly shared moral norms. The reliance on ethical principlism (Beauchamp & Childress, 2012 [originally published in 1979]) and the well-known mantra of *respect for autonomy, non-maleficence, beneficence,* and *justice* is the most prominent witness to this approach. These ethical principles were touted as mid-level principles, not foundational ones. The grounds (epistemological, metaphysical, and religious) for these principles typically were unaddressed in the canonical bioethics monographs. Religious and theological grounds were suspect because they were sectarian and were based on faith, doctrine, tradition, and religious authority in addition to reason. The demise of religion and spirituality in theoretical bioethics was confirmed by the rise of postmodernism, which undercut all claims to universality. H. Tristam Englehardt (1991 and other works) is known for accepting the implications of postmodernism for bioethics and concluding that normativity is not possible.

The demise of religion and spirituality within academic bioethics was paralleled by the hardening of clinical role distinctions that effectively marginalized those practicing in the religious and spiritual dimensions of healthcare. Chaplains were to provide spiritual care and sectarian religious views, not ethical insight. Their role was ancillary to the primary goals of medicine and healthcare. At best, they served as an adjuvant to medical care in that they might better prepare patients for accepting the rigors (and the failures) of modern medical treatment. As a result, the religious and spiritual dimension of healthcare was typically dissociated and relegated to the attention of nonmedical professionals.

It can be argued that the cultural shift which moved religious and spiritual concerns to the periphery was also apparent in the field of mental health. The social segregation of mental healthcare, reinforced by differential payment structures, compounded the shift. Religious and spiritual manifestations of belief and practice were sometimes treated as behavioral abnormalities, approached by means of a clinical reductionism of the religious and spiritual to what is amenable to a scientific paradigm.

THE REEMERGENCE OF THE RELIGIOUS AND SPIRITUAL IN MEDICINE AND HEALTHCARE

There has been a renascence of attention to religion and spirituality in the academic and clinical fields in the last 20 years, prompted by articulate critical perspectives and persistent clinicians. (The critiques of Brody [2009] and Callahan [2012] are notable.)

Proper attention to the religious and spiritual dimension of healthcare and the importance of religion and spirituality to the work of ethics committees have been reaffirmed. Where have these points of convergence occurred, and why?

When approaching the limits of one's discipline or life, religious and spiritual questions often emerge. When the curative powers of medicine are ineffective and a scientific approach to illness and disease has been exhausted, there is still a dimension of the patient and the professional–patient relationship that endures and points beyond these limits. Concerns about the meaning and significance of one's life are frequently prompted when the limits of the ability to control and manage that life are placed in question. Although those limits have been pushed farther than ever in the last century, they are nonetheless still encountered in healthcare settings. Religion and spirituality are the common means by which we address that which transcends these limits. There are at least two areas in which medicine and bioethics have come to recognize the importance of religion and spirituality as constitutive of health and values.

First, when medical science fails to diagnose or cure, we still have a professional and personal relationship that requires us to care for the patient and family. Caring for a person requires attention to all that the person is, and the religious and spiritual dimension of that person must be considered if we are to care rightly. How a patient and family make sense of illness, disability, and death is in part a religious project. Their religious and spiritual resources, or the lack thereof, often are directly correlated to the value of the outcome.

Second, at the end of life, the modalities of care are not primarily focused on curative means. The emergence of palliative care and hospice have opened the door to the religious and spiritual as necessary components of healthcare. Although resistance remains, especially from those specialties that are more oriented to curative ends, the proliferation of palliative care teams with psychological and spiritual disciplines equally represented has brought renewed credibility to the religious and spiritual in clinical settings.

INTEGRATING THE RELIGIOUS
AND SPIRITUAL IN ETHICS COMMITTEES—I

The central practices of ethics committees—consultation, education, and policy development—also reflect the historical developments in biomedical ethics. The religious and spiritual dimensions of the individual patient-provider relationship and the practice of medical care are increasingly regarded as essential to both. However, how to integrate these dimensions honestly and effectively remains a challenge for a variety of reasons.

Another case illustrates a conundrum that often arises for an ethics consultation that aims to incorporate the patient's religious values into its scope. The patient, Mr. Harris, is nearing the end of his life. At 88 years old, his Parkinson's disease, diagnosed many years earlier, is exacting its expected toll. He is now ventilator dependent, receiving his nutrition and fluids by means of a feeding tube, catheterized subsequent to urinary and fecal incontinence, and treated aggressively each time an infection occurs. He has decubitus ulcers that will not heal and contractures of his limbs. He is not consciously interacting with others, although he does open his eyes occasionally and grimaces when procedures are performed. Pain medications assuage the distress he sometimes exhibits. His family are his surrogate decision makers, and there is no advance directive stating what Mr. Harris would want in terms of medical treatment at this point in his life. His family have repeatedly said that he would want "everything done" because he valued life above all else. According to them, Mr. Harris thought death was the worst evil and that enduring pain and suffering is what one has to do to respect life. They are persistent in demanding that, should he experience cardiac arrest, all resuscitation efforts should be attempted. When asked about the grounds for Mr. Harris's beliefs, which his family share, they note that they are members of a conservative Christian church and that their beliefs are grounded in their religious community.

The consensus medical opinion is that the goals of care for Mr. Harris should be preserving his comfort, hygiene, and dignity and that, consistent with these goals, nonbeneficial and possibly harmful treatments should be discontinued. Resuscitation attempts would not be consistent with these goals, and in fact would be harmful to Mr. Harris without any compensatory benefit. An ethics consultation is requested by Mr. Harris's providers due to the moral distress they are experiencing in being required to do what they think is morally wrong. In fleshing out the case, the ethics consultant notes the religious grounds for the family's position and respect them. However, when the beliefs and standards of their Christian denomination are explored, it is clear that the family's position is discordant. Their church specifically states that "when the God-given powers of the body to sustain its own life can no longer function and doctors in their professional judgment conclude that there is no real hope for recovery even with life-support instruments, a Christian may in good conscience 'let nature take its course.'" (*Christian Care at Life's End*. A Report of the Commission on Theology and Church Relations of the Lutheran Church—Missouri Synod, February 1993, p. 4).

In this case, the values of Mr. Harris's caregivers do not diverge from the values of the religious community to which Mr. Harris's family belong. The family's self-identified religious values appear to be idiosyncratic, not shared by their larger religious community. Do idiosyncratic religious beliefs have the same moral weight as those shared by a religious community? Are the motivations of the family grounded in psychologically troubling or pathological states? Professional psychiatric consultation regarding the family's stance may help to answer these questions and offer ethics recommendations regarding the patient's care. If the family's position is motivated by ungrounded fears or dysfunctional relationships that can be surfaced and addressed by skillful psychiatric therapy, their professed religious beliefs may be amenable to revision in the light of their critical assessment. Even if uncovering the psychological dynamics behind their professed religious beliefs does not lead to such revision, the warrant for respecting their treatment goals is diminished by evidence that those wishes are not concordant with what most determine to be in Mr. Harris's best interest at the end of his life.

This case shows that respect for a patient's or family's religious values does not entail acceptance of those values as the primary moral criteria pertaining to a patient's care. Whereas the religious and spiritual dimensions of a patient and family must be acknowledged, they are not an ethical trump for that reason alone. Professional values grounded in shared practices may serve as *prima facie* grounds for refusing to honor the patient's or family's religious values. Considerations of benefit and burden to the patient may also warrant a challenge to those religious values. Respect for religious and spiritual beliefs and values requires due consideration, not acquiescence.

INTEGRATING THE RELIGIOUS AND SPIRITUAL IN ETHICS COMMITTEES—II

The case of Mr. Fayed is an example of the challenges to the professional integrity of caregivers posed by a patient whose religious values entail acceptance of suffering and prolonged dying. Mr. Fayed, a Muslim, is chronically ventilator dependent. His fluid and nutritional needs are provided for by medical means. His condition has progressed to the point at which pain medications are only marginally effective. He is completely dependent on others for all of his care and has been so for almost a year. His caregivers, especially the nurse practitioner at the skilled nursing facility where he now resides, see their efforts as not only medically futile but inconsistent with their professional and personal values. To them, prolonging Mr. Fayed's life so that he can suffer violates their professional integrity. To Mr. Fayed, who is intermittently conscious, and his family, supported by their mullah, enduring suffering is a way of purifying oneself before death and exhibiting one's religious devotion. His caregivers express their moral distress as increasing the longer they have to care for Mr. Fayed. Their professional and personal values cannot condone willful suffering without a meaningful end—and for them, faring well in the afterlife is not such an end. What ethical weight does respect for Mr. Fayed's religious values carry in the face of professional and personal distress?

In response to a request for a consultation initiated by Mr. Fayed's caregivers, the ethics consultant suggests viewing Mr. Fayed's current state in the light of his long-term life project. He has consistently followed what he took to be his Muslim religious calling. Although not everyone in his religious tradition would concur with his interpretation of what that requires, there nonetheless have been examples of the faithful that accord with Mr. Fayed's understanding. He has accepted suffering in the past, which was episodic and followed by return to health. Although such an outcome is not possible at the end of his life, his approach to suffering is consistent. He wants to live the last chapter of his life in a way that substantially connects to all that has gone before. Is his acceptance of suffering a form of self-mutilation? Is it psychologically defective? A psychiatry consultation could address these questions, but if these values are authentic for Mr. Fayed and his family (i.e., not rooted in pathological states or in response to unreasonable social pressures), then they are presumptive grounds for developing an end-of-life care plan for Mr. Fayed.

Mediating the deep moral and religious differences between family members and providers may lead to a compromise wherein the integrity of all can be preserved even if the outcome is less than ideal for both. Negotiating limits to further aggressive treatments that will not alter the outcome for the patient's life may be a possible integrity-preserving compromise for his caregivers, whereas continuing current life-sustaining treatments may honor Mr. Fayed and his family's religious and spiritual values.

INTEGRATING THE RELIGIOUS AND SPIRITUAL IN ETHICS COMMITTEES—III

Another instance in which religious and spiritual values may conflict with the professional and social practices of medicine and medical care occurs when a patient and family may be "waiting for a miracle" in the face of a life-threatening, irreversible prognosis. Continuing aggressive treatments focused on prolonging life, regardless of the costs of doing so, in order to allow for Divine curative intervention is not an uncommon demand. Professional recommendations to move to comfort care as the primary goal, given the futility of curative interventions, are often met with this apparently religiously motivated response. To the patient and family, the crux of the difference is failure on the part of the medical professionals to share their deep-seated religious beliefs expressed in what they see as a test of their faith. Medical professionals, while admitting that unexpected outcomes do occur (an empirical observation, not a claim of faith), nonetheless rely on their best judgment informed by experience and knowledge. What does it require to take these religious beliefs and practices into account when caring for such a patient? Is this an irreconcilable clash of the medical and religious paradigms? What could an ethics consultation bring to this sort of case?

One possible response is to suggest that waiting for a miracle is not an expression of religious faith but a demand on the Divine to subvert the course of nature for one's personal vision of the good. Religious faith is not a project in which one is rewarded for one's persistence in pursuing one's own ends. Properly exercised, religious faith is trust that one's life project is grounded in a vision of the good that is shared and transcendent, not a cosmic projection of one's wishes or needs. To wait for a miracle may be a form of hubris, an expression of the failure to come to terms with the reality of one's contingent existence. Claims of religious faith may be psychologically and theologically defective. An ethics consultant may respectfully suggest this critical perspective because false hopes or beliefs are not adequate grounds for reliable moral judgments.

In contrast to the first response, which is to critically reflect on the religious paradigm being invoked, a further response might look to the ends or goals that inform medical practices. Medicine is a social practice grounded in a larger vision of the goods of a community. Medical treatments are most likely to be of benefit when they are evidence based. A central criterion for excellence in medical practice is reliance on empirical grounds for warranted beliefs. By definition, a miracle is that for which one has no consistent or replicable empirical evidence. Although the unexpected outcome is not uncommon in medicine, it is the basis for more rigorous research and analysis leading to more effective treatments. In response, then, medical practice is not intended to produce miracles, and demands that it not become something other than what it is intended to be. Or, as one physician put it, "We're not in the miracles business." Whereas the religious and spiritual beliefs of patients and families are to be respected by medical professionals, the structural values and practices of medicine are also to be respected by patients and their families.

A final response to the "waiting for a miracle" claim relies on the social and community nature of medical and healthcare practices. Like all social practices, medicine and healthcare are ultimately grounded in and constrained by a larger vision of the goods of the community. Respecting the religious and spiritual practices of its members is one of the goods of a progressive community, and devoting a share of the community's resources to doing so is warranted. However, the single-minded pursuit of one good at the expense of other worthy goods is unjust. It is necessary to place limitations on the resources devoted to one social practice in order to secure other goods. In this case, there are justifiable external limitations imposed on the practices of medicine and healthcare for the overall good of the community. There are reasonable limitations on aggressive life-sustaining treatments when the likelihood that they will succeed is minimal. In the face of an irreversible condition with a grim prognosis, demands that aggressive treatments be continued in order to wait for a miracle yield to the demands of justice that resources be fairly and wisely deployed. To expect medical practices to conform to one's personal religious and spiritual beliefs when doing so would sacrifice other essential communal goods is to treat oneself as an exception to the requirements of justice.

What do these ethics-based responses to the demand to wait for a miracle reveal about the larger questions concerning the relationship of medicine and healthcare to the religious and spiritual dimensions of personal and communal life?

First, whereas respect for religious and spiritual beliefs and values is one element of the basic ethical respect owed to all persons, appeal to those beliefs and values is a presumption that may be overridden in light of further critical appraisal. Conflicting or contradictory beliefs and values may be evidence of a need for honest, sustained reflection leading to a coherent resolution and greater self-insight. Beliefs and values that are in direct contradiction to current realities may reflect mechanisms of denial or delusions that would be better off recognized and replaced.

This is not to say that the invoked religious and spiritual beliefs and values are illicit, only that their meanings and implications would benefit from critical reflection. There is a philosophical dimension to biomedical ethics, and sensitive, thoughtful critique of all professed beliefs and values is part of the examined and presumably good life.

Second, the importance of recognizing value-laden social practices as ethically relevant is highlighted by noting that medical and healthcare practices constitute the social domain for personal healthcare choices. Within this domain, there are standards of excellence that provide criteria for pursuit of the goods of a practice and for the character traits to be developed by its practitioners. Religious practices constitute another such domain, replete with their own criteria for excellence and virtue. When the parameters of the former restrict what practitioners of the latter pursue, negotiation is necessary. To expect either to simply be subordinate to the standards of the other is too simplistic; both embody pathways to personal and social good. In cases of conflict, ethics mandates a process by which an integrity-preserving compromise can be pursued, although this may not always be the actual result.

Finally, because these practices are embedded in a particular community, justice-related concerns may be relevant to considerations of religion and spirituality. The extent to which religious and spiritual practices are accepted or tolerated in a community hinges in part on the contribution they make to the goods of that community or, at a minimum, the lack of harm they do to the community. Justice requires equal consideration of the rights and interests of all, but this consideration will not necessarily yield equal shares or support of the projects of all. In fact, justice may require differential treatment due to relevant ethical and nonethical factors. For example, protection of the rights of those who practice Christian Science does not entail that communal resources be devoted to Christian Science healing practices or institutions, although members of this religious community may fund such endeavors privately. Further, competent adults who opt for faith healing and not for allopathic medicine in the face of illness and disease are protected in their exercise of this basic liberty right. However, the larger community's interest in the lives and well-being of children justifies overriding parental rights when children are threatened by life-limiting or life-threatening medical conditions. Contextualizing the practice of religion and spirituality within the larger community requires that the demands of justice be fulfilled.

INTEGRATING THE RELIGIOUS AND SPIRITUAL IN ETHICS COMMITTEES WITH PSYCHIATRY

Waiting for a miracle when treatment is medically futile. Prolonging pain and suffering for religious sanctification (Mr. Fayed). Providing aggressive life-sustaining treatments when a family's religious beliefs may reflect family and personal dysfunction (Mr. Harris). Determining whether self-harming behaviors based on professed religious beliefs are to be respected (Mr. Abdullah). Each of these cases is situated within the nexus at which ethics, psychiatry, and religious and spiritual beliefs and practices connect. How do ethics committees advance a proper appreciation for this nexus within healthcare practices? How, in particular, do they integrate these religious and spiritual dimensions with the practice of psychiatry?

Recalling the first typical role of ethics committees, ethics consultation, it is important to temper the sometimes abstract, objective, and rational approach to ethics consultation with sensitivity to the existential, religious, and spiritual dimensions of the referred cases. Resolving a conflict of moral values may require consideration of these religious and spiritual dimensions. To understand the stance of a patient or family, consideration of their religious practices may be essential. The degree to which ethics recommendations can be instrumental in working toward an integrity-preserving resolution may hinge on how well those recommendations accord with the religious and spiritual practices of the patient or family. However, critical appraisal of these practices is necessary to assign them their proper weight or bearing on the issues at hand. A coordinated psychiatric consultation may be an effective way to understand this dimension of the case. A complete psychiatric consultation will not be limited to determination of individual decision-making capacity, although that is often assumed to be the only reason for such a consultation. Rather, a consulting psychiatrist may provide insight into the workings of the patient's and family's beliefs, needs, and capacities, including the role played by religious and spiritual beliefs in that specific case. Finding that proper appreciation is akin to pursuing Aristotle's Golden Mean—avoiding the extremes of both wholesale endorsement and skeptical dismissal of the religious and spiritual. Proper appreciation of the religious and spiritual dimension of an ethics consultation may require integration of psychiatric and ethical perspectives in the manner suggested by the cases considered in this chapter.

With regard to ethics education, the work of ethics committees should include cultivation of respect for a range of religious and spiritual beliefs and practices. As a focus of ethics education, these practices are as important to consider as diverse cultural and ethnic practices. They are not incidental to the practice of ethics but are essential to developing expertise in ethics. Cultural competency requires both awareness of the diversity of cultural practices and the cultural humility that is requisite to correct for possible cultural imperialism. Sensitivity to and appreciation for diverse religious and spiritual practices is an analogous prerequisite for robust ethics education efforts of ethics committees. Critical consideration of these practices as they pertain to ethics and health is an equally necessary element of ethics education. When these practices stifle, hinder, or oppress human flourishing, they should be critiqued from a balanced ethics perspective. Psychiatric perspectives on these practices are an important element of this critique, for the ways in which they are oppressive or harmful are often brought to light by an informed, experienced psychiatric analysis. Distinguishing genuine religious self-denial from self-flagellation, for example, requires an astute, nuanced psychiatric diagnosis. Knowing the proper limits of moral tolerance for diverse religious and spiritual practices requires insight into the psychiatric workings and underpinnings of these practices. Drawing that moral line must also be informed by the understanding of mental health and illness provided by psychiatry. Competent ethics education regarding the nature and extent of moral tolerance for religious diversity depends in part on the critical reflection of ethics and psychiatry.

Some of the ethics-related policies generated and reviewed by ethics committees may be informed by critical awareness of religion and spirituality enriched by psychiatric insight. One example pertains to the refusal of beneficial or life-prolonging medical treatments based on religious beliefs and practices. A refusal of beneficial treatment grounded in religious beliefs is an exercise of an individual right to bodily integrity and personal autonomy if those beliefs are authentic—that is, if they are genuine expressions of the person's central commitments and are voluntarily acquired and endorsed. Astute psychiatric insight is required as part of the evidence for the genuine nature of such beliefs, and a policy articulating the process by which treatment refusal is to be considered must incorporate ethical and psychiatric dimensions. When the individual refusing a beneficial or life-prolonging treatment clearly lacks authentic religious beliefs, because of either age (e.g., children) or deficient capacity (e.g., psychosis), this policy will sanction interventions to protect the best interests of the individual until his or her beliefs are the result of mature, sound choices.

Such a policy becomes more complex with regard to borderline cases. For example, an adolescent may articulate clear religious beliefs, but the voluntary nature of their acquisition may be in question (e.g., the individual is a member of a religious group with cultic features). Psychiatry will assist in determining the genuine nature of the adolescent's religious beliefs. Ethical deliberation regarding the balance between respecting individual autonomy and society's interest in protecting and preserving the lives of its members is also required. The considerations laid out in a policy focused on treatment refusals occur in that nexus where ethics, psychiatry, and religious and spiritual beliefs and practices converge.

CONCLUSIONS

To conclude, let's re-visit the case of Mr. Abdullah, with which this chapter opened. How does an ethics consultation incorporate the interplay between ethics, psychiatry, and religious and spiritual beliefs and practices? Mr. Abdullah invokes his religious beliefs as fundamental to his refusal to accept medical treatment and appropriate nutrition. Should his refusal be respected because it is so grounded? Or is he displaying "hyperreligious behaviors" coupled with "beliefs that are inaccurate and out of step with good evidence-based practices," in which case his refusal should not be respected?

Rather than beginning with the pressing question of treatment refusal, an ethics consultant takes a step back and attempts to see this event in the larger narrative that is Mr. Abdullah's life. His medical record notes not only a decline in his physical health but a progressive disengagement from his local Somali community. Not being able to manage all of the activities of daily living on his own because of his disability (blindness), reliance on dialysis, and need to manage his diabetes, he is increasingly reliant on others. Because of the loss of his former professional position in his own community, coupled with the subsequent failure of his alternate career plan, he has grown apart from that community and is now dependent on the larger society. When assisted living seemed his only viable option and there were none in his community to whom he could turn for such assistance, he was placed in an assisted living facility where he was isolated culturally and socially. The generic diet served in the facility was unappealing at least, and objectionable at worst, to Mr. Abdullah. His religious practices were tolerated, but not understood or appreciated by the staff. His decline from his former life was almost complete, and he was thrown back on his own diminishing personal resources and religious beliefs to sustain him. Because those beliefs are clearly central to his current decisions regarding medical treatment and care, it is tempting to reduce him to being a psychotic martyr for his Muslim faith, a religious fanatic out of touch with the realities of his life (i.e., hyperreligious).

From the standpoint of narrative ethics, the current chapter of Mr. Abdullah's life represents a dire break with the moral continuity of his existence. He has lost almost all control over his life, at least in its basic contours regarding where he lives and what he eats. His moral autonomy is greatly diminished. His refusal of dialysis, food, and other medical treatments is the only way he now has to exercise his autonomy, and resistance to that refusal only seems to intensify his resolve. Invoking his religious beliefs is a way of grounding his autonomy in the absence of personal and social supports for his choices.

Clearly, the moral, religious, and psychological dimensions of Mr. Abdullah's case are intertwined. From an ethics perspective, attempts to restore some degree of moral autonomy for Mr. Abdullah are recommended. Searching for assisted living sites at which his cultural and religious practices would be appreciated and supported may yield a choice he would find consistent with his own practices and values. Remaining in hospital and pursuing dietary options that better match his tastes and preferences may also heighten his sense that his choices are effective. Reliance on self-monitoring of his own health status with respect to his renal function and diabetes might be a step in the direction of shared decision-making for managing these medical conditions. Enlarging the scope of his moral autonomy and reconnecting his narrative path to that of his earlier life are worthy ethical goals.

From a psychological perspective, Mr. Abdullah's case is certainly complex. Some of his empirical beliefs are inaccurate. His estimation of his own capacities is inflated. His attachment to his religious beliefs may now serve to facilitate denial of his current condition. Nonetheless, these are symptoms of an underlying state in which Mr. Abdullah has not come to terms with the diminished life prospects that are now his. What is to be done?

Conferring with another clinician who is Somali and requesting his opinion on this case is enlightening. Mr. Abdullah is well-known in the local Somali community but has recently self-exiled himself from that community, in part because of his physical decline and in part because of the failure of his most recent project. Although his Muslim tradition does require devotion to Allah, his Muslim community strongly endorses reliance on medical treatments to sustain and improve life. Mr. Abdullah's refusal of medical treatment would not be seen as an expression of genuine faith but rather as evidence of his social and psychological decline. His religious and spiritual beliefs and practices, although central to his self-identity, are not synchronous with those of his larger faith community.

What emerges from ethics consultation as a comprehensive set of recommendations reflects the many dimensions of this case. Restoring Mr. Abdullah's moral autonomy, in large and small ways, requires coordination of his care across a spectrum including the medical and the social. Reconnecting Mr. Abdullah with his Somali community is essential. This would provide social support for his current needs consistent with his values and routines. It would also provide an opportunity for critical refinement of his religious beliefs so as to be more consistent with Muslim practices and traditions. If this project is feasible, and if Mr. Abdullah finds it to be amenable, then his cooperation with current medical treatment may increase because he knows it is an essential part of an effort to restore the narrative continuity of his life.

Ethics consultations and the work of ethics committees must incorporate the moral, psychological, and religious and spiritual dimensions of care for the whole patient. To neglect any of these dimensions is to fail to rightly pursue the good for caregivers, patients, and their families.

REFERENCES

Beauchamp, T., & Childress, J. (2012). *Principles of biomedical ethics* (7th ed.). New York, NY: Oxford University Press.

Brody, H. (2009). *The future of bioethics*. New York, NY: Oxford University Press.

Callahan, D. (2012). *In search of the good*. Cambridge, MA: MIT Press.

Englehardt, H. T. (1991). *Bioethics and secular humanism: The search for a common morality*. Norwich, UK: SCM Press.

Fletcher, J. (1954). *Morals and medicine*. Princeton, NJ: Princeton University Press.

Jonsen, A. (1998). *The birth of bioethics*. New York, NY: Oxford University Press.

Post, L., & Blustein, J. (2015). *Handbook for healthcare ethics committees* (2nd ed.). Baltimore, MD: Johns Hopkins Press.

Ramsey, P. (1970). *The patient as person*. New Haven, CT: Yale University Press.

NINE

Practical Implications
of Personal Spirituality

James W. Lomax, M.D., and Nathan Carlin, Ph.D.

INTRODUCTION

In this chapter, we review transference and countertransference processes with a particular focus on how the outpatient psychotherapist and the university professor should handle ultimate, deep, and core matters when they arise in clinical and educational settings. Often these matters dealing with personal values include or are related to spirituality and religiosity. The chapter examines various forms of fundamentalism because these can be the most difficult to deal with.

The chapter is divided into three parts. In part one, we begin with a discussion of the origins of fundamentalism in the 20th century, leading up to psychoanalytic commentary on fundamentalism in contemporary culture. In part two, we discuss basic issues of transference and countertransference from a psychoanalytic perspective. In part three, we offer three vignettes—two clinical and one educational—that demonstrate the adaptive value of fundamentalism from a dynamic perspective and the importance of awareness of one's own internal states in order to avoid, or at least to manage, countertransference errors.

PART ONE: ORIGINS AND EXPRESSIONS
OF FUNDAMENTALISMS

Fundamentalism: Religious Studies Perspectives

What is fundamentalism? Fundamentalism, often associated with Christianity, is also associated with terms such as "conservative," "orthodox," "evangelical," and "radical." In *Bible Believers: Fundamentalists in the Modern World*, Nancy Ammerman (1988) provides a thoughtful and concise history of the origins of fundamentalism. As a typical expression of fundamentalism, she offers this quotation from Jerry Falwell (1971–2007), an influential Southern Baptist televangelist:

The Bible is absolutely infallible, without error in all matters pertaining to faith and practice, as well as in areas such as geography, science, history, etc. The disintegration of our social order can be easily explained. Men and women are disobeying the clear instructions God gave in His Word (p. 1).

Among Christians, Ammerman observes that there are differences between fundamentalists and evangelicals, and she describes these differences both in terms of beliefs and in terms of tone. Whereas evangelicals are willing to compromise on some matters, fundamentalists refuse, quite aggressively, to yield any ground whatsoever. Evangelicals, for instance, believe that the Bible is God's Word (i.e., that the Bible is true), but they are, in contrast to fundamentalists like Falwell, less certain that the Bible is infallible in terms of what it reports about history or science. Another key difference is that fundamentalists often insist that there is only one true translation of the Bible—the King James Version—whereas evangelicals are open to a variety of translations. As a result of this difference, evangelicals are, in principle, open to matters of interpretation, whereas fundamentalists are not (Ammerman, 1988, pp. 3–6). Still, to be sure, neither category is monolithic. There are variations across lines of geographical region, age, educational level, socioeconomic class, and so on. Therefore, in terms of clinical practice, it would seem to be best to let patients articulate their religious identification and to ask them to define what these terms mean to them.

Why did fundamentalism emerge? Ammerman (1988) suggests a number of reasons. During the late 19th century, "Old assumptions (mostly Protestant) were replaced by new dogmas of industrialism, historicism, and secularism . . . . Religion gradually became compartmentalized in the private, family, and leisure spheres, leaving political, scientific, and economic affairs to the secular experts" (p. 18). Ammerman (1988) continues:

In the human sciences, psychology and sociology began to question the nature of human responsibility, destiny, and free will. In the natural sciences, Charles Darwin's ideas began to change the way scholars viewed the physical universe. In political science, Karl Marx's ideas led people to look for the hidden meanings in religion, politics, and philosophy. And in theology itself, scholars began to analyze biblical material as if it were ordinary ancient literature that reported events that might also be explained in natural, human terms. From every direction, the world was changing (pp. 18–19).

In this context, fundamentalism emerged as a way of fighting back against all of these changes, even while liberal theologians began writing metaphorically about doctrines such as the virgin birth and the resurrection. (An example of such a contemporary liberal Christian writer is Marcus Borg [1994 and other works].)

Religious studies scholars today sometimes think about fundamentalism more broadly, beyond Christianity and even beyond any particular religious tradition (Strozier, Terman, & Jones, 2010). In the introduction to *The Fundamentalist Mindset*, Charles Stozier and David Terman argue that the psychology of fundamentalism involves "a mindset that transcends its particularity in contemporary religious movements" and add that fundamentalists can be found in any religious tradition because "the mindset of fundamentalism is something more deeply ingrained in the self that finds expression in a variety of human institutions, including religion but by no means restricted to it" (Strozier & Terman, 2010, pp. 3–4). Citing Martin Marty's *The Fundamentalism Project* (Marty & Appleby, 1995), they note that fundamentalism is not orthodoxy because, while orthodoxy seeks to *preserve*, fundamentalism seeks to *change*. In recent years, the Islamic State of Iraq and the Levant (ISIL) has emerged as a fundamentalist, or radical, group that is not seeking to *preserve* Islam (which would be an expression of orthodoxy) but rather to *change* the world by means of violence, ushering in a new world order.

In "Definitions and Dualisms," also a chapter in *The Fundamentalist Mindset*, Charles Strozier and Katharine Boyd (2010) offer the following definition of the fundamentalist mindset:

> The fundamentalist mindset, wherever it occurs, is composed of distinct characteristics, including dualistic thinking; paranoia and rage in a group context; an apocalyptic orientation that incorporates distinctive perspectives on time, death, and violence; a relationship to charismatic leadership; and a totalized conversion experience (p. 11).

Again, this kind of thinking can also be found outside of religious contexts. For example, the terror inflicted during the French Revolution or the Russian Revolution (which were secular movements) was just as brutal and just as totalizing as any religious movement. So it is worth stating what should be obvious: A world without religion would not be a world without fundamentalism; the problem of terrorism cannot be solved by making the world secular.

Building on this insight—that fundamentalism can be found outside of religious contexts— our understanding of fundamentalism includes not only religious fundamentalisms, but also political fundamentalisms and personal fundamentalisms. Our understanding of fundamentalism is highly influenced by the British psychoanalyst Adam Phillips (2010 and other works), as will become clear in the next section. The vignettes offered in part three explore religious and political fundamentalisms.

Fundamentalism: A Psychoanalytic Perspective

In the chapter, "On What is Fundamental," Phillips (2010) argues that "we are all fundamentalists about something" (p. 51). This is an important point to make in psychoanalytic circles, Phillips observes, because psychoanalysts, who tend to be modern, secular, and liberal, often assume that fundamentalists suffer from some kind of regressive fixation, that in other words, fundamentalists are stuck to the past, stuck to their childhoods, and therefore unable to grow up. Fundamentalists, psychoanalysts often assume, are *someone else*, someone in need of analysis. But Phillips points out that Freud's modern individual is pitted against the superego and the id and that both agencies are "without skepticism about their own commitments" (p. 61). So a fundamentalist, for Phillips, is someone without skepticism about his or her own commitments—*and this includes all of us.* Why? Because we all are struggling to live with two fanatics who have no skepticism about their commitments: the id and the superego.

Describing the ego (in contrast to the id and the superego) as having the capacity of self-observation as well as the ability to *restrict* (but not the ability to *control*) the id or the superego, Phillips (2010) writes:

> Rather like us secular, liberal moderns observing in some trepidation the fundamentalisms of the East and the West, the ego sees itself as the one who establishes—who looks for—the most harmonious relations possible; like the ego we see ourselves as the only ones capable of observation and

reflection while they blindly go their violent, self-righteous ways. A democrat in a world of fascists, the ego wants, indeed needs, everyone to have a voice without anyone taking over; a "victory" for the ego is not the defeat of the id or the super-ego but merely their restriction (pp. 67–68).

He adds—paraphrasing Freud's phrase, "Where id was, let ego be"—that the modern liberal's hope for coexisting with fundamentalists is, "Where fundamentalism was, there rationality can be; where revelation and scripture was, there conversation can be" (p. 68).

Yet Phillips does not think that psychoanalysis can cure the problem of fundamentalism. He thinks that the answer that university professors often give to this problem—"dialogue"—seems quite disconnected from reality:

> What kind of compromise would we hope to reach with a convicted racist? How might we per-suade a Palestinian that the Israelis are well-meaning? What would we discuss with a suicide bomber? (p. 76).

He continues: "It is as though we have had the wrong picture of what people are really like . . . [and] of what people are really like about those things that they take to be fundamental" (p. 76). Although Phillips does not provide an answer to the problem of fundamentalism, he ends his essay with a warning: Simply being optimistic about the problem of fundamentalism endangers us, in that being optimistic is not enough.

In "Zombie Alleluias: Learning to Live in the Space Between Worlds," pastoral theologian Robert Dykstra (2014) draws on this essay by Phillips. Reflecting on the fact that Phillips did not offer an answer to the problem of fundamentalism, Dykstra writes: "I realized that the notion that there may be a single, dramatic, or 'fundamental' response to phenomena as widespread and complex as these is, of course, a fundamentalist assumption" (p. 612). He humorously adds, "Fundamentalists, it must say somewhere in the Bible, will always be with you" (p. 612). And he also adds that he came to the realization that not only will fundamentalism always be *with* us but also that fundamentalism will always be *in* us:

> I have come to realize that in many ways I too am a fundamentalist. At least part of how we might confront and perhaps alleviate some of the mischief that fundamentalist religious and political movements are generating all around us is by coming to recognize something of our own inner fundamentalist, coming to understand and accept the fundamentalist within, especially as a path to garnering greater *empathy* with fundamentalist individuals, communities, and movements (p. 612).

Dykstra, to be sure, does not think that empathy alone will solve the problem of fundamental-ism, but he does think that it is a promising way to begin. We will return to this insight below and also in the conclusion of this chapter.

PART TWO: TRANSFERENCE
AND COUNTERTRANSFERENCE

In *Psychoanalytic Terms and Concepts*, a dictionary edited by Burness Moore and Bernard Fine (1990), *transference* is defined as a "displacement of patterns of feelings, thoughts, and behavior, originally experienced in relation to significant figures during childhood [especially parents], onto a person involved in a current interpersonal relationship" (p. 196). It also is noted that this process is mostly unconscious and is therefore different from a therapeutic alliance, which is conscious. Additionally, transference is ubiquitous, routinely occurring in a variety of settings, including work relationships, friendships, and romantic relationships. Employees may experience, for example, a displacement of feelings from one's father onto one's boss. During analysis, transference experiences may be particularly intense, if, as so commonly happens, the patient falls in love with the analyst. Experiences such as love are described in the dictionary as positive transferences, whereas experiences such as hate are negative transferences. When the patient recognizes the transferences, a key moment has occurred in therapy, because now the patient can observe the validity of the work (Moore & Fine, 1990, pp. 196–197).

Countertransference also is defined in *Psychoanalytic Terms and Concepts*: "A situation in which an analyst's feelings and attitudes toward a patient are derived from earlier situations in the analyst's life that have been displaced onto the patient" (Moore & Fine, 1990, p. 47). This process, like transference, is mostly unconscious. This dictionary also notes that countertransference, narrowly defined, refers to the analyst's transference in reaction to the patient's transference, and adds that countertransference

> is likely to appear when the analyst identifies with the patient, reacts to material produced by the patient, or reacts to aspects of the analytic setting. In these circumstances unconscious strivings underlying character traits of the analyst are stimulated, and their derivatives appear in the analyst's thoughts, feelings, and actions (p. 47).

On the one hand, it is warned that countertransference can lead to blind spots in therapy and sometimes even to acting out. On the other hand, self-scrutiny, especially during training analysis, can facilitate even greater empathy for and understanding of patients.

In "Transference, Countertransference, and the Real Relationship," a chapter in *Textbook of Psychoanalysis*, Adrienne Harris offers a brief overview of the development of ideas about transference and countertransference, beginning with Freud and also including various schools of psychoanalysis: American ego psychology, the Kleinian tradition, the British object relations tradition, Lacanian psychoanalysis, the interpersonal tradition, the self-psychology tradition, and relational psychoanalysis (Harris, 2005, p. 213). She observes that, at its heart, psychoanalysis is fundamentally a talking cure and that both transference and countertransference are critical components of the analytic relationship; all schools of psychoanalysis agree on this, yet various schools of psychoanalysis understand transference and countertransference differently in subtle ways. Although there is not space to review these differences in this chapter (interested readers should refer to Harris's chapter), it can be noted that countertransference has received considerably more attention in recent decades and that Harris offers an insightful and helpful list of questions that summarize contemporary debates regarding transference and countertransference:

> Does analysis cure by experience or by interpretation? Are analytic cures cures by love or cures by widening the ego? Does psychic change or mutative action come as a byproduct of enhanced reflection or from the "now" moments of affective link between analyst and analysand? Can these differences become more interdependent? (p. 213).

These questions will not be resolved in the following cases, but we are now in a position to observe instances of transference and countertransference in clinical and educational settings, having reviewed common definitions of these terms.

PART THREE: ILLUSTRATIVE VIGNETTES

In what follows, three cases of fundamentalism are explored in light of transference and countertransference. In each case, the adaptive value of fundamentalism is recognized. By viewing fundamentalism in this light, we are embracing Dykstra's suggestion that empathy is a promising way to begin dealing with the problems and challenges of fundamentalism.

Disclosures of Influence

Given that this chapter focuses on transference and countertransference, especially as they relate to personal spirituality, religiosity, and values, some discussion of our own influences in this regard is in order.

Lomax Disclosure. My personal development did *not* include any consistent participation in a faith community. In fact, my mother's religiosity—which was greater at times of her Bipolar II Disorder–related mood disturbances—probably generated a tendency in me toward anxious avoidance of religious activity and participation. A second influence is that in my early 20s I became "Presbyterian by choice": I chose to get married, and my wife chose for me to become a Presbyterian. When I made a similar comment once at a grand rounds at St. Vincent's Hospital in New York, Dr. Dan Sulmasy (a distinguished internist and medical ethicist and also a Franciscan) commented from the audience: "Jim, in our tradition we call that Grace." An implicit theme in my subsequent disclosures is that Dr. Sulmasy probably made an important point.

Also "accidently," my professional participation in the interface between medicine, religion, and spirituality began when I was asked to take the place of the retiring director of medical student education at Baylor College of Medicine as a voluntary/adjunct faculty member for what is now the Institute for Spirituality and Health (ISH) in Houston, Texas. My role there includes chairing the Planning Committee of our Psychotherapy and Faith Conference. The 26th annual meeting was held in 2017. Our conferences have showcased the works particularly of Drs. Annette Mahoney and Ken Pargament as well as George Vaillant, Ethel Person, Peter Fonagy, and Phil Shaver. Mahoney's and Pargament's works have been influential in my thinking about how to conceptualize religious and spiritual coping, to anticipate positive and negative consequences of religious coping on health, and to appreciate that spiritual struggles may produce clinical psychopathology.

A third influence is that I am a graduate of the Houston-Galveston Psychoanalytic Institute (now Houston's Center for Psychoanalytic Studies) and remain a training analyst there. Psychoanalytic psychotherapy or psychoanalysis accounts for most of my 20-hour a week clinical practice. A final disclosure has to do with my political participation, which is rather far to the left by U.S. standards, in that the last candidate for President I could fully endorse was George McGovern.

Some of my religious "cognitions" resulting from these influences are that I endorse more "hopes" than "beliefs" and that I think it is important to consider truth, like hope, as a thing with feathers (Dickinson, 1960, p. 116) that should be held gently and lovingly (and also that when truth is "squeezed," a variety of problems follow). My spiritual pursuits are manifested in a spectrum of activities and relationships in which I make a fairly consistent effort to "seek the sacred" (Pargament, 2013) while being aware of (and taking a mostly accepting attitude toward) a variety of inconvenient and unwanted internal urges and dispositions. I try to renounce, sublimate, or express those urges in ways that do not excessively complicate my life or the lives of those I love and value. My religious/spiritual activities are carried out in the form of teaching and mentorship jobs as well as roles within a relatively progressive Presbyterian congregation I attend. I also communicate in presentations and in publications like this one.

Carlin Disclosure. My personal development did include consistent participation in a faith community, a small church in western, rural Pennsylvania. I have been a lifelong member of the Presbyterian Church (USA), and today I am an ordained minister in that denomination. I attended a liberal arts college affiliated with the PCUSA (Westminster College) as well as one of the vocational schools of the PCUSA (Princeton Theological Seminary).

I would describe my early years as being raised in a fundamentalist context. My church struggled with the idea that women could be leaders in the church, and my church also taught me that homosexuality is a sin. My father is considerably conservative, politically speaking. In the mornings while I was waiting for the school bus, my father would listen to Rush Limbaugh on the radio (so, by default, I would listen to the show as well). Yet, because my father worked in a steel mill, he is a registered Democrat and he strongly disliked Ronald Reagan for closing down so many of the steel mills during the 1980s. Still, he is pro-gun, pro-death penalty, anti-gay, and anti-Obamacare.

During my teenage years, because of my involvement with my church (specifically, several mission trips), I believed God was calling me to become a minister. So my goal in going to college was to prepare for seminary so that I could follow God's call. I decided to major in history so that I could discover, by means of my studies, which Christian denomination represented the true church; my plan was to convert to that denomination and become a minister in that tradition.

College changed me. Learning about the historical critical method of reading the Bible was very challenging. Specifically, the fact that Moses did not write the first five books of the Bible and the fact that there are two creation stories in Genesis greatly disturbed me. The more I learned, the more complicated everything seemed to be, and it became apparent to me that my plan to discover the true church was quaint. So my faith took on a new shape, and my politics departed from my father's politics: I became pro-gay and liberal on almost all issues. Now I am a registered Democrat, and my faith is informed by liberal theologians such as Paul Tillich. I practice my faith by participating in the life of a Presbyterian church in Houston, Texas; by writing theological essays and books; and by serving as a volunteer chaplain in an inpatient psychiatric hospital in Houston, Texas. I like to joke now that Tillich, not Jesus, saved me, but no one ever laughs at the joke.

Case 1: Arnold

Arnold was a 64-year-old male laborer whose wife developed rapidly progressive Alzheimer's disease a year before their long anticipated retirement. He consulted the psychiatrist member of an Alzheimer's caregivers team when the team chaplain became concerned about comments

Arnold had made about the better times he would have together with his wife in the near future. The chaplain worried these were indirect references to suicidal plans. As his wife's memory and orientation difficulties escalated, Arnold said that he could feel the future his wife and he had planned slipping away. He was furious and depressed about the "unfairness" of these events. In an effort to find solace, he had switched from a conservative, nondenominational church to worship as part of a Jehovah's Witness community. In this new religious participation, he "knew God's name as Jehovah for the first time." He found his solace in the "promised new order to come" in which good and decent people like himself and his wife would be restored and rewarded, while the wicked would be punished. He was also welcomed by a community that provided both a caring interest in his personal distress and practical support for his family.

The specifics of Arnold's faith community were not well known to me when I was asked to do a consultation/suicide assessment. My role consisted mostly of active listening and supportive interventions for Arnold's ideas that involved positive religious coping (God loved him and wanted good things for him and his wife) and healthy religious activity (Arnold's role as a teacher in his faith community as a generative activity). Interventions were largely clarifications without significant interpretation of either defensive ideas or the sublimated aggression involved in his view of "the new order." Arnold seemed convinced that the new order would be a time for him and his wife to enjoy the good experiences they had earned. Furthermore, in the new order, evil people who seemed to be "getting away with" their bad behavior would have a much more enduring period of suffering than they had experienced in human or earthly time. In this new order, he and his wife would be valued, enduring, and appreciated partners of God. Although Arnold's coping seemed fragile and rigid, he expressed his hope as having "everything to live for and nothing to die for" after coming to know Jehovah.

INTERPRETATION

Arnold experienced life challenges that threw him into spiritual struggle. His wife's progressive loss of memory and cognitive function represented a profound threat to his most fundamental beliefs in the ultimate justice of this world. These struggles were accompanied by depression and rage. Arnold sought a new religious direction to cope with his struggles, and a religious conversion did just that. His change in religious identification and participation was highly dependent on specific religious cognitions that allowed him to hold onto his beliefs in ultimate justice, an ultimate reunion with his wife, and a loving God.

There was a health-promoting synergy between Arnold's beliefs and his faith community. He was chosen quickly to be an elder in the faith community. This allowed him to serve as a teacher and leader, which provided significance to his remaining life. This was especially important because he had lost the long-treasured retirement years of travel and co-grandparenting he had planned with his wife.

Arnold's spiritual struggle was resolved in a way that was quite complex. His openness to an exploratory form of psychotherapy in which he might have addressed his underlying spiritual struggles seemed minimal. Exploring the defensive aspects of his religious beliefs and conversion in becoming a Jehovah's Witness seemed ill-advised because his beliefs were not only egosyntonic, but also affirmed by a community in which he was valued. The group members shared a vision of God in which he and the group not only "knew God's name" but also felt known and to-be-rewarded by God in God's time. For similar reasons, a cognitive-behavioral therapy (CBT) approach was not appropriate. Moreover, his religious cognitions did not produce distress, and therefore a therapeutic alliance to address them was not feasible. Instead, a supportive psychotherapy approach helped Arnold to use his beliefs to suppress certain emotions (such as anger at earthly injustices) that might have been mobilized with insight in ways that were unlikely to be beneficial in an available time frame. His desire to be a model of resilience and to use his God-given strength (through his religious beliefs) seemed to be a significant protective factor against suicide.

For me, an ongoing treatment relationship would have been quite challenging. Some of Arnold's vision for the new world order was at great variance with my own values. It was fairly easy to be curious about his faith community and his role in it in a brief evaluation. However, Arnold's religious beliefs would predictably create longer-term countertransference challenges. His religious world and the new order of his anticipated afterlife included intensely dichotomous outcomes for people based on their adherence to narrowly defined, religiously based commitments and behaviors. His religious beliefs about evil were also expressed as racial prejudices and highly discriminatory beliefs about differences in sexual orientation which would create significant countertransference distancing, dismissiveness, and overt or implicit expressions of disapproval that would challenge the therapeutic alliance. Although a therapist will often be able to deflect or attempt to "extinguish" hateful comments by neglecting them, Arnold's passionate disapproval of "niggers" and "queers" would no doubt generate strong negative countertransference responses in me as his therapist (JL). I was interested in Arnold and his situation but grateful that our relationship was limited to the consultation.

Case 2: Dr. A.

A rather different countertransference/personal influence became evident for me (JL) in the case of Dr. A. as I was preparing to write this chapter. Dr. A., a long-term patient of mine, is unusual in my practice because he was referred by a prominent Houston defense attorney after an Agreed Upon Order of the Texas Medical Board as part of a traumatic, career-altering series of legal and court proceedings based on what the attorney was convinced was a wrongful series of actions by a criminal court and unfair (if more understandable) actions by the Texas Medical Board.

On the professional side, Dr. A. grew up in a rural Texas town and was somewhat of an underachiever during high school and his first years of college. But he eventually achieved both an M.D. and a Ph.D. and matched into a respectable neurosurgery program. He was in his early mid-career and doing spectacularly well professionally when a series of painfully traumatic events occurred.

On the personal level, Dr. A. had grown up in a fairly conventional Roman Catholic family and was selected to be an altar boy, but he never found the religious services to be very engaging. During undergraduate school, he met and married a woman who was the daughter of a prominent Pentecostal minister. An unfortunate intersection of his public and private lives occurred when his wife's brother successfully pursued a rather complicated series of legal actions against both his father-in-law and Dr. A. himself, resulting in significant financial and professional losses for both of them, including the wrongful judicial outcomes that led Dr. A. to consult with me.

We had been meeting for several years at the time I was writing this chapter. I had always been greatly impressed by his resilience in the face of enormous adversity and what seemed like betrayals within relationships that were very important to him—which, from the perspectives of the work of Mahoney and Pargament, Dr. A. had "sanctified" (Pargament & Mahoney, 2005).

In his relationships with his brother-in-law and niece, Dr. A. had certainly invested more time, energy, and resources than what was required of him "because that is what Christians are required to do." An important part of his identity (and a shared identity with his wife) was to help others do things. From his perspective (and from the perspective I gained from interviews with his wife, father-in-law, and mother-in-law), the response from an emotionally important relative he was trying to help was not gratitude but exploitation. Yet Dr. A. had somehow maintained a powerful and meaningful affiliation with his new faith community. His father-in-law also found acceptance and tremendous affirmation from national and international activities within that same faith community.

Dr. A.'s version of his religious life was motivated by a strong belief that life events are God-given, either as rewards or as tests. I was also aware that this seemed to work satisfactorily for Dr. A., even though similar types of beliefs have led to spiritual struggles when other persons felt that "no loving God" could let horrific things happen to innocent people—whether painful and disfiguring lethal illnesses in children, hatred-based prejudices toward a variety of minority groups, or betrayals within their sacred relationships and community.

INTERPRETATION

The downside of Dr. A.'s religious participation from my perspective (informed by my own values) is that he is extremely uncharitable with people who ask for special help because of adversity. This dismissiveness results in his making pronouncements that are difficult for me to accept in both his religious worldview and his political worldview. His pronouncements are passionately endorsed by far-to-the-right politicians, so I try to avoid any entry by Dr. A. into political speculations.

What I became more aware of in writing this chapter is that I have not been as curious as I might have been about how Dr. A. receives strength from his religious views and that I might have asked about them in order to be supportive in the type of therapeutic relationship that we have. I have not, for example, asked him about his conversations with God or whether he has found in the Biblical text, which he so treasures, any elements that seem to be in conflict with some of the positions he takes on both the individual and the social level (although I realize this line of questioning could threaten our therapeutic alliance). However, my recent awareness of this countertransference struggle has allowed me to have a new set of conversations about Dr. A.'s identity as a sort of contemporary Job and a clearer understanding of the importance of his belief in an afterlife where a new spiritual justice will be served. Although I cannot personally imagine myself "getting to peace" with Dr. A.'s beliefs, my admiration for his persistence, sublimatory abilities, and resilience has allowed me to be a more helpful therapist by accepting and compensating for these countertransference interferences with our therapeutic alliance.

Case 3: Ms. B.

Our third case is educational. One of us (NC) serves as the Director of a medical humanities program at McGovern Medical School, formerly The University of Texas Medical School, one of the health professional schools of The University of Texas Health Science Center at Houston

(UTHealth). As a part of regular program activities, national experts are invited to campus to give talks. One year, Dr. Steven Miles, a respected bioethicist who has served as the President of the American Society for Bioethics and Humanities, was invited to campus to give several talks. One of these talks was at the UTHealth School of Public Health, and the topic was gun violence—specifically, understanding gun violence from an epidemiological point of view.

I walked to the lecture with a group of students. On the way, we were making small talk, mostly about the upcoming lecture. Ms. B., a 25-year-old student from Texas, mentioned that everyone in her family has a gun and that she has a National Rifle Association (NRA) sticker on her car, so she was very interested in what the speaker had to say. This made me uncomfortable because I knew quite a bit about the speaker and suspected that the talk would be pro–gun control.

I sat next to Ms. B. during the lecture, anxious to see how she was going to respond to the presentation. As I suspected, the speaker engaged the best data that we have on the epidemiology of gun violence. Indeed, he did virtually nothing but discuss data for a whole hour—it was a truly remarkable presentation. He treated guns just like any other risk factor for disease (e.g., smoking tobacco), and the conclusion was clear: It is best, from a public health perspective, to keep guns out of households. Some of the most poignant statistics that he cited involved the death rate of children in the United States due to accidental shootings as well as so-called "successful suicides." As remarkable as the presentation was, the student's response was even more so. The first words out of her mouth were: "I need to take the NRA sticker off of my car. Every medical student should be required to listen to this lecture."

INTERPRETATION

I had never before witnessed anyone changing their mind on any issue, let alone one as emotional as gun control, so quickly. Indeed, my own change of thinking with regard to my religious fundamentalism took years, and it occurred with much struggle, both internal and external. Yet this student, who was raised to *love* guns, who indeed *did* love guns, changed her mind in just under an hour. How?

When I asked the student how and why she had changed her mind, her response was simple: "This is what the data show." To the mind of a medical student, formed to be evidence based and empirically driven, numbers answer questions. When presented with such impressive data, this medical student was convinced immediately, and she was convinced that these numbers would convince others. For her, the issue of gun control, at least for health professionals, was simply a matter of getting the information out.

What shocked me as a humanities-trained person was that I knew a humanities scholar would never be convinced by numbers alone. I knew that if a humanities scholar were presented with a mound of empirical data that flew in the face of his or her deeply held political views, the humanities scholar would mutter something about the fallibility of statistics (e.g., "There are lies, damn lies, and statistics")—or, if they were trendy and postmodern, something about Michel Foucault and the relationship of knowledge to power. But, to the medical student mind, numbers are truth.

As I reflected on this experience, I was reminded of an insight by William James, America's first psychologist, who argued that change, which to an outside observer often seems radical, is more often than not quite conservative (James, 2003, pp. 26–29). Change takes place slowly, and conversions usually are not radical departures but rather ways of shoring up what is already there or what has already happened. In Ms. B.'s case, she was a senior in medical school and her identity at this point in her life was centered to a very great extent on her professional self. Because she had been educated for more than three years in empirical ways of thinking, it would have been *more* remarkable if she had held onto her pro-gun beliefs, because this would have meant a suspension of her now more deeply held beliefs in science. Her identity was as a physician-scientist. To reject science now would be to reject the identity she had been building for her entire young adult life, an identity that had cost her much—quite literally in terms of educational loans and also in the emotional tolls of medical school. What was fundamental to her now was science. So this change of mind for her was quite adaptive. With regard to my own countertransference, I identified with her, and admired her, for her journey was not unlike my own.

CONCLUSION

In conclusion, we would like to offer several insights based on these vignettes for clinicians and educators, in the form of a list:

1. It is helpful to begin with the assumption that, as Phillips argues, we are all fundamentalists about something, whether we are religious or not; there is no us/them dichotomy.
2. It is an important developmental achievement to discover the things in life that are fundamental to us.
3. It is an important interpersonal achievement, as Dykstra intimated in his comments about empathy, to recognize the value of someone else's fundamentals.
4. In both clinical and educational settings, it is not appropriate to evangelize in any form, religiously or politically.
5. Sometimes, as in the case of Arnold, it is wise for therapists to know their limits and to keep interventions focused on the short term (e.g., prevention of suicide) rather than the long term, because countertransference issues are too great to navigate.
6. Other times, as in the case of Dr. A., therapists are able to overcome significant countertransference issues if they are able to admire something about the client (e.g., remarkable resiliency).
7. What is fundamental—what is thought to be universal—can change, and the role of both clinicians and educators is to open up the possibility of change for individuals by providing a safe place for growth without setting the agenda for or the direction of growth.

REFERENCES

Ammerman, N. T. (1988). *Bible believers: Fundamentalists in the modern world*. New Brunswick, NJ: Rutgers University Press.

Borg, M. J. (1994). *Meeting Jesus again for the first time: The historical Jesus and the heart of contemporary faith*. San Francisco, CA: Harper San Francisco.

Dickinson, E. (1960). *The complete poems of Emily Dickinson* (T. H. Johnson, Ed.). Boston, MA: Little, Brown.

Dykstra, R. C. (2014). Zombie alleluias: Learning to live in the space between worlds. *Pastoral Psychology, 63,* 611–624.

Harris, A. (2005). Transference, countertransference, and the real relationship. In E. S. Person, A. M. Cooper, & G. O. Gabbard (Eds.). *Textbook of psychoanalysis.* Washington, DC: American Psychiatric Publishing, Inc.

James, W. (2003). *Pragmatism: A new name for some old ways of thinking.* New York, NY: Barnes and Noble Press.

Marty, M. E., & Appleby, R. S. (Eds.). (1995). *Fundamentalism comprehended* (vol. 5). Chicago, IL: University of Chicago Press.

Moore, B. E., & Fine, B. D. (Eds.). (1990). *Psychoanalytic terms and concepts.* New Haven, CT: The American Psychoanalytic Association and Yale University Press.

Pargament, K. I. (2013). Searching for the sacred: Toward a nonreductionistic theory of spirituality. In K. I. Pargament (Ed.), *APA handbook of psychology, religion, and spirituality* (vol. 1, pp. 257–274). Washington, DC: American Psychological Association.

Pargament, K. I., & Mahoney, A. (2005). Sacred matters: Sanctification as a vital topic for the psychology of religion. *The International Journal for the Psychology of Religion, 15,* 179–198.

Phillips, A. (2010). *On balance.* New York, NY: Farrar, Straus and Giroux.

Strozier, C. B., & Boyd, K. A. (2010). Definitions and dualisms. In C. B. Strozier, D. M. Terman, & J. W. Jones (Eds.). *The fundamentalist mindset: Psychological perspectives on religion, violence, and history* (p. 11). New York, NY: Oxford University Press.

Strozier, C. B., & Terman, D. M. (2010). Introduction. In C. B. Strozier, D. M. Terman, & J. W. Jones (Eds.). *The fundamentalist mindset: Psychological perspectives on religion, violence, and history* (pp. 3–4). New York, NY: Oxford University Press.

Strozier, C. B., Terman, D. M., & Jones, J. W. (Eds.). (2010). *The fundamentalist mindset: Psychological perspectives on religion, violence, and history.* New York, NY: Oxford University Press.

PART TWO

SPECIFIC CLINICAL CONTEXTS

TEN

Outpatient Psychiatry

Morgan M. Medlock, M.D., M.Div., and David H. Rosmarin, Ph.D., ABPP

INTRODUCTION

The prevalence of spirituality and religion among psychiatric outpatients approaches that of the general population, where roughly 60% of individuals report that spirituality/religion is very important in their lives and regularly engage in spiritual practice (Pew Research Center, 2014). In a survey of more than 250 patients at McLean Hospital, Harvard Medical School, 60.5% reported affiliation with a religious group, 70.8% reported "fairly" or greater belief in God, and 58.6% reported "fairly" or greater interest in integrating spirituality into their treatment (Rosmarin, Forester, Shassian, Webb, & Björgvinsson, 2015). These data suggest that clinicians must develop approaches to spiritual assessment and intervention, especially because these issues may have a significant impact on clinical outcomes.

In this chapter, we present a case vignette from our practice to discuss the clinical, cultural, and ethical issues that impact spiritually integrated treatment in outpatient settings. Common dilemmas, such as the role of providers in addressing spiritual issues, determining what aspects of patients' spirituality are relevant to treatment, and when and how to involve faith leaders in resolving patients' spiritual struggles, are addressed. We hope that our discussion will provide a framework for systematically addressing patient spirituality in treatment and will dispel the myth that spiritually integrated treatments are less impactful than secular approaches. As will be shown, addressing patient spirituality is not only worthwhile but can be life-saving in some cases.

CLINICAL VIGNETTE

A 38-year-old woman with a history of bipolar disorder presented to our clinic in the throes of a major depressive episode. Since her twenties, she had struggled with recurrent mood swings, but she was averse to taking medications. Counseling alone was her treatment of choice for many years, but her circumstances had changed. Managing life as a single mother with serious mental illness had proved exhausting. On intake, she reported a plan to commit suicide once her teenage son graduated from high school.

Our work together involved initiating the patient's first trial of lithium while addressing her existential despair in weekly psychotherapy sessions. Early in her treatment, she revealed that her religious beliefs made her feel ambivalent about committing suicide. On one hand, she felt that suicide was a reasonable way to emancipate herself from a lifetime of pain and struggle. On the other hand, she wrestled to reconcile her death wish with her Christian upbringing, which instilled in her the belief that individuals who commit suicide are condemned to eternal suffering.

Her religiosity was supported in treatment because it provided strong leverage against her suicidal plan. She shared that at one time, being involved in a local congregation had helped her cope with her symptoms. She had since withdrawn from her religious community, and we wondered whether this action was correlated with (i.e., was caused by or contributed to) her worsening depression. With her permission, we engaged the patient in a plan to resume the spiritual activities (e.g., prayer, Scripture reading, church attendance) that had supported her in the past. As she became more active in religious and spiritual practices, her suicidal thoughts weakened. Gradually, her hope was restored.

QUESTIONS AND DECISION POINTS

The first decision point we faced with this case was whether to broach the topic of spirituality/religion with the patient and, if so, to what degree. Recognizing that most outpatients today have an interest in addressing spiritual issues in treatment, including a significant minority of religiously unaffiliated psychiatric patients (Rose, Westefeld, & Ansely, 2001; Rosmarin et al., 2015), our practice is to initiate discussions with *all* patients about spiritual/religious matters. However, the extent to which spiritual matters should be focused on in treatment is a function of two primary factors: patient interest (including informed consent), and whether it is clinically indicated to do so. To these ends, we employed the following approach in this case.

At the patient's intake assessment, the topic of spirituality/religion was raised as subject matter through a series of simple questions, such as: "Is spirituality/religion important in your life?" "How so?" "What are some of your religious beliefs and practices?" These questions were not posed simply to gather information about the patient's spiritual life. Their purpose was two-fold. The first purpose is to open the topic for discussion. Many patients today are aware that the history of psychiatry is replete with anti-religious sentiment, and some are reluctant to approach this subject in the context of treatment for fear of being judged or criticized for their beliefs. It is therefore important for practitioners to convey, in both word and deed, that this domain can be discussed in treatment just like any other sensitive topic (e.g., sexuality, finances, politics) inasmuch as it is relevant to patient care. The second purpose of asking these questions is to observe the patient's engagement with the material. By asking questions about spirituality/religion, practitioners can determine through nonverbal cues whether a patient has an affinity with or interest in this subject matter. In this particular case, the patient was immediately forthcoming with information about her spiritual and religious life. In fact, given her depressed state, her engagement with the material produced a palpable shift in the session; she seemed genuinely excited to discuss her faith.

We thus arrived at our next decision point: Now that the patient was clearly interested in discussing her spirituality/religion in treatment, how would we respond? Would we simply validate the personal relevance of this domain? Would we file away the information obtained and change

TABLE 10.1 The FICA Tool for Spiritual Assessment	
Faith and belief	Do you have spiritual beliefs that help you cope with stress?
Importance	What role do your beliefs have in regaining health?
Community	Are you part of a religious or spiritual community? If so, is this of support to you and how?
Address in care	How would you like me as a healthcare professional to address these issues in your care?

From Puchalski, C., & Romer, A. (2000). Taking a spiritual history allows clinicians to understand patients more fully. *Journal of Palliative Medicine, 3*, 129–137.

the subject? Or would we seek to gather more information, and if so, what would our focus be? Puchalski has developed a simple tool, the FICA (Table 10.1), which provides a template for integrating spiritual assessment into mental health treatment (Puchalski & Romer, 2000). Our general approach to spiritual assessment in outpatient practice differs from Puchalski's in that we tend to focus on the *functions* of spiritual and religious life in the context of patients' presenting symptoms. That is to say, the primary goal of spiritual assessment is not to yield a comprehensive account of spirituality and religion across the lifespan, or even to take a spiritual history per se, but rather to assess the interplay between spirituality/religion and the patient's psychosocial functioning. The main thrust of this approach is to identify the clinical relevance of the patient's spirituality/religion: Is this domain a resource to the patient? If so, in what way? Does the patient draw on spiritual/religious beliefs in a psychologically functional and adaptive manner? Do his or her practices help create behavioral consistency or inspire hope? Is a religious community a source of support and social engagement? Alternatively (or in many cases, additionally), are spiritual/religious beliefs maladaptive and dysfunctional from a psychiatric perspective? Does the patient utilize his or her faith in a negative way that exacerbates feelings of guilt, shame, anxiety, or sadness? Has the patient had an interpersonal struggle occurring in a spiritual/religious context, such as a falling out with clergy or members of his or her faith community? Most of all, how are all of these potential factors clinically relevant to the patient's presenting problem? Do they functionally contribute to the patient's distress, or its alleviation, in some way?

To these ends, we continued with our assessment of the patient's spirituality along these lines. Specifically, we commenced with the following question: "How is your spirituality/religion related to the symptoms for which you are currently seeking help?" We have used this approach with more than 500 patients to date (Rosmarin, Forester, & Björgvinsson, 2016), and this particular patient's response was strikingly similar to that of many others. After a long, pensive pause, the patient remarked that the question at hand was "thought provoking" and then proceeded to articulate quite cogently how at one point in her life, religion was very important and had "kept depression at bay" through "inculcating a spirit of hope and meaning" in her life. The ensuing discussion revealed that the patient used to engage in daily prayer—primarily of a petitional nature (requesting prayer) but also prayers of gratitude and praise—as well as regular reading of the Scriptures and weekly attendance at church services. The patient reflected wistfully about this period in her life and expressed a longing to reconnect while simultaneously feeling incapable of being consistent in her practice due to her symptoms. The latter point proved important as well: The patient had experienced several acute depressive episodes during her life, and she felt intensely guilty for the suicidality she had experienced in the context of these episodes.

However, even in that context, religion served an adaptive function in that the patient stated she was terrified that she would go to hell were she to end her own life. Therefore, religion was a double-edged sword for this patient—on one hand, it appeared to be a resource she could use to regulate her emotions and create a sense of hope, meaning, and peace and fend off suicidal ideation. On the other hand, it was a source of strain, which exacerbated her tendency to wax depressive and suicidal.

The discussion brought us to yet another series of decision points: As practitioners, how should we address these spiritual issues in treatment? Should we actively encourage the patient to engage in religious practice to help bolster her remedial resources? Should we discuss her religious beliefs in treatment and/or try to cultivate a religious perspective that would be benefi-cial? Should we use her fear of hell as a contingency to help keep her safe? To what extent should we delve into this domain ourselves, rather than referring the patient to clergy to address these issues, however pertinent they may be to the clinical picture? At each step of the way, our over-arching guiding principle when faced with these decision points was simply to do what was in the patient's best *clinical* interest. As such, our primary duty is to help reduce symptomatology and restore functionality to our patients' lives, irrespective of our personal comfort with the sub-ject matter of spirituality/religion. In this case, it appeared that the spiritual domain could be a catalyst to achieve our aims. Therefore, we decided to approach—and not avoid—the subject of religion in this case, ultimately to the patient's benefit.

POSSIBLE OUTCOMES

As with any assessment or intervention, there are potential benefits and drawbacks of approach-ing the subject of spirituality/religion in the context of treatment. Typically, practitioners fail to fully assess for the clinical relevance of this domain due to a lack of training (Rosmarin, Green, Pirutinsky, & McKay, 2013). Overall, this is disadvantageous to clinicians and patients alike because it relegates the domain of spirituality/religion to the outskirts of treatment and sometimes precludes any inclusion of this subject in the provision of psychiatric care. On the surface, it may seem reasonable, even prudent, for practitioners who feel ill equipped to assess for this domain to refrain from doing so and simply refer patients to clergy. However, given the sheer prevalence of spiritual/religious beliefs in the general population and the extent to which patients profess a desire to discuss spiritual matters in treatment, it seems much more reasonable and prudent for practitioners to prepare themselves for the likely scenario of having to address this domain.

It was admittedly fortunate in this case that we were familiar with the extant literature on the clinical relevance of spirituality/religion to mental health and had spent hundreds of hours assessing for spiritual/religious matters with patients. This prior training and experience was invaluable in providing spiritually sensitive care for this patient in particular. One concern that some practitioners raise about addressing spirituality/religion with patients is that it can seem disingenuous when practitioners themselves do not have a religious affiliation or hold religious practice in high esteem. Although this issue can serve as a countertransference factor that requires management, current research suggests that the implications for patient care do not seem to be significant. In the most cited randomized, controlled trial of religiously informed psychotherapy (for depression among religious patients), religious cognitive-behavioral ther-apy was found to outperform nonreligious cognitive-behavioral therapy. However, the differ-ence was due largely to the superior performance of nonreligious therapists, who held values

---

Box 10.1. Key Readings for Clinicians

- Weber, S. R., & Pargament, K. I. (2014). The role of religion and spirituality in mental health. *Current Opinion in Psychiatry, 27,* 358–363.
- Pargament, K. I. (Ed.). (2013). *APA handbook of psychology, religion & spirituality.* Washington, DC: American Psychological Association.
- Pargament, K. I. (1997). *The psychology of religion and coping: Theory, research practice.* New York, NY: Guilford.
- Pargament, K. I. (2007). *Spiritually integrated psychotherapy: Understanding and addressing the sacred.* New York, NY: Guilford.

---

dissimilar to those of their patients (Propst, Ostrom, Watkins, Dean, & Mashburn, 1992). This suggests that nonreligious practitioners can be trained to provide spiritually sensitive treatment and that they may be more effective in doing so than religious practitioners. It therefore behooves practitioners to become familiar with the literature on the clinical relevance of spiritual/religious life, which will help them conceptualize ways of approaching this domain with patients. See Box 10.1 for a list of key readings on this subject.

MULTIDISCIPLINARY DISCUSSION

The biopsychosocial approach to formulating psychiatric problems, now the standard in our field, importantly highlights the roles of genetics, medical and psychiatric illness, character structure and personality vulnerabilities, and the patient's social and cultural milieus as being potential areas of intervention in clinical practice. It must be recognized that spirituality/religion is overwhelmingly similar to any other domain of life—social, occupational, and cultural factors can all benefit and/or harm psychiatric functioning. In our work with patients, we use an expanded biopsychosocial-spiritual framework of treatment in which spiritual and religious issues are given the same clinical focus as the psychological, somatic, and social domains. Furthermore, the *influence* of religion and spirituality on each of these domains is considered: How does the patient's spirituality impact their target symptoms (biological), coping style (psychological), and support system (social)?

Spiritual and religious practices have been strongly validated as having a generally positive impact on psychological well-being, which in turn contributes to improved health outcomes. From a medical perspective, engaging our suicidal patient in spiritual discussion may have saved her life. Patients suffering from bipolar disorder are at significantly higher risk of committing suicide that people in the general population; some experts have estimated a 60 times greater risk (Simpson & Redfield, 1999). Bipolar depression, in particular, often contributes to hopelessness and suicidality that can be unremitting despite aggressive medical treatment. In the context of significant medical and psychiatric risk factors, our patient's religious beliefs were a potent therapeutic tool for mitigating depression and dissuading her from self-harm. Had spirituality not been explored in treatment, the patient might have succumbed to depression and even committed suicide.

Another benefit of addressing spirituality and religion in treatment is the potential for strengthening the therapeutic alliance. Our patient expressed a strong preference for non-pharmacological interventions in her treatment. When we asked about her religious background, she was initially surprised but welcomed a treatment approach that emphasized reliance on spiritual resources rather than medications. It is often the case among individuals with strong religious backgrounds that psychotropic medications are stigmatized. Some view having a mental illness as a sin and taking medications as a lack of faith. Religious patients often feel guilty for seeing a psychiatrist, sometimes believing that seeking professional treatment represents failure to trust God for healing. When these concerns arise, it is often helpful to explain that medications assist in healing and do not negate religious experience. Furthermore, for patients who prefer psychotherapy but for whom medications are also recommended, it can be explained that medications are a great adjunct to counseling because they combat neurobiological imbalances that can interfere with effective psychotherapy.

Despite the inherent challenges involved in discussing patient spirituality/religion in treatment, we believe that in the final analysis approaching—and not avoiding—this subject matter in outpatient practice is well worthwhile. Some practitioners may feel differently. They may believe that discussing spiritual life with patients is not worth their time or not part of their job. We urge such practitioners to consider that inasmuch as we are committed to helping patients heal, we also ought to be concerned with helping patients live the most fulfilling lives possible. If spirituality/religion is a part of a patient's life and is perceived to help her achieve a desired quality of life, how can it not be part of our job to assist her in exploring the therapeutic value of these resources? With our patient in particular, it meant the world that her treatment team supported and encouraged the practice of private prayer for symptom relief. This not only provided a greater sense of mood stability but strengthened the therapeutic alliance, helped facilitate compliance with medications, and also had auxiliary benefits of improving the patient's ability to cope with parenting and financial stressors. Furthermore, reconnecting with a local church added a sense of community and social support, ultimately lightening the patient's burdens, which had previously felt unbearable. In a similar vein, Koenig (2008) suggested five activities that may help religiously inclined patients and may be appropriate for outpatient treatment settings (Box 10.2). Activities such as praying with patients or challenging beliefs should obviously be done only within the realm of a strong therapeutic alliance but may have a place in outpatient psychiatric care when clinically indicated. Allowing the needs and preferences of the patient—as opposed to our own perspectives and biases—to guide the inclusion of spirituality/religion in our interventions is the best general rule of thumb in protecting against unwanted or negative outcomes.

CULTURAL ELEMENTS

When our patient disclosed her belief in hell as a place of punishment for those who take their own lives, a door was opened to explore how her religion might function as a protective factor against suicide. Similar to many other religious patients we have treated, she believed that the act of destroying life (whether committed against self or others) was offensive to God.

Although it was not the case here, patients may at times disclose beliefs that are at variance with the orthodox teachings of their religion. For providers, staying abreast of the myriad

---

Box 10.2. Proposed Activities for Mental Health Providers in a Religiously Competent Clinical Consultation

1. Taking a spiritual history
2. Respecting and supporting spiritual beliefs
3. Challenging beliefs (when appropriate)
4. Praying with patients (when appropriate)
5. Consultation with clergy (when appropriate)

Note: Activities 3 through 5 should generally be conducted at the initiation of the patient and definitely with patient permission.

From Koenig, H. G. (2008). Religion and mental health: What should psychiatrists do? *Psychiatric Bulletin, 32*, 201–203.

---

cultural nuances of religious practice can prove challenging. Especially when treating psychotic disorders, questions may arise about whether a patient's spirituality is a symptom or a solution. In these situations, providers should be diligent in the involvement of faith leaders and/or family members in discussion of whether patients' beliefs are normative for their religion and culture. Failure to obtain collateral information may lead to misattribution of less well-known beliefs and practices to mental pathology. Engaging patients in spiritual discussion and seeking to clarify the context of their religious beliefs is a form of cultural competency that will ultimately assist in accurate diagnosis and treatment.

DISCUSSION OF RELIGIOUS/ SPIRITUAL ELEMENTS

When patients utilize their spirituality to cope with psychological distress, there is often a strongly positive impact on mental wellness (Pargament, Koenig, & Perez, 2000). With our patient, the investigation of the role of spirituality in mitigating her depressive symptoms, followed by the integration of spirituality into her treatment, proved to be life-saving. But what path should be taken when patients' religious beliefs seem to have a deleterious effect on their well-being? Certainly, religious patients may experience spiritual elation as well as spiritual distress. It is important to explore both positive and negative religious experiences in treatment (Ano & Vasconcelles, 2005). Patients who are positively attuned with their religious faith can be led to utilize spiritual resources in treatment. Similarly, patients in distress can be led to explore the source of spiritual conflict and whether it is related to their symptoms. In either case, patients will likely benefit from discussion that is aimed at uncovering how their spiritual experiences are relevant to treatment.

Not only did spirituality play a role in improving our patient's psychological well-being, but it also enhanced her social support. When she resumed church attendance, she was able to rebuild supportive friendships, which ultimately served to improve her mood and functioning. Most religions have a strong communal emphasis in which weekly (or more frequent) gatherings are encouraged for the purpose of worship and prayer. Being part of a religious congregation often mitigates loneliness and provides a caring community for patients suffering from mental illness. By helping patients build and sustain meaningful relationships, religious services can function as an adjunct to professional treatment, especially by reducing patient isolation and providing spiritual encouragement and coping strategies for dealing with difficult circumstances.

Although our patient did not desire this, it would have been appropriate, with her consent, to engage her pastor in a discussion regarding church-based ministries that could be utilized for additional support. Rather than delegating all spiritual discussion to the pastor or faith leader, it is recommended that providers seek to collaborate with faith leaders in order to brainstorm about adjunctive, faith-based therapies. Here are a few practical suggestions for how to engage faith leaders in the care of religious patients: (1) contact faith leaders to learn more about normative beliefs within patients' identified religion; (2) invite faith leaders to visit with you and your patients as you form a comprehensive treatment plan that may include spiritual interventions; and (3) arrange for faith leaders to meet individually with patients to address spiritually oriented treatment goals, as a supplement to professional treatment. For additional reading on the topic of spiritual care and mental health collaboration, visit the "Mental Health and Faith Community Partnership" Web page of the American Psychiatric Association (2015).

ETHICAL ISSUES AT THE INTERFACE OF MEDICAL AND RELIGIOUS/SPIRITUAL CARE

An important aspect of this case was deciding which components of the patient's spirituality should be supported in treatment. Her religious beliefs regarding hell were felt to be a strong deterrent to suicide, and without explicitly agreeing or disagreeing with her beliefs, we found a way to acknowledge them as important because they were relevant to her symptoms. In a similar way, the patient was encouraged to resume church attendance and spiritual practices because of their presumed positive impact on her well-being. Yet, patients may come to us with beliefs that cannot easily be supported in treatment. What if our patient's church had been teaching her to rely on prayer instead of medication? How does one decide which aspects of a patient's spirituality to encourage and which not to? The answers to these questions should be based on the *clinical relevance* of the patient's spirituality. As providers, we should support spiritual and religious practices that are likely to reduce symptoms and improve functioning. In contrast, practices that worsen symptoms or contribute to a decline in functioning should not be supported (although an effort to understand the patient's religious framework is still helpful, even if it is believed to have a negative clinical impact). In instances in which patient spirituality is felt to have a negative impact on clinical care, it may be appropriate to challenge spiritual beliefs, as discussed earlier.

What about self-disclosure? How much should providers share about their own faith in psychotherapy? This question was recently posed to us by a PGY-3 Psychiatry resident who attended a lecture we gave on how to address patient spirituality in outpatient treatment. The resident felt that a provider's religious background belonged to a "special" category of demographic information and suggested that self-disclosure would enhance the therapeutic alliance and likely settle patients in religious discussion, especially if there was a shared background. Readers may be more comfortable disclosing their religious background to patients who have similar histories. However, we suggest exercising caution with this approach. The assumption that a stronger therapeutic alliance is fostered when provider and patient share similar religious backgrounds is fallacious. In fact, even with a shared background, there is often a significant difference in the personal beliefs and practices of provider and patient. Providers of similar backgrounds may assume that they understand their patient's religious perspective when, in fact, a stark contrast may exist. Contrary to strengthening the alliance, self-disclosure may actually weaken it if patients feel ashamed to reveal their spiritual struggles to someone with a similar background. (The provider in that case may be viewed as critical or judgmental rather than empathic.) Therefore, we do not routinely disclose our religious background to our patients, and if asked to do so, we tend to remind them that we are interested in their spirituality because of its potential clinical impact, not necessarily to compare or challenge individual belief systems. We emphasize the reality of having a safe space to discuss spiritual issues and struggles, regardless of religious background.

We should also say a word about how to handle dual relationships (e.g., treating a member of your own faith community). In general, we discourage treating members of one's own faith community, especially in smaller congregations, where members are closely knit and privacy is even more tenuous. There are several reasons for this suggestion, primary among them being that mental health providers—and especially those who are likely to be deeply invested in their work with patients—can quickly experience burnout, and it can be very stressful for practitioners to have their own spirituality encroached upon by professional obligations. It is important for professionals who have spiritual/religious beliefs and practices to have a protected space, such as a religious community, where they can feel unencumbered by clinical responsibilities. Additionally, patient privacy can be harder to protect in the context of faith communities; innocent questions from fellow community members can easily lead to awkward moments and sometimes even to conflicts of interest. Similarly, patients may understandably feel monitored and critiqued when attending the same church as their provider, and it is important for them to believe that their place of worship is not being used for clinical evaluation. In situations in which providing treatment to fellow faith community members is unavoidable (e.g., in rural areas where such individuals may otherwise have no access to any treatment), it is important for the clinician and the patient to explore potential scenarios that may arise and have a clear plan of action in place.

Finally, how does spiritually integrated care affect how we view our work as clinicians? Our comments thus far may challenge readers who view their work as "public" or "secular," in that the suggestion that clinicians embark upon spiritually integrated treatment may seem to be shifting the frame into a spiritual or religious domain. Yet, we return to our often repeated maxim, that addressing spirituality in treatment is a *clinical* activity, not a religious one. We care about patient spirituality because it is often relevant to patient care. Harnessing this domain in treatment can reduce symptoms and improve functioning—and even save lives! In this case, the willingness of our patient to evaluate her spiritual practices as clinical factors ultimately changed the trajectory of her treatment in a most powerful way. This argues for the conceptualization of spiritual interventions as beneficent rather than intrusive or overreaching. In other cases, addressing and validating spiritual struggles may similarly be a catalyst for emotional and behavioral change. Rather than causing ethical dilemmas, we have consistently found that spiritual engagement strengthens the therapeutic alliance and is a powerful aid to healing. We therefore believe that there are many patients who can experience clinical improvement through spiritually integrated care, and our work in this area falls squarely within our responsibilities and duties as providers of mental health care.

REFERENCES

American Psychiatric Association. (2015). Mental health and faith community partnership. Retrieved from http://www.psychiatry.org/psychiatrists/cultural-competency/faith-community-partnership.

Ano, G. G., & Vasconcelles, E. B. (2005). Religious coping and psychological adjustment to stress: A meta analysis. *Journal of Clinical Psychology*, *61*, 461–480.

Koenig, H. G. (2008). Religion and mental health: What should psychiatrists do? *Psychiatric Bulletin*, *32*, 201–203.

Pargament, K. I., Koenig, H. G., & Perez, L. M. (2000). The many methods of religious coping: Development and initial validation of the RCOPE. *Journal of Clinical Psychology, 56*, 519–543.

Pew Research Center. (2014). Religious Landscape Study, conducted June 4–September 30 2014. Retrieved from http://www.pewforum.org/religious-landscape-study/.

Propst, L. R., Ostrom, R., Watkins, P., Dean, T., & Mashburn, D. (1992). Comparative efficacy of religious and nonreligious cognitive-behavioral therapy for the treatment of clinical depression in religious individuals. *Journal of Consulting and Clinical Psychology, 60*, 94–103.

Puchalski, C., & Romer, A. (2000). Taking a spiritual history allows clinicians to understand patients more fully. *Journal of Palliative Medicine, 3*, 129–137.

Rose, E. M., Westefeld, J. S., & Ansely, T. N. (2001). Spiritual issues in counseling: Clients' beliefs and preferences. *Journal of Counseling Psychology, 48*, 61–71.

Rosmarin, D. H., Forester, B., & Björgvinsson, T. (2016). Spirituality and religion: Initiating a discussion with patients [Letter to editor]. *Psychiatric Services, 67*, 359. doi:10.1176/appi.ps.670301

Rosmarin, D. H., Forester, B. P., Shassian, D. M., Webb, C., & Björgvinsson, T. (2015). Interest in spiritually-integrated psychotherapy among acute psychiatric patients. *Journal of Consulting and Clinical Psychology, 83*, 1149–1153.

Rosmarin, D. H., Green, D., Pirutinsky, S., & McKay, D. (2013). Attitudes toward spirituality/religion among members of the Association for Behavioral and Cognitive Therapies. *Professional Psychology, Research and Practice, 44*, 424–433.

Simpson, S., & Redfield, J. K. (1999). The risk of suicide in patients with bipolar disorders. *Journal of Clinical Psychology, 60*, 53–56.

ELEVEN

Inpatient Psychiatry

Shad S. Ali, M.D., and Abraham M. Nussbaum, M.D., M.T.S.

TO WRITE BROADLY ABOUT THE ETHICAL CONSIDERATIONS AT THE intersection of psychiatric hospitalization and religious and spiritual practices is to risk generalities, platitudes, and bromides. Everyone wants culturally competent care. Everyone desires care that is specific to his or her own faith. Everyone deserves ethical care.

For those who dare to practice at these interstices, such principles are as useful as a featureless map. It is often said that becoming ill is a journey into an uncharted territory. If so, then setting out with only vague principles is insufficient. You need a sense of the country, the details of a person equivalent to the scale, contour lines, and legends that make a map fitting for a journey.

So the journey of caring for people on an inpatient psychiatric ward begins by seeking your bearings. When you first meet a person in an inpatient psychiatric ward, it helps to understand how she came to be hospitalized. Did she enter voluntarily, or was she hospitalized against her will, either explicitly through a coercive legal mechanism or implicitly by the persuasion of other people? Then it helps to ask the patient to orient you to her situation; ask her what she likes to be called.

As we set out with a person, we find it helpful to use open-ended questions that allow a person to explain her own understanding of health and illness as they relate to her cultural background and practices. Several structured interview guides exist, but we often use the questions shown in Box 11.1, which we abstracted from Kleinman's seminal 1978 article (Kleinman, Eisenberg, & Good, 1978), or questions from the Cultural Formulation Interview (CFI) published in Section III of the *Diagnostic and Statistical Manual of Mental Disorders: DSM-5* (American Psychiatric Association, 2013). The CFI is a structured tool for assessing the role that culture plays in a person's experience of mental distress and illness. The CFI includes several domains—Cultural Definition of the Problem; Cultural Perceptions of Cause, Context, and Support; Cultural Factors Affecting Self-Coping and Past Help Seeking; and Cultural Factors Affecting Current Help Seeking—and, as a model for future iterations of our profession's diagnostic manual, it includes interview prompts to guide a practitioner (American Psychiatric Association, 2013).

Both of these tools help a practitioner to get her bearings during an interview, but each has, like all tools, limitations. Cultural-based assessments engage religion and spirituality as cultural phenomena that aid or imperil health rather than as practices and beliefs distinct from health. For example, within the CFI, religious and spiritual practices are assessed in relationship to

---

Box 11.1. Questions from Kleinman's Patient Model

1. What do you think caused your problem?
2. Why do you think it started when it did?
3. What do you think your sickness does to you?
4. How does it work?
5. How severe is your sickness?
6. Will it have a short or long course?
7. What kind of treatment do you think you should receive?
8. What are the most important results you hope to receive from this treatment?
9. What are the chief problems your sickness has caused for you?
10. What do you fear most about your sickness?

From Kleinman, A., Eisenberg, L., & Good, B. (1978). Culture, illness, and care: Clinical lessons from anthropologic and cross-cultural research. *Annals of Internal Medicine, 88*(2), 251–258.

---

a problem the person is experiencing; they are understood as being interesting to a clinical encounter only to the extent to which they aid or hinder health. For interviewers who are interested in more detail, the authors of the CFI created a 16-item supplement—Module 5: Spirituality, Religion, and Moral Traditions—which includes questions about a person's religious and spiritual traditions and identity, both in and of themselves and as they relate to the problem the person is experiencing (Lewis-Fernández et al., 2016). Although the interview prompts on these tools are helpful, they are a poor substitute for being interested in a person's religious and spiritual practices in and of themselves. After all, religious and spiritual practices are sometimes a support, sometimes a stressor, but often something quite different. So while we use validated instruments to assess religious and spiritual practices as part of a person's cultural background, we try to remember that such instruments are analogous to the map, not the territory itself.

Because medicine is a narrative practice, we offer two stories from our experiences with patients hospitalized in inpatient psychiatric facilities to illustrate our approach to religious and spiritual practices as they relate to a person's mental health and the attendant ethical implications.

Case 1: Akram

Akram was a 52-year-old, HIV-positive Arab American with a history of schizophrenia who was admitted to an inpatient psychiatric unit with recurrent psychosis. As his mental illness had progressed, Akram had become dependent on others. For the last 10 years, he had been residing in a nursing home. Three months before admission, he began gradually refusing medications, acting oddly, accusing staff of trying to kill him, and demonstrating paranoia consistent with decompensated schizophrenia. Akram stopped showering and began refusing meals. Finally, while a staff member was encouraging him to eat, Akram acted out, assaulting a staff member whom he believed was poisoning his food. Staff members called for an ambulance, which transported Akram to the Psychiatric Emergency Service at an academic medical center, where he was evaluated and admitted to an inpatient psychiatric unit.

On that unit, Akram exhibited disorganized thinking, severe delusions, and auditory hallucinations. He demonstrated hyperreligious delusions, believing that he could directly communicate to *Allah Subhanahu Wa Ta'ala*, meaning "Allah, the most glorified, the most high." He experienced paranoid and persecutory delusions, reporting that the staff, along with all nonbelievers, was conspiring to harm him. Staff members tried to reassure Akram, but his level of disorganization made it difficult to engage him in an organized conversation about either the events preceding his arrival at the hospital or the risks and benefits of treatment for schizophrenia and HIV. Akram also appeared to be responding to internal stimuli, and the staff often observed him conversing with invisible others. He admitted to hearing the words of *Allah Subhanahu Wa Ta'ala* conveyed through *Jibrail*, the angel Gabriel who delivered divine messages to Muhammad. Shortly after his first meeting with his interdisciplinary care team, Akram refused all medications, both psychotropic and antiretroviral; he remained firm in his refusal for over a month.

Akram's mental status subsequently declined. As his thinking remained disorganized, he spontaneously endorsed delusional content, and staff often observed him responding to internal stimuli. His treatment team eventually petitioned the local court for permission to administer involuntary treatment. At the court proceedings, his psychiatrist testified that Akram required involuntary treatment to achieve his previous level of health. After the court agreed, Akram began receiving involuntary medications. Akram responded within days after initiation of medications; his thinking became progressively less disorganized, his paranoia dissipated, and he gradually stopped responding to internal stimuli. A week later, he began to participate in his own care and eventually developed excellent rapport with his treatment team. To explain our process and Akram's progress, we can use Jonsen's Four Quadrant Model to analyze ethical issues according to medical indications, patient preferences, quality of life, and contextual features (Jonsen, Siegler, & Winslade, 2015).

Case 1 Analysis Using Jonsen's Four Quadrant Approach

Medical Indications: Akram experienced a recurrent episode of psychosis, with both positive and negative symptoms of his chronic schizophrenia. Given his symptoms, functional decline, and resulting assault, his presentation was an indication for hospitalization and administration of a D2 dopamine antagonist. He had no medical contraindications to this intervention. Because of his long history of noncompliance, he was an ideal candidate for a long-acting depot formulation of a D2 dopamine antagonist. He also had a 10-year history of an HIV diagnosis, which was previously well controlled on highly active antiretroviral therapy (HAART), but Akram had self-discontinued this regimen 3 months before admission. Upon and during admission, Akram refused any physical or laboratory examinations to assess the status of his HIV infection. Without a clear sense of his HIV stage, the treatment team considered HIV-associated dementia as a cause for his symptoms and functional decline, remembering that cognitive deficits and mood symptoms are common to both schizophrenia and HIV-associated dementia.

Patient's Preferences: Akram requested spiritual support but refused to meet with a hospital-employed, nondenominational chaplain. Akram desired only to speak to an *imam*, a term that in Sunni communities refers to a worship leader and, in Shiite communities, to a spiritual leader whose authority derives directly from Muhammad. Akram, a Sunni, asked specifically for Imam Ahmed, the imam at the mosque Akram had been a part of for several years. Akram asked Imam Ahmed to visit frequently.

As he improved, Akram asked his treatment team to communicate with his imam. At several inflection points during his hospitalization, Akram refused to make a treatment decision without first conferring with Imam Ahmed. As they observed this pattern, the treatment team found it useful to align themselves with Imam Ahmed, both to gain insight into Akram's spiritual beliefs and to strengthen their therapeutic alliance with Akram. Akram asked the treatment team to accommodate his spiritual practices—praying five times daily at prescribed times and cleansing himself ritually before each prayer. To accommodate Akram's practices, hospital staff provided him a quiet, clean, and relatively private space, usually his bedroom, to perform daily prayers. Daily prayer and active communication with Imam Ahmed, who represented the greater Muslim community, became central values informing Akram's treatment.

Quality of Life: Before being hospitalized, Akram had lived at the same nursing home for 10 years. He lived in the nursing home peaceably, but his quality of life fluctuated with his adherence to medications. At times, Akram took medications voluntarily, but at other times, he received court-ordered involuntary medications. When not taking medications, he became paranoid and confrontational with peers and staff at his nursing home. He isolated himself and began refusing offers to attend ṣalāt al-jum'ah (Friday prayer) with friends from the mosque. In time, the nursing home staff observed that when Akram stopped performing his daily prayers, it signaled a recurrence of his psychosis.

When Akram arrived on the inpatient psychiatric unit, he neither prayed nor engaged with his religious community, even though he spontaneously endorsed hyperreligious delusions. When Akram finally received medications, some of the first signs of his journey back toward health related to his faith. He reached out to his imam and his religious community. After eventually reconnecting with his imam, Akram began performing his daily prayers routinely and attending to his hygiene in accordance with his Sunni Muslim beliefs.

Contextual Feature #1: *How does being a Muslim in a non-Muslim society affect a person's care?* Akram was a son of Egyptian immigrants. He was born in Ohio but had spent most of his life in Colorado. He self-identified as an Arab American and both read and spoke Arabic. Akram recalled feeling different during his childhood but felt singled out after the September 11th attacks. Akram's paranoid symptoms included themes of persecution because of his religious beliefs and practices. These themes are reflected in the medical literature, where researchers such as Padela have reported that "post-9/11 discrimination and abusive behaviors toward Muslims may lead to increased psychological distress and mistrust of the healthcare system, which in turn may have negative consequences for health" (Padela, Killawi, Heisler, Demonner, & Fetters, 2011, p. 360). Such findings raise an important point regarding paranoia experienced by Muslims living in America. Medical and mental health practitioners often identify suspicion of discrimination and profiling as signs or symptoms of psychosis, but these suspicions are often reality-based for Muslims. To distinguish between warranted fears of surveillance and discrimination and paranoia, practitioners must remember the cultural context. In a culture that often characterizes Muslims as religious extremists or terrorists, many members of the Muslim community experience discrimination. Akram perseverated on the possibility that he was being persecuted by being perceived as a terrorist or extremist.

To care for Akram, the treatment team had to be aware of Akram's cultural background and empathize with his experience as a Muslim living in America. At present, very little clinical research has distinguished fears of discrimination from frank psychosis among Muslim populations residing in the United States. While we await better data, we also receive every case as an opportunity to connect isolated patients to culturally competent systems of care. Often, especially during periods when patients are refusing care, we can effectively develop a therapeutic alliance by exhibiting cultural awareness and acknowledging the patient's cultural background. For Akram, the treatment team would often greet him by saying *as-salamu alaykum*, an Arabic greeting which translates to "peace be upon you." This simple gesture showed respect for Akram's cultural background while allowing him to feel less disenfranchised. Meeting Akram where he was, without forcing him to conform to the biomedical values of contemporary mental health treatment, embodied our respect for his personhood, his practices, and his identity.

Contextual Feature #2: *How does a diagnosis of HIV affect inpatient psychiatric care?* Akram was HIV-positive. Although he identified as heterosexual, he had contracted HIV through male-to-male sexual encounters. Akram experienced a significant conflict between his HIV diagnosis and his Islamic faith. As his treatment team observed this conflict, we struggled to explore it fully. It is one thing to know how to greet a practicing Muslim; it is quite a bit more challenging to help a practicing Muslim reconcile his behavior with his faith. As practitioners, we remember the nature of our relationship: We are interested in the behaviors that affect health, and HIV clearly affects health. So, even though his feelings about HIV status were entangled with taboos about his sexual practices, we broached the subject with Akram. Unfortunately, Akram was never willing to discuss his HIV diagnosis or his sexual activities. Even after restarting medications and experiencing a reduction in his psychotic symptoms, Akram remained convinced that "Allah had cured" his HIV and declined any medical workup. The treatment team was never able to overcome Akram's delusion. We were able to engage infectious disease consultants to speak with Akram on the importance of HAART medications and provide further patient education regarding his medical disease. Although Akram resisted our attempts to treat his HIV infection, we repeatedly tried to engage him around his HIV status because of its importance to his health, and we encouraged his outpatient practitioners to continue these conversations.

Cultural Element #1: *Religious identity as a Sunni Muslim. Discussing difference between Sunni and Shiite Islam. What does is mean to be Sunni Muslim? Is this divide significant for clinicians to keep in mind?* Akram identified as a Sunni Muslim. The Sunni and Shiite communities are the largest branches within Islam, and the adherents of both are bound by the same Qur'an, the same Five Pillars of Islam (i.e., belief in one God, daily prayer, fasting, charity, and hajj or pilgrimage), and reverence for the Prophet Muhammad, who founded Islam in 620 C.E. Sunnism, the larger of the two branches, is followed by approximately 87% to 90% of all Muslims and is dominant in Saudi Arabia, Egypt, North Africa, Turkey, Pakistan, Bangladesh, and Indonesia. Shiism is smaller representing approximately 10% to 13% of all Muslims, including almost all of the populations of Iran and Bahrain as well as parts of Iraq, Yemen, Lebanon, Azerbaijan, and Afghanistan (Pew Research Center, 2009, p. 1). The chief theological difference between the two is that Sunnism holds that the Islamic prophet Muhammad's first caliph was his father-in-law Abu Bakr, whereas Shiism holds that Muhammad's son-in-law and cousin Ali ibn Abi Talib, not Abu Bakr, was his first caliph (Rogerson, 2006). Many commentators make a rough, and admittedly imperfect, analogy between these two Islamic branches and the divisions between

Protestant, Catholic, and Orthodox Christians. Adherents of each group are Christian, but they have diverging views on theology, leadership, leadership, and worship (Esposito, 2002). In the medical literature, the question of if or how the different denominations of Islam influence health care and health outcomes remain unanswered. Most current studies examine Muslims as a single group rather than a collection of heterogeneous but related groups of believers. Still, it can be helpful to clarify a patient's denomination when he or she identifies as Muslim, because this identification will likely impact the spiritual care they prefer to receive and may also influence their health outcomes.

Cultural Element #2: *What is an imam? What is an imam's function and role? What influence does an imam have on individual Muslims? How can an imam be best engaged on an inpatient psychiatric unit?* In contemporary hospitals, it is common to defer spiritual care to nondenominational chaplains employed by the institution. Akram refused to meet with our hospital's chaplain because he believed his spiritual needs could be met only by a leader of his own faith. Instead of immediately equating Akram's request for spiritual care with a referral to our hospital's nondenominational chaplain, we could have better engaged Akram by asking him, from the beginning, more details about what kind of spiritual care he desired and from whom he desired to receive it. If we had, he would likely have asked for his imam. An imam's role within Islam is analogous to the role that a priest or rabbi plays in Catholicism or Judaism, respectively. An imam, like any religious leader identified as such by a patient, can be an effective patient advocate and a critical ally of a treatment team. Patients typically already have a therapeutic alliance with a religious leader, one that extends beyond their immediate health. Consequently, working alongside religious leaders identified by a patient can enable treatment teams to make clinical gains with patients that they could not otherwise achieve. This can be acutely true in inpatient psychiatry, where many patients are skeptical of the treatment team or even, like Akram, receive them as persecutors. Akram did not regard his imam as a persecutor, and he often refused to make medical decisions without consulting with his imam.

Imams have many roles in a Muslim community, and we find it helpful to follow Padela and his colleagues, who defined an imam as "the individual who is a prayer leader, chief sermon giver, and spiritual advisor to the congregation of a mosque. As sources of Islamic knowledge, imams interpret for the Muslim community how Islam informs healthcare provision and behaviors. They also serve as confidants providing counseling to ill-stricken congregants and as religious adjudicators on ethical challenges" (Padela, 2011, p. 361). As such, imams can help communicate treatment goals and interpret treatment implications for patients. At Akram's suggestion, our treatment team met often with his imam, both with and without Akram present. By engaging with Akram's imam, the treatment team not only was able to better connect and provide care to Akram but also demonstrated a respect for his beliefs and decision-making process.

Cultural Element #3: *Discussing the importance of all issues surrounding prayer. What is the significance of daily prayer in Islam? What can be done to accommodate prayer requirements on an inpatient psychiatric unit?* Salah (prayer) is not simply important within Islam; it is essential, one of the Five Pillars of the faith. Like *salah*, the other four pillars are practices: *hajj* (pilgrimage); *zakah* (charity); *shahada* (testifying that there is no God except Allah and that the Prophet Muhammad is His messenger); and *soum* (fasting during the month of Ramadan) (Hamdan, 2010). In Islam, *salah* helps believers remember God and protects them, as illustrated by the following verse from the Quran (Al-Ankabut 29:45): "Recite that which has been revealed to you of the Book and keep up prayer; surely prayer keeps one away from indecency and evil, and certainly the remembrance of Allah is the greatest, and Allah knows what you do." Muslims are obliged to perform ritual prayers at five proscribed times daily: dawn, noon, afternoon, sunset, and evening (Hamdan, 2010). Adherents believe that following this schedule forms them as punctual and disciplined people who appreciate the value of time (Siddiqui, 2008). Muslims are also required to perform the act of ablution, the cleansing of the body, before praying (Hamdan, 2010). Ablution includes the washing of the head, hands, arms, face, nostrils, mouth, and feet, as well as the inside and outside of the ear (Henry, 2015).

There is literature suggesting that Islamic prayers may yield many psychological benefits, such as amelioration of stress and improvement in subjective well-being, interpersonal sensitivity, and mastery (Henry, 2015). Islam encourages *salah* to be performed in the company of other Muslims as a congregation, but this can be challenging in contemporary hospitals, especially on inpatient psychiatric units, which are often locked. Many contemporary hospitals provide interfaith chapels which accommodate Muslim patients and visitors who desire to perform daily prayers. If a patient cannot access such a space, *salah* can be performed anywhere as long as the person prays in the direction of the *Kaaba*, the building at the center of Islam's most sacred site in Mecca. For Akram, his desire to pray was a proxy for his mental health; as he became less psychotic, he rediscovered his desire to pray, so the treatment team allowed him to perform his daily prayers in his room. Allowing *salah* on a psychiatric unit requires minimal accommodation by a treatment team but can increase a patient's therapeutic alliance with the treatment team.

Ethical Issue #1: *Is Akram hyperreligious or a devout Muslim? Can we reconcile the two, or are they mutually exclusive?* It is often difficult to delineate between expressions of religious fervor and the hyperreligious delusions of psychosis. This distinction was unclear in Akram's case, so the treatment team contextualized Akram's behavior in relation to his religious background. Whether well or ill, Akram was always a faithful believer in Islam, so it was unsurprising that his beliefs became source material for his delusions. His religious practices changed during the periods where he was most psychotic: Akram did not pray, read the Qur'an or participate in the routines of his religious practices when psychotic. Distinctions between hyperreligious delusions and devotion to one's faith are often blurred, but they can be distinguished when a treatment team takes a balanced approach and retains an objective perspective about what is mental illness and what is religious conviction.

Case 1 Conclusion: Like many people we meet as patients, Akram belonged to several clinical populations (i.e., he had a chronic psychotic disorder and was HIV positive) and several cultural populations (i.e., he was a Sunni Muslim and a member of a religious minority group). Like many patients, Akram belonged to so many groups that it would be difficult to train practitioners to care for someone else precisely like him. Instead of following a strict ethical rule, we believe that Akram, like all patients, deserves culturally competent care that accounts for all aspects of his life that affect his health, including his faith. On an inpatient psychiatric ward, especially a locked ward, it can be especially challenging to provide spiritual support to patients who are often isolated from their faith community, its leaders, and constituent practices. Consequently, it is essential that the inpatient psychiatric treatment team provide a patient access to his or her faith community, albeit without compromising psychiatric treatment. With Akram, we worked alongside his imam and tried to accommodate his prayer requirements. We learned that, even on an inpatient psychiatric unit where patients have limited freedoms and are restricted for their own safety and the safety of others, we can make spiritual accommodations that advance a patient's well-being.

Case 2: Christopher

Christopher, a 24-year-old man with a history of bipolar II disorder, was admitted on an involuntary hold after he attempted to hang himself with his own belt in a hotel room. Christopher was an Italian-American who had lived his entire life in the Boston metropolitan area. While on vacation with his girlfriend Stephanie in Colorado, he discovered that she had recently been sexually active with another man. Wounded by her infidelity, Christopher stayed in their hotel room while Stephanie went out on a hike. In her absence, he ruminated over Stephanie's betrayal and decided to kill himself. However, the belt broke under his weight. While falling to the floor, Christopher hit his head on the hotel room furniture, lost consciousness briefly and woke up to find himself bleeding from a superficial scalp laceration. Dazed by the fall and the sight of his blood, he called Stephanie. Christopher told her that the attempt was premeditated, saying, "I waited for you to walk out the door so I could get my revenge." Stephanie called emergency services, and Christopher was eventually admitted to an inpatient psychiatric unit.

During admission interviews, Christopher reported that Stephanie's infidelity had sparked a long-smoldering desire to commit suicide, and he admitted several episodes of practicing hanging himself so that he could kill himself in the "same way Robin Williams, the greatest comedian ever, did." With little prompting, Christopher spoke at length about his relationship with Stephanie and his fear she would abandon him. In discussing his life, Christopher described multiple intense relationships, an enduring fear of abandonment, long-term depressed moods, poor sense of self, and chronic feelings of emptiness. Christopher was notably intelligent, articulate, and very talkative but interruptible. Strangely, Christopher's affect did not match his mood; he laughed inappropriately while deploying humor as a defense mechanism. He exhibited no signs of anxiety, mania, or psychosis. Instead, he described intermittent but intense feelings of suicidality even while seeming to do well, with a stable job and a supportive extended family. Christopher acknowledged being previously diagnosed with bipolar II disorder but could not describe any past or present manic or hypomanic episodes. However, his treatment team suspected that his hyperverbal and interruptible speech could be confused with pressured speech. Christopher had not been previously diagnosed with a personality disorder, but during serial interviews he met most of the criteria for borderline personality disorder, including a fear of abandonment, poor sense of self, history of self-mutilating behavior, intense relationships, and brief dissociation when stressed. Christopher reported multiple depressive symptoms that had been constant for several years but attributed his suicidal behavior to conflicts with Stephanie. He admitted that he would have likely died had the belt not broken.

Case Analysis Using Jonsen's Four Quadrant Approach

Medical Indications: Despite his previous diagnosis, Christopher's condition was most consistent with major depressive disorder because he endorsed or exhibited all nine of the DSM-5 criteria, accompanied by pervasive maladaptive character traits consistent with borderline personality disorder. Despite having a psychotherapist, Christopher could not recall being diagnosed with borderline personality disorder. He was otherwise in good health, and a thorough physical examination revealed no significant medical sequelae from his suicide attempt. The treatment team believed that Christopher would benefit from a combination of pharmacotherapy and psychotherapy. Christopher had previously been prescribed mood stabilizers, which caused sedation without therapeutic benefit. Given his revised diagnoses, the treatment team helped Christopher select an antidepressant to target his depressive symptoms but titrated the medication slowly to avoid inducing a manic or hypomanic episode. To treat borderline personality disorder, the team began psychoeducation and psychotherapy including dialectical behavioral therapy (DBT) among other approaches. Christopher had never participated in DBT but appeared to be an ideal candidate because of his presentation and psychological-mindedness.

Patient Preferences: Christopher had a long history of intense and dysfunctional romantic relationships with women. His self-harming and impulsive behaviors occurred in the context of failed relationships or unrequited feelings toward a woman. Interestingly, Christopher had always sought out female practitioners for healthcare, believing they would be more sympathetic to his concerns; he appreciated attention from women, even if it occurred within a therapeutic setting. What Christopher could not tolerate was any treatment modality with a spiritual component. Christopher identified as an atheist and strongly condemned people with religious values, saying that he "had nothing but disdain for organized religion." Christopher diluted his strong opinions with frequent injections of humor. Indeed, interviews with him often resembled stand-up comedy routines in which he would fall into extended jokes as a way to avoid painful subjects and defend himself from the possibility of changing his maladaptive perceptions and behaviors. Christopher preferred members of the treatment team who could engage his humor and mocked those members who addressed him in a more stereotypically therapeutic mode.

Quality of Life: Christopher had a superficially high quality of life. He lived in metropolitan Boston and was able to afford to live on his own. He claimed to have several friends and an active social life. He had ample familial support. He was an only child, and his parents had catered to him and rarely held him accountable for any disrespect or harm he caused them. A college graduate, he had a stable job as a soil tester for an engineering company with adequate compensation and full benefits. He denied a previous history of physical, sexual, or emotional abuse. His family structure was intact, and there were no discernible adverse events in childhood or otherwise. In spite of all this apparent stability, Christopher reported several depressive symptoms and recurrent bouts of self-destructive behavior. He was impulsive in interpersonal relationships, skittering from one unhealthy relationship to the next. He had chronic feelings of emptiness and found himself constantly emotionally dysregulated. Although he had seen the same therapist for more than a year and reported a strong therapeutic relationship, his symptoms had not improved because he defended against change by deploying humor and resisted learning adaptive coping skills. In the absence of the appropriate pharmacotherapy and effective psychotherapy, Christopher's quality of life was poor.

Contextual Features: Christopher presented to the hospital after a suicide attempt during a vacation. One challenge of his situation was that he had harmed himself in an unfamiliar environment. He had no local supports, and during his inpatient psychiatric admission, Stephanie announced that she was continuing their road trip without him. In her absence, Christopher had no one to accompany him home, and the treatment team feared discharging him to travel alone because of his low frustration tolerance, impulsive nature, and recent self-harm. Patients admitted to inpatient units often pose unique challenges to treatment teams. In the inpatient environment, treatment teams are tasked with stabilizing a person's acute condition and dispositioning him or her to an effective but less restrictive level of care. Although the stabilization of current psychiatric symptoms is usually straightforward (and, perhaps not coincidentally, the focus of most medical training), practitioners often find it challenging to plan an effective and safe discharge. Practitioners on inpatient psychiatric wards are forever estimating how the stability a patient achieves in a controlled and structured environment will be maintained or ameliorated after discharge to a less-controlled and less-structured environment.

Cultural Element #1: *Christopher was a young man immersed in popular culture. Is it important or even relevant to discuss popular cultural influences on psychiatric patients?* When asked to describe the major figures in his life, Christopher identified celebrities, especially comedians. His identification with celebrities and comedians influenced his behavior. For example, when asked why he chose to hang himself, Christopher claimed that he wanted to kill himself the "same way Robin Williams, the greatest comedian ever, did." Although Christopher could not achieve the cultural status of this celebrity, he could mimic his suicide, which, in Christopher's perception, made his attempt meaningful. Later, when discussing medications for his depressive symptoms, Christopher declared that "Tony Soprano was on Prozac, so I'll take Prozac," using the brand name for fluoxetine. Brand names, like celebrities, supplied Christopher with a sense of self. Christopher was intelligent, but his self-esteem was fragile, and he depended on external evaluation for his identity. In a way, he defined himself by his tastes in popular culture. Treatment teams should strive to understand how elements of culture and popular opinions can affect contemporary patients, many of whom spend their lives immersed in mass media culture. Christopher's treatment team helped him observe the ways in which he allowed popular culture to influence his identity and impair his self-direction. Christopher embraced fantasies of celebrity at the cost of reality and paid the price in impaired personality functioning. Christopher initially resisted staff confrontations of his cognitive distortions, but his level of insight improved. Even in an acute inpatient setting, psychotherapeutic measures can be clinically useful.

Religious/Spiritual Element #1: *Christopher's parents raised him in the Roman Catholic tradition, and they still identified as devout Catholics. Despite his affection for his parents and reports of a happy and uneventful upbringing, Christopher was opposed to organized religion. How does opposition to religious faith figure into psychiatric treatment?* Developmental histories are essential to understanding a patient's background but infrequently account for how a person's experience of faith changes throughout his or her development. When practitioners do discuss faith with patients, they typically ask about current beliefs and practices. However, it is often illuminating to explore the faith traditions and practices a person experienced in the developmental period because early experiences often influence a person's spiritual development and attitudes later in life. Christopher reported being "forced to attend Sunday Mass" weekly until he was 18 years old. His attitude toward Catholicism was extremely negative and often offensive to members of the treatment team. The treatment team understood Christopher's negative comments as an unresolved developmental conflict, an adolescent strategy for individuating from his parents. Although the treatment team believed that Christopher would primarily address this conflict in long-term psychotherapy, they set boundaries around offensive language and used motivational interviewing to help him explore the discrepancy between his affection for his parents and his strong dislike for their spiritual beliefs.

Religious/Spiritual Element #2: *Christopher was an atheist. What is it to be an atheist? Do they have spiritual experiences? How does one engage in spiritual discussions with an atheist?* Atheists typically ascribe to the belief that there is no God or supreme power and no afterlife (Lizardi & Gearing, 2010). *Spirituality* is a term whose boundaries are diffuse and whose meaning varies according to the individual using it, so when a patient describes his or her "spirituality," the concept always requires definition. Unlike other faiths, atheism is defined negatively, by a lack of belief in a supreme being. Like better-recognized faiths, atheists are a heterogeneous group with diverse opinions and practices. Consequently, because people's opinions and experiences cannot be predicted, it is essential for clinicians to ask each patient about his or her spiritual beliefs and practices. Just as Christians vary in their beliefs and practices, the engagement of atheist patients in spirituality needs to be assessed on a case-by-case basis. Otherwise, we risk generalization and incomplete understanding of our patients. That is to say, it would be unfair to decide that our atheist patients should not be engaged in spiritual discussions. Christopher was an atheist, but he considered himself to be spiritual, which he said meant "being interconnected with nature." Although he did not believe in God and did not pray, Christopher was very interested in meditation and mindfulness. He identified these as effective tools for him to regulate his emotions and cope with stress. Based on our experience, we encourage all treatment teams to engage in spiritual discussions with all of their patients because it is an important dimension of person-centered care.

Religious/Spiritual Element #3: *Christopher attended Narcotics Anonymous (NA) and Alcoholics Anonymous (AA) meetings while on the inpatient unit. Christopher was annoyed by these spiritually grounded treatment modalities and eventually interrupted the group with verbal outbursts and threats. What other clinical modalities are available for atheists to engage in substance abuse treatment?* Although the data are conflicting, about the efficacy of faith-based modalities such as NA and AA, these approaches appear to be, on balance, quite effective for treating substance abuse in many patients (Humphreys, Blodgett, & Wagner, 2014). While Christopher's response was extreme and required redirection in psychotherapy, it reminded staff that some patients have very negative feelings toward these modalities precisely because of their spiritual component. Because AA and NA programs are free and substance use disorders are so highly comorbid among persons hospitalized with mental illnesses, inpatient psychiatric wards often encourage (or even require) patients to attend NA and AA meetings while hospitalized. However, some patients are averse to these modalities, so it is essential for treatment teams to identify reasonable alternatives. For instance, secular recovery groups such as LifeRing emphasize human efforts, instead of divine intervention, for treatment of substance abuse. Like AA meetings, LifeRing meetings provide peer support and a communal setting in which members commit to complete abstinence from addictive substances. AA members use a 12-step program and have mentors called sponsors—people who have overcome their addiction through participation in AA. LifeRing utilizes neither. Instead, it uses cognitive behavioral therapy, motivational interviewing, solution-focused therapy, and other clinical approaches to recovery (LifeRing, 2015). This is one example of a secular alternative that staff can offer. To increase adherence, practitioners should evaluate a patient's spiritual and religious practices, even if they initially deny having any, and choose treatment options that accord with those practices.

Ethical Issue #1: *Is atheism a risk factor for suicide?* Religiosity and participation in religious practices are protective factors against suicidal behaviors, attempts, and completed suicide. The correlation varies among adherents of different faiths. For example, on a population basis, Jews have lower rates of completed suicide than Protestants. Determining the rate of suicidal behaviors, attempts, and completed suicide among atheists is more complicated because it is challenging to determine the prevalence of atheists. Because atheists are comparably less organized than adherents of other faiths, it is not surprising that only a few studies have investigated the influence of atheism on suicidality (Lizardi & Gearing, 2010). Clearly, this is an area of study that requires further research, because atheists are a growing population in contemporary life.

Case 2 Conclusion: Christopher was a 24-year-old atheist with major depressive and borderline personality disorders who was hospitalized after a serious suicide attempt. Christopher
had several contradictions that were initially difficult to understand. He was an independent
adult but endorsed an adolescent's fascination with celebrities. He loved his parents but reacted
strongly to their faith. He described himself as an atheist but also as spiritual. His case taught
us that atheism does not preclude spirituality and that it is important to approach all patients
without assumptions. Spirituality has a broad definition and consequently a broad application
which, for better or worse, needs to defined for each patient. On inpatient psychiatry units, the
journey to mental health for each patient often requires developing a map particular to his or
her own territory. Population-validated assessment tools like the CFI can be useful guides, but
ultimately clinicians need a person-centered understanding of each patient and the many ways
his or her faith affects mental health.

CONCLUSION

Caring for Akram and Christopher, along with many other people with mental illness, has
taught us that each person deserves consideration of the religious, spiritual, and ethical aspects
of their illness, care, and recovery. And yet, there are obstacles to doing so. On inpatient psychiatric units, dangerousness is often an explicit component of the criteria for admission, so
these units prioritize patient and staff safety, often at the expense of understanding each patient
as a person. Further, while working on inpatient units, it can become easy for practitioners to
write off religious statements, by, say, attributing one patient's strong religious belief to delusions
while dismissing another patient's atheism as a sign of intoxication. These obstacles are real, but
we receive them as motivation for redoubling our efforts to approach each person as a territory
unto themselves, one that deserves to be explored, appreciated, and understood. We use structured tools such as Kleinman's Patient Model and the CFI but also analytic frameworks such as
Jonsen's Four Quadrant Model as we approach each person with curiosity and a desire to serve
their unique needs.

REFERENCES

American Psychiatric Association. (2013). *Diagnostic and Statistical Manual of Mental Disorders: DSM-
    5.* Washington, DC: American Psychiatric Publishing, Inc.

Esposito, J. (2002). *What everyone needs to know about Islam.* New York, NY: Oxford University Press.

Hamdan, A. (2010). A comprehensive contemplative approach from the Islamic tradition. In T. Plante
    (Ed.), *Contemplative practices in action: Spirituality, meditation, and health* (pp. 122–142). Santa
    Barbara, CA: Praeger.

Henry, H. (2015). Spiritual energy of Islamic prayers as a catalyst for psychotherapy. *Journal of Religion
    and Health, 54,* 387–398.

Humphreys, K., Blodgett, J. C., & Wagner, T. H. (2014). Estimating the efficacy of Alcoholics Anonymous
    without self-selection bias: An instrumental variables re-analysis of randomized clinical trials.
    Alcoholism, Clinical and Experimental Research, 38(11), 2688–2694.

Jonsen, A. R., Siegler, M., and Winslade, W. J. (2015). *Clinical ethics: A practical approach to ethical deci-
    sions in clinical medicine* (8th ed.). New York, NY: McGraw-Hill Education.

Kleinman, A., Eisenberg, L., & Good, B. (1978). Culture, illness, and care: Clinical lessons from anthropologic and cross-cultural research. *Annals of Internal Medicine, 88*(2), 251–258.

Lewis-Fernández, R., Aggarwal, N., Hinton, L., Hinton, D., Kirmayer, L., & American Psychiatric Association. (2016). *DSM-5 Handbook on the Cultural Formulation Interview.* Washington, DC: American Psychiatric Publishing, Inc.

LifeRing Secular Recovery. (2017). Retrieved from http://lifering.org/.

Lizardi, D., & Gearing, R. (2010). Religion and suicide: Buddhism, Native American and African religions, atheism, and agnosticism. *Journal of Religious Health, 49*, 377–384.

Padela, A. I., Killawi, A., Heisler, M., Demonner, S., & Fetters, M. (2011). The role of imams in American Muslim health: Perspectives of Muslim community leaders in southeast Michigan. *Journal of Religion and Health,* 50, 359–373.

Pew Research Center. (2009). Mapping the Global Muslim Population: A Report on the Size and Distribution of the World's Muslim Population. Retrieved from http://www.pewforum.org/2009/10/07/mapping-the-global-muslim-population/.

Rogerson, B. (2006). *The heirs of the Prophet Muhammed: And the roots of the Sunni-Shia schism.* London, England: Hachette Digital.

Siddiqui, H. (2008). *Groundwork guides: Being Muslim.* Toronto, Canada: Groundhood Books.

TWELVE

Consultation-Liaison Psychiatry

Marta Herschkopf, M.D., M.St., and John R. Peteet, M.D.

CONSULTATION-LIAISON PSYCHIATRISTS, WORKING AT THE INTERFACE between psychiatry and other medical specialties, frequently receive consultation requests reflecting tensions among the values of the clinical team, the patient, and the patient's family (Hayes, 1986). Yet little attention has been devoted to the religious and spiritual dimensions of these challenges. This chapter, using brief clinical case examples, reviews the relevance of religion/spirituality for ethical conflicts in several domains of consultation-liaison psychiatry. These areas of conflict include (1) the appropriate scope of the consulting psychiatrist's role in diagnosis and treatment, (2) religious/spiritual aspects of capacity and candidacy evaluations, (3) patient and family values that conflict with those of the medical care team, and (4) a psychiatrist's own values that conflict with the patient's or society's values. The chapter concludes by discussing in more depth a case involving several of these themes, analyzing it according to the Jonsen Four Quadrant Model (discussed in Chapter 1).

AREAS OF ETHICAL CONFLICT

Appropriate Scope

Offering a useful psychiatric diagnostic assessment in the medical setting is a value-laden task. Many consultation requests are explicitly or implicitly prompted by behaviors that raise concern for psychopathology that may be amenable to psychopharmacology or psychotherapy. This may be more subtly phrased as a request to evaluate a patient's "coping" in the face of significant medical illness or by simply asking for a "psychiatric evaluation" or "medication recommendations" while a patient is hospitalized on a medical service. Thus, a psychiatric consultant is asked to comment on the appropriateness of a patient's response, in a given moment, to profound suffering.

A 55-year-old man from Nepal comes to the hospital for a chronic cough and is diagnosed with advanced idiopathic pulmonary fibrosis, with an expected survival time of 1 to 3 years. Psychiatry is consulted to evaluate his "coping" because the team is concerned that he does not understand his prognosis, describing him as "flat" and "seemingly unconcerned." The man explains to the psychiatrist that according to his Buddhist beliefs, it is best not to be overly attached to things in life that are inevitably impermanent, and he is hoping to practice this ideal in the face of his illness. The psychiatrist offers to have the hospital Buddhist chaplain see the patient, but he declines and says that he prefers to engage his own Buddhist community.

The ethical question arises, what is the appropriate scope of a psychiatric formulation? Arguably, a comprehensive formulation would include relevant religious and spiritual elements of a patient's coping. Yet psychiatrists are clinical experts with a focus on clinical issues and on diagnosis based on the *Diagnostic and Statistical Manual of Mental Disorders*, not necessarily on spiritual matters. The latter may be more appropriately the domain of hospital chaplaincy or palliative care teams, who explicitly aim to address spiritual distress. However, these other consulting services may not be available in all practice settings, or teams may not be as open to using them.

Whether or not spiritual consultants are involved, consulting psychiatrists need to consider the implications of including religious and spiritual elements in their formulations. For example, when a psychiatrist comments on a patient's coping, there is often an assessment of whether that coping is adaptive or maladaptive. This question can become ethically fraught when elements of that coping are religious or spiritual in nature. Physicians may be reticent to question or challenge purportedly religious/spiritual coping behaviors. In this case, the psychiatrist did not question the patient's attribution of his coping style to normative Buddhist practice; another clinician might have sought collateral to corroborate the patient's account, at least if the stakes were higher. Although some researchers have started to formulate tools to evaluate religious aspects of coping (Pargament, Koenig, & Perez, 2000), there is no evidence to suggest that psychiatry residencies have started emphasizing religion/spirituality in their curricula since the last national surveys on this topic (Sansone, Khatain, & Rodenhause, 1990). It could be argued both that commenting on religious/spiritual aspects of coping is beyond the average psychiatrist's realm of expertise and that psychiatrists need to educate themselves well enough in this area to address the often intertwined emotional and religious/spiritual needs of the patient as a whole person. One possible means to this end is to include a chaplain on psychiatry and/or multidisciplinary rounds to facilitate discussion of patients who have been seen by both services. Another is to reach out to a member of the patient's religious congregation. The next section describes a capacity evaluation in which knowledge of a patient's religious beliefs is necessary to inform clinical decision making.

Including religion and spirituality in a formulation leads to questions about how much to incorporate spiritual goals and interventions in the work at the bedside. Should a clinician respond in the moment to spiritual distress as a problem in its own right, suggest a referral to a chaplain, or offer psychological interpretations of spiritual material? What is the distinction between spiritually-based interventions that have become part of the standard psychiatric armamentarium, such as mindfulness and 12-step programs, and those that have not? Should a clinician disclose his or her spiritual orientation or agree to pray with a patient if asked? The answers to these questions will vary by clinician and context. Relevant considerations in making this clinical decision ethically include the patient's primary need from the clinician in a given context, the availability of other resources, and the clinician's own experience and comfort (Peteet, 1994).

Capacity and Candidacy Evaluations

Medical and surgical providers regularly consult psychiatrists when patients refuse recommended medical treatment, usually to help evaluate capacity but also often to help facilitate negotiation toward a plan. Many capacity evaluations are prompted by ethical rather than clinical concerns: Rather than doubting a patient's capacity to make a decision, consulting teams or the patient's family may feel uncomfortable about the content of that decision (Kontos, Freudenreich, & Querques, 2013). Therefore, psychiatrists may implicitly be requested to comment on matters outside their clinical domain. In the realm of medical decision making, medical ethics in the past several decades has moved from a prior stance that privileged the principle of beneficence (now referred to pejoratively as "paternalism") to one that emphasizes the importance of respecting patient autonomy (Stirrat & Gill, 2005). In this context, the role of the consulting psychiatrist often becomes one of evaluating whether the patient understands the relevant medical information and whether the patient's decision is consistent with his or her authentic values (Kontos, Querques, & Freudenreich, 2015).

Some treatment refusals involve canonized religious tenets—for example, rejection of the "medical" by Christian Scientists and refusal of blood products by Jehovah's Witnesses (Stotland, 1999). In recent years, healthcare professionals have become more familiar with such objections and more comfortable accommodating them. That said, by virtue of being involved in capacity evaluations, consultation-liaison psychiatrists often have more knowledge and experience in these topics and can guide the team accordingly, even if such expertise is not strictly psychiatric. For example, in situations involving the refusal of blood products by Jehovah's Witnesses, the psychiatrist can assist in opening up potential options by explaining that Jehovah's Witnesses are asked to sign a card documenting their wishes in advance, that centers and procedures for bloodless surgery exist, and that Hospital Committees of Jehovah's Witnesses are often available to help clarify and negotiate difficult situations.

Even with this increased familiarity, ethical concerns frequently arise. What are the ethical implications of encouraging a patient to find emotional and spiritual support in his or her faith community if that community is supporting the patient's refusal of care? One could argue that it is incumbent on medical professionals to make the strongest case possible to encourage evidence-based care, including pointing out the limitations of faith-based healing, while at the same time acknowledging the importance of respecting a patient's values.

A 45-year-old woman is brought to the hospital after fainting. Head imaging reveals a large, well-circumscribed mass that is concerning for meningioma. When the patient regains consciousness, she explains that she is a Christian Scientist and wishes to be discharged from the hospital to seek healing in her community. Her physicians explain to her that without treatment, her neurologic symptoms are likely to progress to the point of coma and death, but that she could potentially have a full recovery with surgery. Psychiatric consultation is requested to evaluate the patient's capacity to leave against medical advice. The patient explains to the psychiatrist that she understands her prognosis is poor without medical treatment. However, she also states that her faith has been an important part of her values and identity for many years and that she would rather risk death than betray her ideals. While the psychiatrist is gathering collateral information from the patient's family, several members of the patient's church come to visit her. Her nurse overhears one of these friends encouraging the patient to elope from the hospital, and the patient is placed on elopement precautions. The team also considers instituting visitor restrictions. The patient's parents tell the psychiatrist that they are not Christian Scientists but that the patient has been part of that community since college. They report that she has consistently held a strict understanding of the tenets as disallowing medical interventions under any and all circumstances, although she does have some friends who allow for interventions as a supplement to prayer. Her mother spontaneously states that she would not want to make decisions on the patient's behalf because she could not in good conscience deprive her daughter of life-saving medical care even knowing that it is against her religious convictions. Ultimately, the patient is found to have capacity to leave against medical advice and is discharged.

In this case, it became clear that members of the Christian Science community have a range of interpretations regarding the circumstances under which medical treatment may be permissible, and the psychiatrist appropriately sought collateral information to clarify the longitudinal nature of the patient's beliefs. The psychiatrist's assessment of the patient's capacity also helped temper the team's inclination to restrict access to members of her faith community who had encouraged her to take matters into her own hands.

This case also brings up the question of who is the appropriate person to serve as a health-care proxy. If healthcare proxies are meant to exercise substituted judgment, one could argue that a member of a patient's faith community may be better equipped to do so. How does one weigh the effects of a patient's decision on others, such as loved ones who have a practical or emotional stake in the patient's health? Moreover, a parent's religious convictions may prevent minor children from receiving recommended medical care. This issue has been considered in a number of court cases in which Christian Scientist parents refused medical care for their children (Merrick, 1994). Psychiatrists are sometimes asked to assess the decision-making capacity of healthcare proxies, particularly when the proxies are making or supporting decisions with which the medical team disagrees. Because the health-care proxy is not the identified patient, such questions are beyond the practice scope of a consultation service and are better deferred to social work professionals or the hospital legal department.

Other reservations involve religious convictions that are not as clearly doctrinal and therefore are in some ways less understandable to medical providers. These may include belief in miracles, in the power of prayer, or in various folk healing rituals. Such approaches may appear to be subjective and therefore open to challenge or interpretation. Religious individuals who believe in miracles sometimes refuse treatment recommendations or, alternatively, pursue more aggressive care at the end of life, when physicians may feel that such care is futile (Phelps et al., 2009). Sulmasy (2006) highlighted the tendency of some secular clinicians to be put off by patients' belief in miracles and, in the process, to make assumptions about their goals of care, thus missing the opportunity to provide them with options such as hospice care. At times, such convictions are interpreted by providers as denial or as another form of maladaptive coping.

A 42-year-old, unmarried teacher with breast cancer metastatic to bone entered clinical remission after an experimental treatment. One year later, she asks her oncologist to provide a medical report to an adoption agency in support of her application for an international adoption. Her nurse requests a psychiatric consultation because of her concern that the patient does not appreciate the risk to the child of losing a mother to cancer. Others on the team express concern that the adoption agency might not appreciate the patient's risk of recurrence from a medical report that indicates she is in remission. The patient explains that she realizes her disease could recur, but as a devout Christian, she also believes that God can heal her and would want her to care for a child who might not have a home. A psychiatric consultant finds the patient able to relate her beliefs to her personal motivations and prognosis. An ethics consultant clarifies that the oncology team's responsibility is to provide a medical report to the adoption agency, not an opinion about the patient's suitability to adopt.

This case demonstrates the participation of psychiatrists in evaluations of medical fitness for various societal roles. At times, the question of capacity is a stand-in for issues that might be better addressed by other members of a multidisciplinary team, such as social workers or other consultants.

Psychiatrists are also frequently involved in determining a patient's candidacy for particular medical treatments, such as the transplantation of scarce organs. Part of such an evaluation is assessing whether a patient will comply with recommended medical treatment so as to help "safeguard" this limited resource after the transplant. In allocating organs, a transplantation team considers not only the needs of a given patient but also the abstract yet very real needs of other patients waiting for the same organ.

A 35-year-old man is being evaluated for liver transplantation. His liver has failed due to a combination of hepatitis C infection (presumably contracted during intravenous drug use) and alcoholism. In the past few years, he tried and failed several times to stop drinking, but now he has been sober for 4 months, since learning of his need for transplantation. In the psychiatric candidacy interview, he tells the psychiatrist that he is not concerned about his ability to stay sober after transplantation, explaining that he has always maintained the ability to quit when he really wanted to. He says that his illness has been a wake-up call and that he has recently rejoined his childhood church and been re-baptized. "With God's help, I won't need any alcohol or drug treatment; all I need is church." The psychiatrist is concerned about the patient's insight into his addictions and recommends ongoing substance abuse treatment as part of his candidacy requirements.

In both of these cases, the patients' faith-based optimism may play an important role in their healing and coping but also has implications for others should their prognosis prove poorer than anticipated. These cases also demonstrate ways in which an emphasis on respecting individual autonomy can compromise other ethical principles, such as justice. Is it fair to allocate medical resources—be they organs, intensive care unit beds, or expensive drug regimens—to patients with less likelihood of benefitting from them, simply because these patients or their families choose to be optimistic? Should that optimism be taken more or less seriously because it is purportedly predicated on religious/spiritual beliefs? In what situation is it permissible to challenge those beliefs and suggest alternative or supplementary motivations such as self-interest?

On the other hand, perceived or actual religious reservations about organ donation can contribute to organ shortages. Israel, for example, has one of the lowest rates of organ donation among developed countries, a statistic that is partially related to different understandings of Jewish definitions of brain death (Quigley, Wright, & Ravitsky, 2012). Consultation psychiatrists usually are not involved in decisions for postmortem donation, but they may be involved in the evaluation of living donors. This evaluation includes assessing the ability of the potential donors to cope psychologically with the stress of donation as well as their capacity to make the decision, with an emphasis on ensuring that the decision is not coerced.

A 25-year-old man volunteers to donate one of his kidneys to a member of his mosque, saying that his imam told him that Allah commands him to do so. During the psychosocial evaluation, the psychiatrist discerns that the volunteer has a history of schizophrenia, has recently converted to Islam, and does not have social supports beyond his mosque community. The psychiatrist is not sure whether Islam mandates organ donation and is concerned that the volunteer lacks capacity or is being coerced by his imam. The psychiatrist seeks the advice of a Muslim colleague, who suggests contacting the imam to engage in the discussion. The imam clarifies that he made a public plea to the congregation looking for a donor, which the volunteer misinterpreted. The imam tells the volunteer that he is under no obligation from Allah to donate his kidney and that although the congregation would do its best to support him in his recovery should he wish to donate, the imam would advise him not to be a donor because his lack of social supports makes the risk too great. The man decides not to donate.

In this case, the man's decision was based on a misunderstanding of his imam's teaching, potentially informed by his social isolation and desire for a community. In capacity evaluations, a psychiatrist may be asked to help the members of a medical team ascertain whether a patient's decision is motivated by religious/cultural values, psychopathology, or both. Many individuals are ignorant or misinformed regarding their own religion's stances on bioethical issues. Although it is arguably not within the scope of practice of the consulting psychiatrist to evaluate a patient's religious beliefs or to educate a patient about religious tenets, the psychiatrist can reach out to members of the same faith community to clarify whether a patient's beliefs are consistent with doctrine and/or to engage in a discussion to help the patient come to a religiously informed decision. Such overtures may be complicated by concerns for confidentiality. As previously mentioned, educating psychiatrists about these issues can help them recognize when such overtures are needed. Whereas the imam in this case appears to have encouraged a decision that is in the patient's best interest, other patients may be vulnerable to exploitation by members of their religious or spiritual communities.

Conflicting Values 1: Patients' Values

At times, psychiatric consultations are prompted when cultural values of patients conflict with those of their clinicians. A common example is religiously justified domination or abusive treatment of female patients by male spouses.

A 19-year-old Muslim woman from Saudi Arabia comes to the hospital with abdominal pain. Her middle-aged husband takes the emergency room physician aside and explains that in their culture, all medical decisions are made by the husband, and the physician therefore should be relaying information to him rather than unnecessarily worrying his wife. The physician asks the patient in front of her husband whether she wants to know information about her treatment. She replies that all information should go through her husband and quotes a verse from the Qu'ran which declares that a man is the protector of his wife. A psychiatry consultation is requested with the question: "Is this patient suffering from Stockholm syndrome?"

In this situation, appreciation for the cultural and religious background of the patient and her family is crucial to formulating an appropriate response. Some providers would insist on questioning the woman about her preferences in private, maintaining that it is imperative to ascertain her true wishes even if doing so involves temporarily disrespecting her stated wishes. Others would be concerned that this approach could irretrievably damage the treatment relationship. It can be difficult to engage patients when a consultation is prompted by a medical provider who is at best questioning, and at worst challenging, the patient's cultural values. Furthermore, many religious individuals are suspicious of psychiatric practice and have qualms about any interaction with a mental health professional.

As mentioned previously, the more familiar the psychiatrist can be with the religious culture of the patient, the more helpful she or he is likely to be to the medical team in its attempts to do the right thing. From a virtue ethics perspective, the role of a consulting psychiatrist in helping the team and patient come to a workable consensus in cases involving conflicting values speaks to the importance of the professional traits of flexibility, wisdom, respect, and self-awareness.

Conflicting Values 2: Clinicians' Values

Clinicians' religiously-based values may conflict with those of the treatment establishment, particularly in cases involving issues at the beginning or end of life, such as abortion, euthanasia, or assisted suicide.

An Orthodox Jewish psychiatrist practicing in the Netherlands is asked to evaluate individuals requesting euthanasia in order to certify their appropriateness to proceed. The psychiatrist understands euthanasia to be morally wrong and finds herself in a dilemma: Should she refuse to perform consultations because they might lead to euthanasia, or should she agree in the hope of helping applicants to find meaning in their lives?

Physician-assisted suicide is legally protected and largely accepted in several countries and several U.S. states, but it remains an area of controversy in much of the United States. However, it is likely to become increasingly common and more accepted in coming years. Physicians who have until now not needed to grapple with the ethical implications of being part of this process may find themselves conflicted about what services their role as physicians may entail. There are several cases of Canadian physicians requesting to opt out of participating in physician-assisted suicide as conscientious objectors based on religious beliefs. Some ethicists argue that physicians who voluntarily join a profession that has a monopoly on providing certain types of services are not permitted to conscientiously object to providing them because doing so places their own beliefs above the needs of their patients (Schuklenk & Smalling, 2016). Others hold that moral objections, including those grounded in religious beliefs, should be respected (Weinstock, 2014). Defenders of both views argue that religiously motivated objections do not hold more weight than other moral objections and in some cases may be more difficult to defend as reasonable requests.

Physicians must be vigilant in situations in which they are tempted to impose their own values onto patients. In the first example of conflicting values, the conflict arose because the patient was coming from a minority culture, whereas in the second example, the physician found herself holding a minority moral view. Many physicians intentionally define their scope of practice to limit these conflicts, for example by choosing an obstetrics residency with an option to not perform elective abortions. But questions continue to arise: In a pluralistic society, how can physicians respect the values of their patients if they profoundly conflict with the physician's own values? Are physicians restricted from publicly supporting values that some of their patients and colleagues find offensive (e.g., by attending demonstrations in favor of or against abortion or same-sex relationships)? Similarly thorny dilemmas challenge hospital medical staffs to balance respect for religious beliefs and other deeply held convictions with the effects of expressing them in public and in professional medical contexts.

In summary, consultation-liaison psychiatry, by virtue of its close engagement with conflicts among stakeholders who hold differing values at a time of medical crisis, often touches on religious and spiritual aspects of these values and conflicts. Psychiatric consultants are often asked to comment on areas that are not currently part of formal psychiatric education. The decision of how to address these requests is context- and clinician-dependent. Including members of a patient's spiritual community when such questions arise can be helpful and may be necessary to inform capacity assessments. A greater understanding of the diversity and depth of these commitments will better prepare clinicians to address them.

CASE VIGNETTE

The following case illustrates several of the themes discussed and is followed by a more extensive discussion using the Jonsen Four Quadrant Model.

A 50-year-old woman is diagnosed with early-stage breast cancer. The medical team explains that with aggressive surgery and chemotherapy, her cancer is likely curable. However, the woman declines this treatment and says that she wishes to be discharged from the hospital and go to another state for a program of "detoxification" that she has read about, which was initially recommended to her by a friend from church. Psychiatry consultation is requested to evaluate the patient's capacity to decline surgery and chemotherapy.

During the capacity evaluation, the woman is able to recount her physicians' assessment that surgery and chemotherapy would likely be curative and that without these treatments, the cancer would likely progress and require more invasive treatment. She also repeats her decision to decline such treatment at this time. She says that although her religious beliefs do not comment directly on medical treatment, she feels that God is leading her to have faith in a nontraditional path. She acknowledges that the physicians do not think that this treatment will be curative for her and says that she has not yet decided what steps she would take after the detoxification program is complete. She says, "This is my decision to make. You cannot force me to do something that goes against my religious principles."

The consulting psychiatrist asks the patient about her past psychiatric history. Further exploration reveals a history of childhood sexual abuse, which prompted a period of depression and anxiety with symptoms including panic attacks, anhedonia, and suicidal ideation. She did not engage with mental health treatment but instead became involved in her church community. After an extended period of prayer from the leaders of her church community, her depressive symptoms resolved. She has remained active in her church since that time and says that it helps her "gain control" of her life and mental well-being. The few times that her depressive symptoms have recurred, they have eventually resolved with prayer. When the psychiatrist asks her what she thinks of the medical establishment, she responds, "You probably don't want to know." With gentle encouragement, she declines to say more, other than to comment that "in my time of greatest need, you weren't the ones who helped me."

The psychiatrist asks the patient's husband, who is also her healthcare proxy, what his thoughts are on her treatment. He acknowledges that his wife has always looked to her faith to guide decisions in all aspects of her life. Although he is concerned that the detoxification regimen she proposes will prove ineffective and will delay definitive oncologic treatment, he feels that ultimately she must make the decision that is true to her spiritual values, and he supports her in doing so. The psychiatrist did not reach out to members of the woman's church community, deciding that the patient likely had capacity to make this decision, and that even if she did not, her healthcare proxy supported it.

Summary of the Facts

Medical Indications: Early-stage breast cancer is potentially curable if treatment is offered early. Delaying treatment will likely mean progression of disease and a need for more aggressive treatments later and/or losing the possibility of a cure. It is not known what evidence, if any, supports the proposed detoxification program.

Patient's Preferences: The patent has clearly stated that she wishes to delay treatment, potentially indefinitely, to explore an alternative. She also appears to consistently value the support of her church community over engagement with the medical system.

Quality of Life: The patient's quality of life will likely suffer from medical complications of untreated cancer. Although early treatment and chemotherapy do negatively affect quality of life, the stresses of surgery and side effects of chemotherapy or hormonal therapy are usually temporary. The effects of delayed treatment can be permanent, including disfigurement from mastectomy, lymphedema from radical lymph node dissection, and pain, disfigurement, or death from metastases. However, her quality of life will also suffer if she is coerced into treatment to which she does not consent. Her quality of life is enhanced by living in accordance with her religious and spiritual values and having her decisions respected.

Contextual Features: Religious communities are often a source of support for patients, and they may offer doctrinally based or idiosyncratic information for members about healthcare decisions. In this case, the church's precise stance was unclear and unexplored. Holistic practitioners are often able to propose treatments that appeal to patients for a number of reasons, including alignment with values of "natural" healing or antiestablishment views, having fewer or more benign side effects, offering personalized care and attention, or being supported by people a patient admires. However, holistic treatments are not held to the same evidentiary standard as biomedicine, and they are less regulated in terms of what practitioners can claim to deliver. Some holistic practitioners are genuine, but others may be frankly predatory.

Discussion

The medical facts of this case suggest that it is in this patient's best interest to receive the recommended standard medical treatment of surgery and chemotherapy. Physicians are ethically obligated to offer patients medically indicated, evidence-based care and to educate them about why such care is indicated. One could further argue that even though a physician's expertise generally does not extend to full knowledge of holistic alternatives, he or she is duty-bound to comment on the limitations of such approaches when they would compromise recommended medical care. Acknowledging the limitations of medical certainty and knowing that there is no guarantee the patient's cancer will respond as anticipated, the odds with medical treatment are still in the patient's favor.

However, the patient feels that delaying treatment may in fact be in her best interest. One can speculate as to why the alternative regimen appeals to this patient. She may not wish to accept the idea that she has cancer and may see the detoxification regimen as a way to address a different formulation of her diagnosis. She may fear the practical or symbolic implications of many chemotherapy side effects, including making her feel less womanly by losing her hair, disfiguring her breast, or affecting her hormonal balance. She may feel that it is "unnatural" to pump her body full of chemicals and consider such treatment anathema or one of last resort. She may feel resentful or distrustful of the medical establishment and wish to demonstrate the limitations of her doctors' expertise and, by implication, the validity of alternate viewpoints, including faith-based ones. All of this is speculation because the psychiatrist in this example did not elicit such views from the patient herself. Some of these views might be considered maladaptive coping if they are motivated by anxiety and interfere with definitive medical treatment.

One way to formulate the ethical issues at stake in this case is to say that there is a conflict between the principle of beneficence and that of autonomy. The former principle may indicate that it is in the patient's best interest to receive the recommended medical treatment, but the latter would allow her to choose an alternative that is not in her best interest and that may in fact cause her irreparable harm. The psychiatrist is being asked to evaluate whether her choice is truly autonomous. Such a model, intentionally overly simplistic, assumes that a patient's well-being can be reduced to medical symptomatology. It overlooks the contributions of psychological well-being and living in accordance with one's deeply held values. The patient's husband, although he disagrees with her decision, feels that it is important to allow her to live according to her values. Although this formulation suggests a way of interpreting her decision as maladaptive, it could also be argued that the best thing for this patient's emotional well-being is not to force her into a treatment that she believes conflicts with her faith. And on a practical level, how would one force someone into a months-long chemotherapy regimen?

Alternatively, one could argue that respecting this woman's autonomy will contribute to her psychological well-being and therefore could be considered to be in line with the principle of beneficence; forcing unwanted treatment on her would violate the principle of non-maleficence. A consulting psychiatrist performing a capacity evaluation is in the unique position of considering what is in the patient's interest not just medically but also psychologically. Yet such an argument is similarly problematic: It might be considered a form of psychological paternalism. Furthermore, it is not clear what is in this patient's interest, psychologically or otherwise, in the short term versus the long term. One cannot anticipate what will ultimately be in her best interest. Will she die slowly and painfully of metastatic cancer, despairing and angry that her faith led her astray? Will the detoxification regimen work, leading to her celebration in her church as a living miracle? Or, perhaps less melodramatically, will she have a change of heart after the detoxification treatment when she notices a swollen axillary lymph node, undergo radical mastectomy with lymph node dissection followed by chemotherapy, yet feel satisfied that she acted according to her principles? Patients and physicians all are required to make decisions despite inevitable uncertainty.

In this case, there are several potential avenues that the psychiatrist chose not to explore. The psychiatrist did not attempt to engage a chaplain or members of the patient's religious community. It could potentially have been helpful to clarify whether there were specific church beliefs informing her decision or whether perhaps she had been misinformed about church doctrine by the parishioner who recommended the detoxification regimen. Alternatively, engaging these parties in discussion could have helped build trust in the medical team and potentially convinced the patient to accept the recommended treatment. The psychiatrist similarly did not engage in much discussion of the patient's religious beliefs themselves. Some providers may have chosen to disclose their own religious or spiritual traditions; a psychiatrist coming from the same tradition as the patient might have suggested to her that God sometimes works through physicians.

The psychiatrist may also have sought out a member of the patient's treatment team with similar religious beliefs to see if that person could engage the patient. However, such engagement with the patient's beliefs or with her community would be perceived by some providers as involving boundary crossings or boundary violations.

The psychiatrist also did not explore the full psychological meaning of this patient's decision and her longitudinal relationship with the medical establishment. This choice was informed by the patient's own reluctance to discuss these issues, which itself suggests that she does not have particularly positive views of the healthcare system. It is not clear how invested she is in this particular detoxification regimen or whether her decision might be amenable to change if she had a better relationship with her treatment providers. In some situations, a consulting psychiatrist may have the benefit of time to see the patient on several different occasions and build an alliance. With an understanding of the patient's history, the psychiatrist could help the medical team avoid traumatizing behaviors and regain the patient's trust.

Ultimately, the psychiatrist felt comfortable leaving many of these avenues underexplored because of a combination of practical concerns and the fact that her healthcare proxy supported her decision. The psychiatrist did not try to evaluate the husband's capacity because this was beyond the scope of the capacity evaluation. Although there was a possibility of working to engage the patient and her family and steer them toward an alternate decision, the psychiatrist felt that such an approach was unnecessarily paternalistic and, given the patient's fear of losing control, had the potential to backfire and further estrange the patient from her medical providers.

CONCLUSIONS

The following is a list of take-home points from this discussion:

- When asked to comment on religious or spiritual aspects of hoping, it can be helpful to confer with members of other teams such as chaplaincy or palliative care.
- Appropriate religious/spiritual interventions are determined based on patient need, physician comfort and ability, and availability of other resources.
- Capacity assessments may be prompted by ethical rather than clinical questions; it is helpful for consulting psychiatrists to consider what is within their scope of practice.
- For substituted decision making, the choice that is medically indicated is not necessarily what is in the patient's best interest. What is in the patient's psychological best interest in the short term may not be so in the long term.
- Reaching out to members of a patient's religious or spiritual community may be helpful but can also raise issues of boundaries and confidentiality.
- It is not the role of a consulting psychiatrist to evaluate the capacity of a surrogate decision maker.
- Ethical concerns regarding differing values may arise when a patient or clinician is a member of a cultural or religious minority.

REFERENCES

Hayes, J. R. (1986). Consultation-liaison psychiatry and clinical ethics: A model for consultation and teaching. *General Hospital Psychiatry*, 8, 415–418.

Kontos, N., Freudenreich, O., & Querques, J. (2013). Beyond capacity: Identifying ethical dilemmas underlying capacity evaluation requests. *Psychosomatics, 54*, 103–110.

Kontos, N., Querques, J., & Freudenreich, O. (2015). Capable of more: Some underemphasized aspects of capacity assessment. *Psychosomatics, 56*, 217–226.

Merrick, J. C. (1994). Christian Science healing of minor children: Spiritual exemption statuses, First Amendment rights, and fair notice. *Issues in Law and Medicine, 10*, 321–342.

Pargament, K. I., Koenig, H. G., & Perez, L. M. (2000). The many methods of religious coping: Development and initial validation of the RCOPE. *Journal of Clinical Psychology, 56*, 519–543.

Peteet, J. R. (1994). Approaching spiritual issues in psychotherapy: A conceptual framework. *Journal of Psychotherapy Practice and Research, 3*, 237–245.

Phelps, A. C., Maciejewski, P. K., Nilsson, M., Balboni, T. A., Wright, A. A., Paulk, M. E., . . . & Prigerson, H. G. (2009). Religious coping and use of intensive life-prolonging care near death in patients with advanced cancer. *JAMA, 301*, 1140–1147.

Quigley, M., Wright, L., & Ravitsky, V. (2012). Organ donation and priority points in Israel: An ethical analysis. *Transplantation, 93*, 970–973.

Sansone, R. A., Khatain, K., & Rodenhause, P. (1990). The role of religion in psychiatric education: A national survey. *Academic Psychiatry, 14*, 34–38.

Schuklenk, U., & Smalling, R. (2016). Why medical professionals have no moral claim to conscientious objection accommodation in liberal democracies. *Journal of Medical Ethics.* doi:10.1136/medethics~2016-103560

Stirrat, G. M., & Gill, R. (2005). Autonomy in medical ethics after O'Neill. *Journal of Medical Ethics, 31*, 127–130.

Stotland, N. L. (1999). When religion collides with medicine. *American Journal of Psychiatry, 156*, 304–307.

Sulmasy, D. P. (2006). Spiritual issues in the care of dying patients: ". . . It's okay between me and God." *JAMA, 296*, 1385–1392.

Weinstock, D. (2014). Conscientious refusal and healthcare professionals: Does religion make a difference? *Bioethics, 28*, 8–15.

THIRTEEN

Addiction Psychiatry

Christopher C. H. Cook, M.B., B.S., M.D., M.A., Ph.D.,
Eilish Gilvarry, M.B., M.Ch., B.A.O., and
Andrea Hearn, B.Sc. (hons), Ph.D., M.B., B.S.

ADDICTION PSYCHIATRY PRESENTS ITS OWN PARTICULAR ETHICAL
challenges and opportunities in relation to matters of spirituality and religion. This is, in part,
due to the huge influence of Alcoholics Anonymous (AA) and its spiritual approach to recovery.
However, there is a long history of religious support for recovery from addiction that predates
AA, and faith-based organizations continue to play an important part worldwide in offering
rehabilitation and treatment (Cook, 2009). Perhaps even more importantly, it is in the nature
of addictive disorders that they raise important ethical issues, both for those who are directly
affected and also for the wider society (Cook, 2006).

In this chapter, two cases are presented that illustrate some of the ethical issues arising in
relation to spirituality and religion in the course of clinical practice in addiction psychiatry.
Both cases were encountered during the course of delivering a service for people with addictive
disorders in the National Health Service (NHS) in England. This cultural and political context
is important, both because of the nature of statutory services as compared with services offered
in other contexts and also because of the largely secular nature of United Kingdom (UK) society (notwithstanding the complex constitutional relationship between church and state). Many
UK citizens continue to consider themselves broadly Christian or identify as belonging to the
Church of England even though they do not regularly attend any place of worship or engage in
other religious practices. Others explicitly identify with particular faith traditions (Christian or
other), and yet others identify as agnostic or atheist. Many now say that they are "spiritual but
not religious." In this context, the place of spirituality/religion in current clinical practice is con-
troversial and must be handled with care and sensitivity (Cook, 2013b, 2013a).[1]

Twelve-step groups such as AA and Narcotics Anonymous (NA) are widely available in the
UK and have long provided a spiritual approach to recovery that is utilized both in the community and in many residential rehabilitation programs. They have been less widely accepted

---

1. It is also not entirely clear that the protective benefit of spirituality—as opposed to religion—in relation to substance misuse operates in the same way in UK society as in North America (King, Marston,
McManus, Brugha, Meltzer, & Bebbington, 2013).

in the NHS (the UK state-funded health service, which is available to all citizens), although many NHS addiction services do encourage patients to attend local groups, and some invite closer contact. Similarly, there is a complex relationship between NHS services and faith-based organizations working in this field. Generally speaking, referral for Christian or other religious approaches to rehabilitation has been the exception rather than the rule. Mindfulness-based relapse prevention has been something of an exception, having been effectively detached from its Buddhist roots and now being offered more widely in mental health services, including some addiction services (Mason-John & Groves, 2013).

There is thus something of a disconnection, at least within the UK, between spiritual/religious approaches to treatment and recovery and medical/secular approaches. Both of the following cases illustrate some of the problems that this disconnect might occasion.

Case 1

W. was a 40-year-old man when he first presented to Addiction Services with an opiate addiction (Opiate Dependence Syndrome—F11.2[2]). He gave a history of having been a very nervous child; his mother would give him kaolin and morphine to settle his anxiety. Otherwise, he described an uneventful childhood and upbringing and after school went straight into factory work as an apprentice.

In his early twenties, there was a re-emergence of anxiety with features of panic disorder (F41.0). He had sought medical attention but found treatment with antidepressant therapy unhelpful, and he was unable to engage in psychological therapies. He started to drink heavily to manage his symptoms and within a year had fulfilled the criteria for Alcohol Dependence Syndrome (F10.2).

At this point, W. was living alone. His parents were both dead, and he was socially isolated. He lost his job after a period of poor attendance, and his drinking increased as a result. On the verge of losing his home, he saw his general practitioner, who prescribed a course of medically assisted alcohol detoxification and suggested he attend AA. W. was initially reluctant, particularly given his vulnerability to anxiety in social situations. However, a sponsor was found, and after a few AA meetings, he embraced the concept and remained abstinent from alcohol. He returned to work, and AA remained the focus of his life; he attended meetings at least twice weekly and became a sponsor for others.

In his late thirties, W. noted increasing anxiety. To avoid drinking alcohol, he started to buy kaolin and morphine (available over the counter); as in his childhood, it alleviated his symptoms. Over time, his consumption escalated. Local pharmacists started to question the amount he was buying, and he had to travel further afield to get it. He started to experience symptoms of opiate withdrawal when he was unable to obtain it.

W. then returned to his GP, who referred him to specialist addiction services with a diagnosis of Opiate Dependence Syndrome. He was seen and assessed, and his treatment plan included switching to a long-acting opiate (methadone) with a view to opiate detoxification once the underlying anxiety had been adequately treated.

---

2. Diagnostic categories are taken, throughout, from the *ICD-10 Classification of Mental and Behavioural Disorders* (World Health Organization, 1992).

W. disclosed the situation to his AA sponsor. His sponsor felt that opiate substitution ther-apy was not commensurate with AA principles and that abstinence was the only way forward. W. felt guilty about his perceived lack of adherence to AA principles. This was discussed with his addiction team, who suggested opiate detoxification from methadone with transfer to a 12-step residential rehabilitation facility.

W. continued to report guilt and shame about his use of substances to manage his emotions and was unsure about residential rehabilitation but could see no other way forward at the time. He was detoxified from methadone and admitted to the facility as a priority. Within 2 days of admission, he was found dead in his room, having hanged himself from the curtain rail.

Discussion

W. found the spirituality of AA supportive of recovery for many years. Unfortunately, despite his in-depth knowledge of the 12 Steps and his active involvement with his local AA group, when he relapsed his spiritual beliefs contributed to a sense of guilt and failure which was further reinforced in the course of conversation with his sponsor. A conflict of approaches between his sponsor and his medical team further increased the tension surrounding management of his relapse. Eventually, despite progress that should have been a source of encouragement to him, he committed suicide.

For W., social isolation was relieved primarily by his involvement in the 12-step community. The concerns expressed by his sponsor contributed not only to a sense of spiritual failure but also isolated him from the community that had provided social support so reliably for almost a decade. Although some members of AA also belong to a faith community that provides addi-tional support, W. did not have this resource to fall back on. It is probably true to say that for many in the UK, a "spiritual but not religious" approach to life is very individualistic. Although it may provide coping resources associated with meaning and purpose in life and a sense of relationship with a transcendent order or Higher Power, it does not necessarily offer the social networks and supports associated with traditional religious communities.

The role of the sponsor was crucial for W. At its origins, AA had good relationships with med-ical professionals such as Dr. William D. Silkworth and Dr. Carl Jung (Kurtz, 1991). However, in the UK today, it operates largely independently of medical services. Closer liaison between the sponsor and the medical team in this instance could well have allowed development of a treat-ment plan incorporating both the strengths of AA and those of the medical team and might have avoided the perceived conflict between those seeking to help W, which further contributed to his sense of tension and guilt. However, such liaison is not easily established and in some cases is not welcomed by AA sponsors. Although in this case the medical professionals were very sympathetic to W's spirituality and supportive of it, some atheist doctors find a professional and ethical conflict in recommending or supporting a spiritual approach to treatment with which they cannot personally agree.

W. did not reveal his suicidal thoughts to health professionals before his eventual suicide. Mental health chaplains report one of the most frequently asked questions in their work with patients is what will happen after death by suicide (Cook, 2014). However, many patients are unaware that chaplains now work across traditional religious boundaries and also provide sup-port to those with no formal religious affiliation. Being independent of religious institutions yet affiliated with them, and independent of the medical team yet employed by medical services, chaplains occupy a uniquely independent role that allows them to discuss such matters with patients in a manner that is not open to other professionals.

Case 2

Ms. M. was a 38-year-old woman who sought treatment with Addiction Services. She had a history of heroin use and a diagnosis of Opiate Dependence Syndrome on a clinically supervised maintenance regime (methadone) (F11.22). She described an aversive upbringing and had been exposed to domestic violence between her parents. Her history suggested that her father was probably alcohol dependent. She had spent some time within the care system, as had her two brothers.

Throughout her teenage years, she had had contact with Child and Adolescent Mental Health Services (CAMHS) as a result of episodes of self-harm. She gave a long history of substance use, including use of solvents and Ecstasy in early adolescence, moving on to cocaine and heroin use in late adolescence. She first entered into treatment at the age of 22. She did not use alcohol, blaming it for her difficult upbringing and the violence within her parents' relationship.

At age 28, Ms. M. began a relationship with a man who misused drugs and alcohol. She became pregnant unexpectedly but saw this as an opportunity to turn her life around and give her child the family life that she had wanted. Children's Services was involved throughout the pregnancy because of her history of drug use. Ms. M. did well in treatment during the pregnancy and initially after the birth of her baby. However, over time, the relationship with her partner deteriorated with episodes of domestic violence, and she eventually relapsed into heroin use.

By the time her daughter was 3 years old, Children's Services had intervened; the child was placed in foster care and subsequently adopted. Ms. M. had no contact with her daughter other than through a mail drop with the exchange of gifts and cards at birthdays and Christmas. She struggled with thoughts of being a "not good enough mother," repeating the mistakes of her own parents, and abandoning her child.

Ms. M. continued in treatment. Her recovery was punctuated by periods of crisis with self-harm and sometimes suicidal intent, which were always worse when she was misusing substances. However, her motivating and protective factor throughout was her daughter and the hope that she could resume contact once the child was 16 years old.

When the child was 9 years old, she ran out into the path of a car while in the care of her adoptive mother and was killed. There was a significant delay before Ms. M. was informed of the death because the social worker felt that she was not stable enough to receive the news and might attempt suicide.

Ms. M. did make a significant suicide attempt and was briefly admitted to hospital. She insisted on leaving once she was declared medically fit. She was supported in the aftermath, mainly by the addiction service and social work team. She made good progress with respect to her opiate addiction and talked about the death of her daughter as a catalyst for this improvement.

However, Ms. M. remained unable to come to terms with her guilt at giving up her child to a mother who, in her mind, had allowed the child to die. She felt unable to grieve, and this was compounded by not having played a part in planning or attending the funeral (she was not informed of the death until afterward). She said that there would have been some consolation if arrangements had been made for her daughter to be an organ donor. For her, this would have given meaning to her daughter's life and death, in the sense of offering a kind of life after death.

Discussion

Ms. M. appears to have been nominally a Christian but not an active member of any church community or congregation. Her spirituality did not appear to play a major part in her life, but certain implicit religious beliefs came to the fore when her child was so tragically killed. The funeral would have provided both an important rite of passage and an opportunity to deal with grief and mourning, but these were unhelpfully denied to Ms. M. At such times, even in a post-Christian society, religious ceremonies continue to provide spiritual meaning and support. In this case, an important source of meaning and purpose might also have been provided had possibilities for organ donation been properly explored. Ms. M. found in this domain some way of understanding "life after death" that could have been a source of significant comfort and hope.

Ms. M. did not have any of the resources, either of a traditionally religious kind or based on the principles of the Twelve Steps, to help her deal with her sense of guilt and failure as a mother. Guilt, and the need to forgive and be forgiven, are issues that frequently (perhaps even universally) need to be addressed during the course of recovery from addiction. Within a purely medical context, therapeutic and psychological approaches to addressing these issues can be helpful but are not as universally recognized as within the 12-step programs and most religious approaches to assisting recovery.

Whereas the social worker in this case was clearly operating out of a well-intentioned concern to avoid distressing her client, it was clear that the pain of grief could not ultimately be avoided and that delay in breaking the news of the child's death was likely to cause additional problems rather than resolve existing ones. Closer liaison between social and medical services, and particularly more careful planning of how to support Ms. M. through her receipt of the news of the death of her child and her subsequent grief, might have avoided the eventual distress she experienced.

CONCLUSIONS

The foregoing cases illustrate just some of the ethical issues that arise when working in addiction psychiatry in the UK. We are aware that other contexts, cultures, and subcultures present different, and differently emphasized, concerns. For example, within the context of a strongly religious culture such as that found in many Islamic countries, there are opportunities for greater integration between treatment and religious belief and practice (Abdel-Mawgoud et al., 1995; Ali, 2014), and there is probably also greater uniformity (rather than plurality) of belief within the population served. However, we believe that these different contexts offer mainly differently emphasized ethical issues, rather than a completely different set of issues. In particular, we identify the following issues as among the most important ethical considerations.

First, the professional and the patient may or may not share the same spiritual/religious perspective. Nothing can be taken for granted, and identification with a shared faith tradition (e.g., Islam, Christianity) may conceal greater differences than between a doctor and patient of different traditions. It is therefore important for the professional to have the clinical skills and ethical awareness to explore sensitively and affirm in a patient-centered fashion the beliefs, belonging, and practices of their patient which, generally speaking, may offer hugely positive coping resources. Even if they do not, it is important that the clinician properly understand the conflicts or tensions that a patient may perceive as a result of his or her faith perspective. A treatment professional should not hesitate to offer a spiritual/religious treatment option that may be of benefit to the patient, even if the professional does not personally subscribe to, or agree with, the spiritual or religious tradition concerned.

Second, medical and spiritual/religious approaches to treatment generally need present no conflict with each other. However, in some cases they do, especially when a medical goal of harm reduction accepts that abstinence may not be possible in the short term or even at all (Inciardi & Harrison, 2000). When conflicts are perceived, they can often be negotiated and misunderstandings clarified. It is important (as in Case 1) that possible tensions should not be left unresolved to the detriment of treatment and that patients should be supported in managing them. This may require much patience on the part of the treatment professional.

Third, there are often expressed or unexpressed feelings of guilt on the part of the person receiving treatment that arise from the physical, psychological, and social harm that has been inflicted as a result of addictive behavior. Substance misuse may also have been a way of coping (maladaptively) with unresolved guilt or anger at real or perceived offenses, whether inflicted or sustained. At the heart of the phenomenon of addiction is a struggle within the self which is an inherently spiritual issue. Many such considerations are explicitly addressed within a 12-step approach to treatment, but they are not always identified as important within medical treatment programs. In Case 2, more specific attention to the sense of guilt that Ms. M. carried as a mother might have gone a long way toward preventing the eventual significant distress.

Fourth, there are some specific issues regarding 12-step treatment programs that can lead to ethical concerns. As helpfully summarized by Wendy Dossett (2013), they include the potential dangers of emphasizing powerlessness over addiction (especially for women), as well as particular concerns regarding the Judeo-Christian religious emphasis and the stigma associated with self-identification as an addict or alcoholic. Each of these concerns is associated with valid counterarguments, and they may also impinge differently upon different people. For example, an emphasis on powerlessness for a woman who has been repeatedly abused may be profoundly unhelpful and may be a good reason for considering alternative approaches to recovery, or at least additional support and counseling aimed at addressing the particular dilemmas involved in accepting powerlessness over addition while not accepting powerlessness in relationships with men.

Perhaps the most important ethical consideration of all is simply that the need for treatment should be acknowledged and that treatment should be available equally for all. Patchy geographical availability of treatment (Drummond et al., 2005) and the stigma that prevents access to treatment or labels people as undeserving of treatment are (or should be) important considerations in treatment service planning and in relation to any attempt to inform professional and public attitudes.

REFERENCES

Abdel-Mawgoud, M., Fateem, L., & Al-Sharif, A. I. (1995). Development of a comprehensive treatment program for chemical dependency at Al Amal Hospital, Damman. *Journal of Substance Abuse Treatment, 12*, 369–376.

Ali, M. (2014). Perspectives on drug addiction in Islamic history and theology. *Religions, 5*, 912–928.

Cook, C. C. H. (2006). *Alcohol, addiction and Christian ethics.* Cambridge, England: Cambridge University Press.

Cook, C. C. H. (2009). Substance misuse. In C. C. H. Cook, A. Powell, & A. Sims (Eds.), *Spirituality and psychiatry* (139–168). London, England: Royal College of Psychiatrists Press.

Cook, C. C. H. (2013a). Controversies on the place of spirituality and religion in psychiatric practice. In C. C. H. Cook (Ed.), *Spirituality, theology and mental health* (1–19). London, England: SCM Press.

Cook, C. C. H. (2013b). *Recommendations for psychiatrists on spirituality and religion.* London, England: Royal College of Psychiatrists.

Cook, C. C. H. (2014). Suicide and religion. *The British Journal of Psychiatry, 204*, 254–255.

Dossett, W. (2013). Addiction, spirituality and 12-step programmes. *International Social Work, 56*, 369–383.

Drummond, C., Oyefeso, A., Phillips, T., Cheet, S., Deluca, P., Winfield, H., Jenner, J., ... & Christopolous, A. (2005). *Alcohol Needs Assessment Research Project (ANARP): The 2004 National Alcohol Needs Assessment for England.* London, England: Department of Health.

Inciardi, J. A., & Harrison, L. D. (2000). Introduction: The concept of harm reduction. In J. A. Inciardi & L. D. Harrison (Eds.), *Harm reduction: National and international perspectives* (pp. vii–xix). Thousand Oaks, CA: Sage.

King, M., Marston, L., McManus, S., Brugha, T., Meltzer, H., & Bebbington, P. (2013). Religion, spirituality, and mental health: Results from a national study of English households. *British Journal of Psychiatry, 202*, 68–73.

Kurtz, E. (1991). *Not-God: A history of Alcoholics Anonymous.* Center City, CA: Hazelden.

Mason-John, V., & Groves, P. (2013). *Eight-step recovery: Using the Buddha's teachings to overcome addiction,* Cambridge, England: Windhorse.

World Health Organization. (1992). *The ICD-10 Classification of Mental and Behavioural Disorders.* Geneva, Switzerland: World Health Organization.

FOURTEEN

Geriatric and End-of-Life Psychiatry

John R. Peteet, M.D.

BETWEEN 2013 AND 2040, THE NUMBER OF INDIVIDUALS AGED 85 YEARS and older in the United States is expected to grow from 6 to 14.1 million. The aging of the population makes increasingly insistent several clinical and related ethical challenges that have significant religious/spiritual dimensions. In this chapter, we considers the definition and implications of personhood, the meanings and value of autonomy, optimal care at the end of life, existential challenges and spiritual needs of the elderly, and the needs of caregivers. We conclude by discussing a case with the use of the Four Quadrant Model of Jonsen and Winslade (see Chapter 1).

THE DEFINITION AND IMPLICATIONS OF PERSONHOOD

The daughter of a 75-year-old patient with progressive Alzheimer's dementia described her father as "not there anymore." She reported not only grieving the loss of his capacities but beginning to think of him as already dead.

Personal identity in the post-Enlightenment West is typically grounded in an individual's abilities and accomplishments. The corollary, evident in our attitudes toward the elderly and disabled, is that one is less a person when one has lost important capacities and independence. In other cultures with a greater emphasis on a person's social role as opposed to cognitive capacity, individuals may be protected in the early stages of impairment from the marginalization that is sometimes experienced by those in more developed countries (DeBaggio, 2003; Whitehouse, Gaines, Lindstrom, & Graham, 2005). Spiritual traditions also offer a more relational and transcendent view. For example, Christians believe that every person has value because he or she is known and loved by God. As John Swinton (2012) pointed out, seeing a demented person as "living in the memories of God" both locates the individual and his family within the larger framework of reality and underscores the importance of narrative and community to being human.

Recognizing societal tendencies to marginalize and devalue those who are no longer independent and capable, many religious lay and professional people feel a calling to serve "the least"
of these persons, and faith-based organizations have frequently led the way in the care of the
elderly and disabled (Vanier, 1979).

THE MEANINGS AND VALUE OF AUTONOMY

*An 80-year-old man with end-stage heart disease was re-hospitalized for congestive heart failure
after dietary indiscretion and told his treatment team that he was ready to die. His physicians
agreed to disconnect his implantable defibrillator and designated his code status as DNR/DNI.
His wife objected, arguing that he was in acute distress. Once his fluid status improved, he seemed
ambivalent about dying.*

Understandably, the first question in making difficult decisions with impaired elderly individuals is, "What does the patient want?" The capacity of an individual to make a medical or
other major life decision is often difficult to assess. Frequently, as suggested by this case, cognitive capacity is given more weight than emotional and situational factors. Although respect for
autonomy is generally acknowledged to surpass in importance other ethical principles in our
Western culture (Beauchamp & Childress, 2012), it is less well appreciated that the term has
multiple meanings. For example, *autonomy* can refer to a right (implying duties and claims)
or to a good (a worthwhile object or end). Using the term in bioethics in only the former way,
to refer to a right to self-determination (sometimes termed *personal sovereignty*), can give an
incomplete clinical picture. An individual may have the right of self-determination yet lack
autonomy in several other senses. For instance, if that individual is constrained by external
circumstances from putting his personal sovereignty into action, he lacks autonomy understood
as *liberty*. Or, a patient may lack the capacity to make rational decisions for himself, a critical
test of competency for medical decision making. This condition might be referred to as a lack
of *basic cognitive autonomy*. In discussions of psychotherapy, autonomy often refers to freedom
from undue influence by undesired or ego-alien affects and cognitions. Such freedom may be
termed *intrapsychic autonomy*. And *formal autonomy* is the actual condition of individual self-
government or self-legislation.

These multiple meanings of autonomy become important when considering the ethical
mandate to respect autonomy. Psychiatrists, accustomed to fostering intrapsychic autonomy,
often see this goal as requiring therapeutic neutrality. And yet, as Bishop, Josephson, Thielman,
and Peteet (2007) pointed out, the concept of neutrality itself has several meanings. Like autonomy, it was first used as a political term, denoting nonalignment with other states or political
entities. Later, it came to refer to a means of respecting some form of another's autonomy. The
term *intrapsychic neutrality* refers to a technical stance employed by a psychotherapist to avoid
a countertherapeutic alignment with any of the structures of the patient's intrapsychic world
(i.e., id, ego, and superego) (Gabbard, 1994). As a kind of equipoise with respect to the patient's
conflicts, it creates an important space for examining them together in an evenhanded way. By
comparison, *ethical* (or *conscientious) neutrality* implies the attempt to refrain from allowing
one's morals, values, or worldview to influence another's thinking or actions.

With the pervasive acceptance of psychodynamic understanding within our culture, intrapsychic neutrality—a technical *means* to a therapeutic end—has become conflated with, and

taken on some of the ethical weight of, respect for the *right* to personal sovereignty. The concept has also lent an aura of medical or scientific weight to what had been a purely moral conception. All of this has helped to obscure the ethical role of the clinician in going beyond acquiescence to the patient's wish to be free from constraints to promotion of the patient's individual (formal) autonomy, understood as his fullest possible functioning.

As Bishop et al. (2007) put it, "The idea of formal autonomy recognizes that self-legislation expresses itself in much more than mere individual, isolated decisions. Rather, it implies a relationship between—on the one hand—desires that lead to action and, on the other, commitments, perspectives, and a life narrative that are, in some special way, the individual's own. It also implies some degree of self-mastery" (p. 170).

Autonomy, then, in this formal sense, requires authenticity. My actions are autonomous if they are, in some particular sense, my own. (They can still be authentically mine even if influenced by others. Pure independence is not necessary for autonomy.) Formal autonomy thus involves what has been termed *conditions of authenticity* that cannot be adequately captured by the concept of mere individual autonomy. A number of ethicists have pointed out that, in day-to-day medical practice, autonomy has essentially been reduced to the ritual of informed consent. Such a reduction is consistent with an uncritical tendency to think of autonomy as being expressed primarily in individual, isolated, self-determined decisions. And it fails to take into account the role that trust and delegation of authority play in real-life medical and psychiatric practice. O'Neill (2002) argued that a procedure such as informed consent may increase trustworthiness because compulsion by procedural safeguards can serve to protect certain rights. Therefore, there is real value in such consent-informing procedures. But procedural safeguards do not necessarily thereby increase trust.

Trust, a relational attitude, is dependent on one's surrounding community, and authenticity, a condition of formal autonomy, is dependent on one's narrative and values. Both highlight the religious and spiritual dimension of the task of fostering formal autonomy. Using the case presented earlier as an example, a clinician caring for the patient would want to assess not only the patient's insight into his medical condition and the consistency of his attitudes toward aggressive care but also how his core values and his relationship to his community inform these views. How authentically does he ground them in a religious tradition or comparable set of basic beliefs? Does he need help to clarify these attitudes or to resolve ambivalence? Who in his spiritual life and community is best positioned to provide this resource? Have conversations taken place with his spouse, adult children, or pastor during prior medical hospitalizations or before surgeries regarding his preferences for care that could shed light on his convictions and remaining questions?

OPTIMAL CARE AT THE END OF LIFE

A 70-year-old professor newly diagnosed with lung cancer asked about options for assisted dying.

What values should shape our society's provision of care at the end of life? Recent years have seen increasing interest in quality of life at the end of life, as evidenced by the growth of the specialty of palliative medicine and the reception of Atul Gawande's book, *Being Mortal* (2014), which brought to the fore our culture's neglect of what is most important to the dying.

Somewhat paradoxically, research has correlated the use of religious coping with more aggressive care at the end of life (Phelps et al., 2009), perhaps related to hopes for a miracle or to mistrust of the medical establishment. Receiving spiritual care from the hospital team, on the other hand, is associated with less aggressive care at the end of life (Balboni et al., 2009). Studies are now underway to assess whether information and attitudes of community clergy about end-of-life care could be contributing factors.

A growing number of countries and American states have legalized physician assistance in dying (PAD). Older individuals make up the largest number of those requesting PAD, the vast majority to preserve a sense of dignity and control rather than to escape pain. In Belgium and the Netherlands, the basis for requesting PAD has extended beyond terminal illness to psychiatric diagnoses, with many requesting individuals found to lack support and to feel "tired of living" (Kim, DeVries, & Peteet, 2016). Attitudes toward PAD tend to correspond to worldviews: PAD supporters are often secular humanists committed to the relief of suffering, whereas more traditionally religious individuals are more likely to support comfort, community, and help for individuals to bear and put into perspective their suffering. Psychiatrists, who are accustomed to assisting individuals find meaning in their lives rather than choose suicide, may be opposed to participating directly in PAD but see value in agreeing to work with individuals who are considering this option in order to help them better understand their conditions, motives, and options.

Some religious traditions, not necessarily valuing the extension of physical life for its own sake and seeing death not only as an end but also as a beginning, provide rituals for voluntary stopping of eating and drinking. This process is seen by Jains as death with equanimity, although Indian courts have ruled it equivalent to suicide (Braun, 2008).

All of these considerations highlight the need to explore and take into account the religious/spiritual dimension of a patient's request to end his or her life and of the clinician's own response.

EXISTENTIAL CHALLENGES
AND SPIRITUAL NEEDS OF THE ELDERLY

A 65-year-old, married, retired elementary school teacher required nursing home placement for dementia and intermittent catatonia. His son asked his pastor for the name of a Christian psychiatrist who was unaffiliated with his treatment team. The patient was unspontaneous but, when asked his opinion, said he had been reading a hymnal.

Aging inevitably is accompanied by existential challenges, which can become overwhelming and may bring individuals to psychiatric attention. How should clinicians think about the spiritual resources that patients need to deal with them?

Wisdom in late life reflects a developed inner life, and the continuity of this life frequently reflects a relationship with a larger, spiritual context (Atchley, 2009). Measures of religious faith correlate with longevity, well-being, and resilience, and positive spirituality, with its connection to wisdom, has been suggested as a fourth factor in successful aging (Crowther, Parker, Achenbaum, Larrimore, & Koenig, 2002). At the same time, religious distress (i.e., feeling abandoned by God or questioning God's love) has been associated with greater mortality among hospitalized elders (Pargament, Koenig, Tarakeswar, & Hahn, 2001).

Aging can present existential challenges in relation to identity, hope, meaning or purpose, guilt, and autonomy or connectedness. Identity is frequently threatened by the loss of social role entailed in retirement and in the loss of defining physical and mental capacities—no more poignantly than in progressive dementia. Yet studies have shown that spiritual well-being can be preserved into late stages of dementia. As Swinton (2007) pointed out, demented persons remain in relationship to others, including God. Given that implicit (primarily unconscious, diffused, symbolic, affective and not language-based) memory is often better preserved, ritualized practices may remain accessible and meaningful despite an individual's loss of cognitive capacity. Oliver Sacks (1998, p. 37) described what he saw when a nurse asked him to "watch Jimmie in chapel and judge for yourself":

> I did, and I was moved, profoundly moved and impressed, because I saw here an intensity and steadfastness of attention and concentration that I had never seen before in him or conceived him capable of . . . . Fully, intensely, quietly, in the quietude of absolute concentration and attention, he entered and partook of the Holy Communion. He was wholly held, absorbed, by a feeling. There was no forgetting, no Korsakov's then, nor did it seem possible or imaginable that there should be . . . . [C]learly Jimmy found himself, found continuity and reality, in the absoluteness of spiritual attention and act.

Hope becomes more difficult for many aging individuals to preserve as their future becomes truncated, and they become vulnerable to depression. Yet a spiritual perspective can help one to preference *being* over *doing* and to live in the present, "becoming friends of time," feeling less judged by clock time. As Swinton (2007, p. 253) put it:

> We are called to learn what it means to be in the moment, to notice the small things that the world rejects or explains away. We need to learn to live differently with time. To do so requires that we recognize where it is that we are living. If 'the world' is actually creation, then we live in God's created time, and God created time for a purpose. Time doesn't just happen; it is created by God, sustained by God, and if we take time to listen, directed by God. Time matters. Living in God's created time means, if nothing else, that time is intentional, meaningful, and purposeful.

Thus hope gives purpose even at the end of physical life.

Meaning and purpose can be difficult for the elderly to sustain without such a spiritual perspective, and a spiritual perspective can be difficult to sustain in the presence of depression or trauma.

A 70-year-old woman with an abusive childhood and early marriage saw a therapist for years and was vulnerable to traumatic memories and feeling suicidal under stress. Although she had once attended seminary, she had became disappointed in her church and struggled to believe in a God who "could have created me so damaged." Nevertheless, she retained a love of the natural world, which had been her refuge since childhood, and felt sustained by volunteering with children at a nature center.

Therapists may need to lend their own hope in a purposeful life to such patients but must remain mindful of their countertransference-based risk of imposing what is meaningful or important to them onto the patient. Duff Waring has thoughtfully discussed the role of a therapist in helping patients to see what a morally satisfactory life might look like and how the desirable virtues might contribute to it (Waring, 2016, p. 98).

Guilt and regrets over a long life may be prominent concerns of elderly patients, particularly those who are depressed or estranged from family members.

An 83-year-old man took an overdose of pills and required psychiatric hospitalization for stabilization. His chronic depression had been stable on medication for years until his wife developed

Alzheimer's dementia and his daughter took an extended vacation. In retrospect, he described feeling that he had failed to care adequately for his wife. Obtaining outside help for her 3 days a week and providing transportation for the man to his weekly Bible study group were important interventions.

Resources for forgiveness, grounding, and community may lie in faith communities with their familiar prayers, Bible readings, hymns, and attendance at shared worship services. Such experiences can powerfully connect a patients to core aspects of the person he has always been because they tap into procedural or implicit memory. These memory processes, the kind that govern such things as riding a bicycle or playing a musical instrument, are controlled by brain structures below the cerebral cortex (e.g., the cerebellum), which are relatively resistant to Alzheimer's disease in its early and middle stages. A dramatic example was provided by Oliver Sacks's interview with a 92-year-old former musician named Henry who was suffering from dementia and who emerged from his apathetic, abulic state on hearing music from his era (Abdul-Rouf, 2012). A number of resources, including sample worship services, that take this phenomenon into account are now available for fostering the spirituality of individuals with dementia (see, for example, http://www.spiritualityandaging.org/aging-service-professionals/).

THE NEEDS OF CAREGIVERS

A family with three small children took in an elderly grandparent after a stroke left him hemiparetic and somewhat disinhibited. After 3 months, they decided they could no longer care for him despite feeling a religiously based obligation to do so.

The dilemma of how much to sacrifice for an aging relative is becoming increasingly common; often, it is intertwined with the dilemma of how to weigh considerations of safety against the desire of a failing loved one to remain at home. Spirituality can play a central role in making these decisions, as a basis of core values, as a source of support (including through prayer), and as an encouragement to self-reflection (Koenig, 2005). Values typically endorsed by faith traditions include interdependence over individual self-interest, sacrifice consistent with basic self-care, and the practice of caring and hospitality by the community. Pastoral counsel may be helpful for individuals struggling to understand how these values should be interpreted or apply in a given case. Because this struggle can be overwhelming at times (Ewing, 2005), support groups and written resources may also have a role (http://www.spiritualityandaging.org/faith-group-leaders/). In *The Moral Challenge of Alzheimer Disease* (2002), Stephen Post urged church communities to become prepared for and more proactive in the area of dementia caregiving by becoming aware of the realities of the disease; offering support groups for family caregivers; and providing respite care for patients so that the caregivers can rest and rejuvenate.

The following case vignette uses the Jonsen Four Quadrant Model to analyze and discuss ethical aspects of the treatment of an elderly woman who was ambivalent about her faith.

CASE VIGNETTE

A 73-year-old woman diagnosed with lung cancer refused surgery, not only because she feared its limited potential benefit and likely morbidity but because she felt her life was already barely worth living. She was attached to her dog, enjoyed reading to children at her local library, and saw a neighbor regularly, but she was in only occasional contact with her son, who lived out of state. The diagnosis of cancer added to her existing medical problems of chronic back pain and chronic obstructive lung disease.

Medical Indications

Today, a diagnosis of lung cancer needs to be further qualified as to the mutation involved, because immune therapies for some types now provide extended periods of disease control with a good quality of life. This patient's fear of treatment and relative isolation raise the question of whether a psychiatric diagnosis is presenting an obstacle to good care and potential recovery, if not cure. Further history revealed that she had married young to escape a critical and controlling mother, only to find her husband physically and emotionally abusive. In an effort to protect her son from his father, she later felt, she had given him too much, contributing to his attitudes of entitlement and anger. Despite a period early in her life when she had attended a charismatic church and studied theology, she harbored an expectation of being disappointed by God and in life. Although she did not meet criteria for major depression, her vulnerability to demoralization significantly influenced her view of what entrusting herself to the care of others might be like.

Patient Preferences

In favor of accepting treatment was the value she placed on giving to others on her own terms and on managing her own life without interference. Weighing against it were her intolerance for feeling vulnerable, helpless, and out of control as she expected to become in the process. For her, the proposed treatment raised the questions of whether she could trust her caregivers to respect her wishes if she reached the limit of what she could stand and whether God was ultimately interested and good rather than indifferent, if not cruel.

Quality of Life

If the objective of all clinical encounters is to improve, or at least address, quality of life for the patient, as experienced by the patient, how are the unknowns of her prospects to be weighed? Is there a reasonable chance that she could be treated with the prospect of ultimately maintaining her quality of life without making it intolerable for her in the meantime? And if she had an adverse outcome, what could be done to help her feel that her life was still satisfactory?

Contextual Features

In spite of her relative isolation, her decision making was taking place in a wider social context, including not only her physician and her therapist but also her son, the law's provision for her to express advance directives, the fate of her dog, her spiritual views about her ultimate fate, and her ability to afford more care should she need it.

Discussion

Given all of these considerations, what should be the clinician's role in addressing them? From a principle-based perspective, benevolence would incline a clinician to help the patient accept potentially life-saving treatment, whereas avoidance of harm would make one cautious about doing more damage than good, including to the patient's fragile psyche. Respect for autonomy would also impel one to listen to the patient's reservations and her wish to limit interventions. However, promoting formal autonomy would call for a clinician to promote the conditions of trust and perceived safety that could allow the patient to make the most rational decision possible. It is here that virtue ethics can shed some light on what this dilemma could look like from the perspective of a psychotherapist. Waring (2016) described the treatment of the Demoralized Woman in ethical terms of self-regard; the aim was to help her treat and care for herself so as to cultivate a satisfactory life. Put another way, the qualities of self-love and self-respect provided the foundation on which she could engage her critical interests and thus achieve an authentic way of living.

The therapist has a role in helping the patient to see that she is worthy of self-regard, but this responsibility is ultimately the patient's. Positive psychology can contribute a fuller understanding of positive mental health concepts such as attitudes toward the self; growth, development, and self-actualization; integration; perception of reality; and autonomy and environmental mastery (Waring, 2016, p. 83). If spiritual/religious resources are not too conflicted to be readily available (as they might be in this case), they are often significant factors in the therapeutic project of helping the patient approximate her best self. Lacking access to positive aspects of her religious faith, this patient's therapist would do well to attend to the spiritual meaning and purpose in her relationships with others, including her dog.

In summary, elderly individuals face existential challenges in the areas of personal identity, autonomy, mortality, and caregiver burden. The clinical and ethical dilemmas raised by these concerns have religious and spiritual dimensions that are often important for their clinicians to address.

REFERENCES

Abdul-Rouf, M. (2012). *Old man in nursing home reacts to hearing music from his era* [YouTube video]. Retrieved from https://www.youtube.com/watch?v=NKDXuCE7LeQ.

Atchley, R. C. (2009). *Spirituality and aging.* Baltimore, MD: Johns Hopkins University Press.

Balboni, T. A., Paulk, M. E., Balboni, M. J., Phelps, A. C., Loggers, E. T., Wright, A. A., . . . & Prigerson, H. G. (2009). Provision of spiritual care to advanced cancer patients: Associations with medical care and quality of life near death. *Journal of Clinical Oncology, 27,* 1–7.

Beauchamp, T. L., & Childress, J. F. (2012). *Principles of biomedical ethics* (7th ed.). Oxford, England: Oxford University Press.

Bishop, L., Josephson, A., Thielman, S., & Peteet, J. (2007). Neutrality, autonomy and mental health: A closer look. *Bulletin of the Menninger Clinic, 71,* 164–178.

Braun, W. (2008). Sallekhana: The ethicality and legality of religious suicide by starvation in the Jain religious community. *Medicine and Law, 27*(4), 913–924.

Crowther, M. R., Parker, M. W., Achenbaum, W. A., Larrimore, W. L., & Koenig, H. G. (2002). Rowe and Kahn's model of successful aging revisited: Positive spirituality—The forgotten factor. *The Gerontologist, 42.* 613–620.

DeBaggio, T. (2003). *When it gets dark: An enlightened reflection on life with Alzheimer's.* New York, NY: Simon & Schuster Adult Publishing Group.

Ewing, W. A. (2005), Land of forgetfulness: Dementia care as spiritual formation. *Journal of Gerontological Social Work, 45,* 301–311.

Gabbard, G. O. (1994). *Psychodynamic psychiatry in clinical practice: The DSM-IV edition.* Washington, DC: American Psychiatric Press, Inc.

Gawande, A. (2014). *Being mortal: Illness, medicine, and what matters in the end.* New York, NY: Metropolitan Books.

Kim, S. Y. H., DeVries, R., & Peteet, J. R. (2016). Euthanasia and assisted suicide of patients with psychiatric disorders in the Netherlands 2011–2014. *JAMA Psychiatry, 73,* 362–368.

Koenig, T. L. (2005). Caregivers' use of spirituality in ethical decision-making. *Journal of Gerontological Social Work, 45,* 155–172.

O'Neill, O. (2002). *Autonomy and trust in bioethics.* Cambridge, England: Cambridge University Press.

Pargament, K. I., Koenig, H. G., Tarakeswar, N., & Hahn, J. (2001). Religious struggle as a predictor of mortality among medically ill elderly patients: A two-year longitudinal study. *Archives of Internal Medicine, 161,* 1881–1885.

Phelps, A. C., Maciejewski, P. K., Nilsson, M., Balboni, T. A., Wright, A. A., . . . & Prigerson, H. G. (2009). Religious coping and use of intensive life-prolonging care near death among patients with advanced cancer. *JAMA, 301,* 1140–1147.

Post, S. (2002). *The moral challenge of Alzheimer disease: Ethical issues from diagnosis to dying.* Baltimore, MD: Johns Hopkins University Press.

Sacks, O. (1998). *The man who mistook his wife for a hat and other clinical tales.* New York, NY: Touchstone.

Swinton, J. (2007). Forgetting whose we are: Theological reflections on personhood, faith and dementia. *Journal of Religion, Disability & Health, 11,* 37–63.

Swinton, J. (2012). *Dementia: Living in the memories of God.* Grand Rapids, MI: Eerdmans.

Vanier, J. (1979) *Community and growth.* London, England: Darton, Longman & Todd.

Waring, D. R. (2016). *The healing virtues.* Oxford, England: Oxford University Press.

Whitehouse, P. J., Gaines, A. D., Lindstrom, H., & Graham, J. E. (2005). Anthropological contributions to the understanding of age-related cognitive impairment. *Lancet Neurology, 4,* 320–326.

FIFTEEN

Child and Adolescent Psychiatry

Carol L. Kessler, M.D., M.Div., and Mary Lynn Dell, M.D., D.Min.

CONSIDERATIONS AT THE INTERFACE OF ETHICS, RELIGION, AND spirituality are common in the practice of child and adolescent psychiatry. Not every instance is a quandary, a dilemma, a matter of patient safety, or a threat to the clinician's relationship with the child and family. However, when serious matters involving a child's or family's religious and spiritual beliefs and practices do arise, few resources exist to guide mental health clinicians as they manage these often weighty issues. There are publications in the pediatric literature that address ethics and/or religion/spirituality in general pediatrics and in some pediatric subspecialties. An example is the issue of objection to immunizations and certain treatments based on families' religious beliefs or practices (American Academy of Pediatrics [AAP] Committee on Bioethics, 1997, 2013; Kelly, May, & Maurer, 2016). Ethics and religion/spirituality are increasingly the subjects of attention and research in pediatric palliative care (AAP Section on Hospice and Palliative Medicine, 2013; Wiener, McConnell, Latella, & Ludi, 2013). Whereas ethics in child psychiatric practice and research has received considerable attention in the past decade, relatively little has been written about religion and spirituality as a topic separate from ethics (Dell, 2004; Josephson, 2004).

The clinical issues at the interface of ethics, religion/spirituality, and child and adolescent psychiatry are limitless. This chapter seeks to help fill the void in the literature concerning ethics, religion/spirituality, and child mental health in a way that is most helpful to practicing clinicians struggling with these issues in their daily clinical contacts. Three specific areas are addressed that commonly present challenges:

1. Religious/spiritual objections to psychiatric care
2. Ethical issues and the clinician's relationship with children, adolescents, and families
3. Ethical issues that may arise when mental health clinicians work with religious/spiritual professionals and institutions

The religious and spiritual beliefs and practices of both patient populations *and* the mental health clinicians who serve them are becoming increasingly diverse. Therefore, significant attention is given to ethical questions and quandaries that can arise due to the ever-expanding religious, spiritual, and cultural beliefs, rituals, and other practices of mental health providers and religious/spiritual leaders working with children and families.

RELIGIOUS/SPIRITUAL OBJECTIONS TO PSYCHIATRIC CARE

General Themes

A common theme for religious and spiritually-minded patients is fear that mental health providers will be dismissive of their beliefs. Distrust of psychiatry became most acute during the Freudian psychoanalytic era for those religious patients who were aware of Freud's view of religion as an illusion (Freud, 1927). Psychiatry developed a reputation as a discipline of primarily atheists. Theologian Hans Kung spoke of religion as "psychiatry's last taboo" (Kung, 1979). More likely, mental health providers refrained from being open about their own religious identities to avoid stigma. Faced with a "blank screen," patients may refrain from using God-talk to avoid being pathologized by their provider.

More recently, religion/spirituality has gained the respect of mental health providers, who are encouraged to incorporate it into a biopsychosocial and culturally competent perspective (Josephson, 2004). Religion and spirituality may be a critical component of "what's at stake" for patients and may be central to the meaning of their illness (Kleinman & Benson, 2006).

Parents who see a spiritual etiology for their child's emotional or behavioral problem may seek religious guidance and deem psychiatry to be irrelevant. For example, a Guatemalan-American maintenance worker at a children's mental health center in the Bronx shared that his Pentecostal brethren had tried to persuade him that the clinic was a negative influence on the community. The psychiatric clinic was viewed as tempting the distressed to seek help where there is none, because only the Lord heals.

Interviews about religious/spiritual coping among depressed African American youth found a similar sentiment of the primacy of religion in mental health. A qualitative analysis found that "sometimes rigid ideals and values held within faith communities could be a hindrance" to seeking mental health care (Breland-Noble, Wong, Childrens, Jankerson, & Sotomayor, 2015). Songs calling on people to "take everything to God in prayer" and to "wait on the Lord to strengthen your heart" have offered solace and hope since the time of slavery. Many African Americans lean on prayer and on the church; they also have significantly lower rates of mental health service utilization. Whereas some youth in this study by Breland-Noble et al. identified religion as a motivator for seeking mental health care, others voiced the belief that "Christian Black people are usually like, okay, 'All you have to do is take your troubles to God and he'll deal with it.'" One commented, "I think that people, teenagers especially, don't get help because of what other people say about . . . how you should pray . . . and you don't need drugs because all you gotta do is pray." The message that prayer alone is the key encourages a deferential or deferring religious coping style that dissuades active engagement with mental health services (Breland-Noble et al., 2015). Turning to psychiatry may be seen as betraying God and lacking faith (Dein, 2004).

Communities with histories of oppression and marginalization may have rich healing traditions offering indigenous, holistic care that is more trusted than medical/psychiatric services. The black church has been compared to a therapeutic community (McRae, 1998). It serves as a reminder of an ongoing struggle for liberation and provides a place to cry out, sing, pray, and lay one's burdens down. Central American immigrants bring with them spirit-based illnesses of *susto* (trauma-based loss of soul) and *mal de ojo* (the evil eye). Traditional healers called *curanderos* practice in immigrant communities prescribing herbs, prayers, and rituals. Family from one's country of origin may send herbs from the afflicted one's native soil. *Santeros* heal in the Yoruban tradition, which originated in Nigeria and traveled with slaves to the Caribbean, that blends gods of nature with Roman Catholic saints. They prescribe healing baths, beads, and herbs and invite members to dance and chant to the rhythms of the saints (McNeil & Cervantes, 2008). Hindu individuals may seek balance from ayurvedic medicine before venturing to the realm of psychiatry (Black, 2004). If faced with a psychiatric encounter, those immersed in alternative healing may fear judgment of their beliefs and practices.

For recent immigrants from impoverished countries, psychiatry may have terrifying associations.

A 17-year-old Peruvian-American man was referred for a psychiatric consultation by his primary care provider in a federally qualified community health center in Westchester County, New York. He sat trembling before the psychiatrist. When asked why he was so frightened, he said, "If I was sent to see a psychiatrist, I must be in bad shape." In his country of origin, there were no community mental health centers; those seen by psychiatrists were the severely mentally ill in underfunded mental hospitals (Nolan & Whetten, 2011). Perhaps the wealthy had access to quality care. For this young man, to see a psychiatrist meant that his doctor believed him to be "insane." Once the purpose of the consultation was clarified, he settled into a psychiatric evaluation, and at the end he declared, "I feel that my soul has been cleansed."

Most religions do not see psychiatry as a source of care for the soul, and may see manifestations of mental illness as spirit based.

The mother of a 14-year-old girl, Maria, was convinced that she was cutting herself and verbalizing suicidal thoughts because she had been cursed by playing a Ouija board. The mother could not see any role for psychiatry and had difficulty listening to her daughter's report of the family as a source of distress. The depressed teen was more acculturated and less religiously affiliated than her mother; she easily engaged in treatment. She acknowledged fear instilled by her mother's belief that she had been possessed despite doubting that possibility.

CONSIDERATIONS IN PROTESTANTISM AND CATHOLICISM

Mental illnesses, particularly psychotic disorders, are frequently interpreted to be demon possession in certain Protestant denominations. A survey of 500 evangelical Christian church leaders revealed that almost 30% investigated possible demonic influence and prayed for deliverance when made aware of mental illness (Simpson, 2013). Parents facing their child's psychosis may feel torn between recommendations of the church and psychiatric formulations.

A 45-year-old, single Dominican-American mother agreed that her 11-year-old son, Juan, who was responding to command hallucinations, needed inpatient psychiatric care. Because it took time to stabilize Juan, his mother wondered whether her Pentecostal brethren were correct. They were convinced that Juan's problems could be attributed to the Devil, who was attacking him to dissuade her from continuing in her path of becoming a pastor. Referral to a Spanish-speaking National Alliance for Mental Illness (NAMI) parents' group and matching with a parent peer offered support and psychoeducation. However, the woman's church was her only local "family," and she valued her role of child educator and her relationship with a 90-year-old pastor there. Her church began to feel unsafe when Juan returned to the community. Although she taught children, church brethren took it upon themselves to heal and to exorcise demons from Juan. They prayed over him, exhorting the Devil to leave his body. Juan began to have difficulty sleeping. His mother worried that Juan's psychosis was worsening because he said there were devils at night. Juan clarified, "They pray for the devil to leave from me; so it makes me feel that the devil must be inside of me. They squeeze my head when they pray and it hurts. Doesn't Jesus say, 'Let the children come unto me'? So why do they pounce on me?" Juan's mother was torn between loyalty to her pastor and love of teaching and her concern for her son. She decided to have Juan become her teaching assistant so that he would not become prey to her church brethren's good intentions.

Attribution of psychotic symptoms can be found in other Protestant denominations as well.

The Iraq-born Assyrian Christian parents of an 11-year-old girl presented to a Jewish-sponsored community mental health center with concern that their daughter had begun to hear voices of demons that terrified her. Her father was a seminary student, and his mentor had recommended exorcism. He wanted a psychiatric consultation and welcomed the notion that his daughter was suffering from anxiety and that the voices, which occurred primarily at night, might ease with appropriate therapeutic intervention. Indeed, as the psychiatrist and clinical social worker worked with the child and her family to develop her coping skills, the voices faded away.

Acute emotional distress may also be attributed to the spirit world in the tradition of Santeria.

A 12-year-old boy, Gabriel, presented with depressive symptoms as well as compulsions to read the Bible, to obtain holy water to clean the home, and to hold on to a rosary. These symptoms began shortly after Gabriel reached out to his biological father, who had been absent from his life. His father denied paternity. Gabriel's mother was a practicing Roman Catholic who feared that the father, who practiced Santeria, had placed a curse on Gabriel. Although she denied belief in Santeria, she feared its power. She sought support from her religion by requesting a nun's prayers and obtaining a blessed rosary. She also faithfully attended psychiatry and social work sessions at the Bronx Mental Health Center with Gabriel, who responded to antidepressant medication and therapy to address his disappointment with his father.

Some patients are lost to follow-up when they comply with a school's suggestion of a psychiatric evaluation yet ultimately opt for a spiritual cure. For example, a 6-year-old girl presented with her mother and extended family. She had been hearing voices at night and was unable to sleep. The family declared that they would go to their Roman Catholic Church to pray. They never returned to the clinic.

Aside from demon possession or curses, some religious traditions may attribute disturbed behavior or thoughts to a sin-sick soul. The cure is seen as "spiritual work wherein people work harder and harder to achieve a greater level of righteousness that will justify freedom from illness." Those who suffer may be shamed and told, "If you've got a problem, you must not be walking with the Lord" (Simpson, 2013). A depressed and/or anxious adolescent may feel ashamed to come forward to ask for help if it means being labeled "of little faith."

Parents of impulsive, disruptive children may be seen as lacking in discipline in some Christian settings. Parents may feel shamed by their children's behavior. Instead of hearing encouragement to seek professional help, parents may be judged, and their children may be shunned (Mercer, 2004). In some cases, the distorted biblical warning, "Spare the rod, spoil the child," may encourage corporal punishment.

A 5-year-old boy with attention-deficit hyperactivity disorder (ADHD) went Christmas caroling. There was snow on the ground, and he delighted in making snowballs. The organizer of the church event shouted, "Stop!" The child stopped until the next home, where he returned to play in the snow. Incensed, the leader grabbed the child's coat and yelled to his parent, "Can't you control that boy?"

In this case, a message of disciplining the bad trumped the notion of a child with a behavior disorder who is in need of care.

CONSIDERATIONS IN JUDAISM

Unlike Christians, Jews seldom see mental illness as purely spiritually based. Biological and social stressors are acknowledged as contributing factors. Psychiatric medications are accepted by the religion as God-given remedies. The psychiatrist is seen as empowered by God to heal. The Code of Jewish Law advises choosing the most competent medical professional, regardless of religion (Loewenthal, 2006). Nevertheless, psychotherapy may be suspect if not performed by a rabbinically endorsed therapist, particularly in the Orthodox and ultra-Orthodox communities. Judaism is a religion of orthopraxis, of doing right, as defined by the Torah. Laws prescribe behaviors surrounding food, sexuality, and family life. There is emphasis on honoring one's parents and on refraining from gossip and slander. Loyalty to family and community is primary. Secular therapy may be seen as disrespecting the Torah, by permitting expression of negative feelings toward one's parents and by valuing individuation and autonomy. It may risk the "danger of the unguarded tongue," which can harm the speaker, the listener, and the object of discussion. Girls and boys begin to bear adult moral and spiritual responsibility for these transgressions at 12 and 13 years of age, respectively (Loewenthal, 2006). A rabbinically endorsed therapist would respect Jewish religious prohibitions against masturbation and premarital sex and would help the patient accept and cope with the Torah's 613 commandments (Margolese, 1998).

Many Orthodox Jewish families will opt for care outside of the community due to concerns about professionalism and confidentiality. Mental illness is carefully hidden to prevent it from affecting the marriage prospects of the entire family. Providers outside the community may ensure anonymity and protect against stigma (Rube & Kibel, 2004).

Ultra-Orthodox Jewish parents may have difficulty seeking inpatient care for their children. They would accept an inpatient environment only if it allows adherence to the Torah. Respect for ultra-kosher meals, restraint from exposure to unacceptable media, and means of access for parents on the Sabbath would be essential (Sublette & Trappler, 2000).

CONSIDERATIONS IN ISLAM

Concerns that religious values will not be upheld by mental health providers may also dissuade Muslims from seeking psychiatric care. Like Judaism, Islam is a religion of right practice, *orthopraxy*. Sharia paves a path of right-relation between self and neighbor as well as self and God (Pridmore & Pasha, 2004). The Quran offers valued advice regarding anger, panic, and phobia. For help in times of distress, a devout Muslim may feel more comfortable confiding in an imam who is a trusted interpreter of the Quran. Alternatively, a Sufi master might be consulted to indicate a path to God through prayer and worship (Sabry & Vohra, 2013). Western psychotherapy may be seen as too focused on individuation and as permitting unacceptable sexual behavior.

Although religious-based counsel is available, a medical model of mental health care is not incompatible with Islam. In fact, when medieval Europeans were at the height of exorcising demons, the Muslim scholar Ibn Sina claimed mental disorders to be physiologically based (Ciftci, Jones & Corrigan, 2012). As early as 705 C.E., in Baghdad, Iraq, the physician al Razi used psychotherapy and medicine in the world's first psychiatric ward (Sabry & Vohra, 2013). And so, psychopharmacology is an acceptable treatment modality. It is a gift from God who in Muhammad's words provides "a cure even as He has sent down the disease."

Adherence issues may still arise. During the fasts of Ramadan, Islamic patients may stop taking their medications. They may not be aware that they are exempt from fasting should it compromise their health (Sabry & Vohra, 2013). Another barrier to medication adherence may arise if the inert components contain pork products. A gelatin- or stearic acid–containing medication would not be halal or kosher and would be forbidden to both Muslims and Orthodox Jews. Yet, Jewish and Muslim religious leaders have declared animal-derived medication acceptable if it is "the only way to maintain life" (Hoesli & Smith, 2011). Providers demonstrate respect for a patient's religion and the ethic of truth-telling by informing them of any animal products in prescribed medication and seeking an acceptable means of administration.

Although Islam boasts the first psychiatric unit, there is tremendous variation in the treatment of the mentally ill across 50 Muslim-dominant countries from Asia to Africa, with mental health services ranging from Westernized psychiatric hospitals to reliance on traditional exorcism. Spiritual explanations of mental illness include demon possession and divine punishment. Unique to Islam is the notion of possession by Jinn—invisible creatures made of smokeless fire that become visible at will. When visible, these creatures of Islamic folklore have black tails and goats' hooves; they are capable of driving people mad. In a 2012 study in the United Kingdom, many Muslims acknowledged strong belief in Jinn, black magic, and the evil eye (Gholipour, 2014). Traditional healers—shaykh, dervish, or pir—would more likely be consulted than psychiatrists. Prayer, music, dance, and Quran reading would be prescribed. The Jinn might also be beaten out of the afflicted person (Sabry & Vohra, 2013).

Many Muslims avoid interacting with psychiatry out of fear of marginalization within their community. They may refrain from acknowledging depression and suicidality because suicide is a grave sin. Merely acknowledging depressive symptoms may feel unacceptable. A family may hide mental illness for fear that everyone in the family will be labeled as a poor marriage candidate. Men in the Muslim community may have difficulty adhering to the recommendations of a female practitioner. Women may feel uncomfortable being in a therapeutic relationship with a man. It has been found that Muslim parents are more likely to seek professional help for children who have autistic disorders or intellectual disabilities than for those with emotional difficulties (Cifti, Jones & Corrigan 2012).

Since the September 11 attacks, Muslims in distress may also refrain from seeking treatment because of fear of discrimination by providers and being branded as "terrorists." Those who wish to seek help may be unaware of available resources. The British Royal College of Psychiatrists created "Feeling Stressed? A Leaflet for Muslims," to clarify the role of mental health care and to share ways to seek help. It speaks to traditional concepts of mental illness (e.g., Jinn, evil eye) while offering mental health care as an alternative (Ahmed, 2012).

ETHICAL ISSUES AND THE CLINICIAN'S RELATIONSHIP WITH CHILDREN, ADOLESCENTS, AND FAMILIES

The Royal College of Psychiatrists has provided other materials to assists mental health providers attempting to reach across the religiosity gap that is often attributed to Freudian theory . This gap affects day-to-day psychiatric care and compels providers to acknowledge its presence in order to provide effective treatment. Ironically, Freudian notions of transference and countertransference provide a lens to focus on dynamics within and between patient and provider that influence effective communication (Dein, 2004).

Comas-Diaz and Jacobsen (1991) developed the notion of ethnocultural transference and countertransference to examine the influence of a patient's cultural background on the therapist's response and vice versa. Abernathy and Lancia (1998) expanded on their work by discussing religiocultural transference and countertransference—how perceived religious differences or similarities affect the therapeutic relationship. They distinguished interreligious from intrareligious transference and countertransference based on whether the therapist and patient have different or similar religious backgrounds.

Religion, unlike race and gender, is not immediately apparent unless individuals dress or don religious symbols that are indicative of their faith tradition. There may be a temptation to ignore its presence. The first author of this chapter has the last name Kessler, and patients may assume she shares a Jewish background, whereas in reality, she is the daughter of German immigrants and a pastor in the Evangelical Lutheran Church in America. Should such a presumption on the part of a patient be articulated, she may be tempted to remain silent to avoid a possible negative transference. It may not be appropriate for her to clarify her religious identity in a moment of crisis; however, lack of clarification prevents authentic relationship. Similarly, her fluency in Spanish and cultural awareness stemming from immersion in Central and South America may lead a patient to be perplexed about her ethnic and religious identity. Clarification of her German-American roots and Latin American journey provides a roadmap for patients to navigate the relationship. Religious or ethnic identity can be clarified to orient patient and provider (Asnaani & Hofmann, 2012).

Self-awareness is critical in the therapeutic process. When working with religious content, a provider needs to consider several factors. First, one needs to gauge how open one should be to religion so as not to avoid or overemphasize it. There is the danger of feeling immobilized when faced with a patient's powerful beliefs. A provider may avoid discussion of religion due to insecurity, fear of being insensitive, or not being able to address spiritual issues. She may minimize a child's spiritual insights. Second, one needs to be attuned to both one's own as well as the patient's religious orientation. A provider may devalue a patient's faith tradition and fear that those feelings will be apparent. A patient's faith tradition may evoke anger and be seen as harmful. A provider may feel uncomfortable with cultural tension and therefore act as if the patient and provider are of the same group. A provider may struggle with how revealing to be about her own faith tradition. She may be concerned that the power differential will lead to the imposition of her worldview. Alternatively, a provider with conflicted religious experiences may feel uncomfortable navigating spiritual matters. Third, one needs to be open to consultation with peers and/or clergy to clarify a patient's religious practices. A provider may have stereotyped notions of a patient's religion and could benefit from reality testing regarding the "normality" of the patient's beliefs. One may clarify whether a patient's image of God or notion of sin is a distortion of the norms of his community (Dein, 2004).

Dynamics vary depending on whether the patient and provider share a religion. Whereas a provider from a different faith tradition may feel ill-equipped to deal with a patient's religious struggles, the patient may feel safer with someone who is neither a member of his community nor an idealized representative of his faith. Alternatively, both provider and patient might wonder whether someone within the patient's religion would better comprehend his plight. Yet, when religions match, there is the risk of overidentification and of hesitating to critically examine beliefs (Abernathy & Lancia 1998).

Transference issues may readily arise when a provider bears visible signs of a religion. For example, a Mexican-born Orthodox Jewish social worker and therapist wore a yarmulke and worked with a poor Latin American immigrant population in a community mental health center. He reported a stereotyping transference by his clients, who might never have knowingly interacted with a Jewish person before. Some felt compelled to convert him yet were able to agree with a position of mutual respect of different faiths. Others declared, "You're Jewish. I hear that Jews are rich and that they control everything." To this, he responded with humor: "If I were rich, do you think I'd be working here?" On the other hand, when he was working in schools in an ultra-Orthodox Jewish community, parents questioned his value because he was not as observant as they were.

A child psychiatrist and rabbi noted that the relationship between religion and psychiatry became more fluid after she assumed her rabbinical position. She found herself turning to prayer in her work with children at a residential facility and their families. When things reached a standstill and she knew that a family had a faith tradition, she invited them to choose a prayer. Often, the Transcendent was felt to enter the space, and the session could move forward. She was careful to invite only the patient's prayer choice so as not to impose her own tradition.

As a psychiatrist and pastor, one of the authors of this chapter (CK) recalled a time when she was doing clinical pastoral education, developing skills in spiritual counseling. Her pastoral supervisor said, "Don't leave your psychiatry hat at the door." As a novice pastor, she did not want psychiatry to intrude. With time, she came to understand that religion and mental health are interwoven within all of us. She allowed both approaches to inform her interventions while being careful not to impose her worldview on a patient.

It is not uncommon for patients to bear witness to their religion in their language, their beads, their headdress, and so on; the provider's response will determine whether these signs might lead to further understanding of the patient's belief system. God-talk is woven into the speech of many patients from Latin America and from the African American community. "God-willing" is frequently spoken, as well as "Thanks be to God," "God spare us," and "May God bless you."

A session with a 5-year-old girl, Raquel, fleeing the war in El Salvador focused on a prayer. She and her mother had lived in San Salvador, where the guerillas launched an offensive and were met with a military response. The street outside her home became the site of an intense battle. Airstrikes hit her home. Raquel sat in the Long Island office of a Salvadoran community agency where the practitioner was offering psychiatric treatment. She took a toy house, placed a doll inside it, and then grabbed crayons. The crayon "rockets" assaulted the house as Raquel repeatedly cried for Papa Dios/Father God to make the bullets disappear in mid-air. Posttraumatic play in Long Island had recreated an appeal to God in a setting that was not yet safe. Raquel heard the sound of planes and entered panic. Yet she also appealed to a God who promised rescue. God became one who could allow her to imagine a safe ending.

Prayer also became a focus in the treatment of a Turkish-American Muslim woman whose dress signaled her religious affiliation. She had confided in a colleague of the practitioner, who frequented her family deli, that she needed help after the birth of her son. She shared that she was horrified to be having thoughts or hearing a voice telling her to hurt her child. These ideas were ego-dystonic, and she was sure that she would not act on them. The colleague referred her to the community health center. She accepted antipsychotic and antidepressant medication. She also stated that she would pray to Allah to help her to cope with the haunting message to hurt her son, whom she adored. A safety plan was implemented, and the importance of her right-relationship with God was validated.

Whereas Raquel and the Turkish-American woman presented boldly with God-talk and prayer, some patients arrive with trinkets or attire that subtly point to their religion. It may be the provider who chooses whether to explore their significance to the patient. For example, a youth who bore the colorful beads of Santeria. was asked about them. He said they were a gift from a relative and that he wore them for protection but didn't know much more about them.

A 17-year-old Indian-American young man was brought by his mother due to concerns that he lacked motivation. They lived in an affluent, predominantly white neighborhood, and she freely shared her concerns about racism. She was upset that her son was presumed to be a supplier of illegal substances. The family practiced primarily Roman Catholicism yet also followed Hindu traditions. The psychiatrist noticed a black thread tied around the young man's neck. He explained that there was a reading when he was born that instructed him to wear the thread, whereas his sister was told to avoid the color red. His mother expressed embarrassment about these "primitive" ideas. She pointed out that he was also wearing a scapular from the Roman Catholic tradition. With encouragement, she shared that the thread was to protect against the evil eye. It remained a sacred object to her son.

ETHICAL ISSUES AND WORKING WITH RELIGIOUS/SPIRITUAL PROFESSIONALS AND INSTITUTIONS

Families can sometimes serve to clarify beliefs, yet there are times when outreach to religious leaders is indicated. Such outreach prevents providers from overstepping their bounds. Consultations may assist in diagnostic dilemmas—for example, to determine whether a child's statements are delusional or normative within his religion. Communication with faith leaders may also expand the patient's support network. Such consultations may be sought only with the consent of the patient's guardians, who may prefer to keep their mental health needs private (Dell, 2004).

Clarification of pathology became paramount when a psychiatrist was asked to consult with pediatric staff at a community hospital. A 13-year-old girl had been admitted to the pediatric unit after ingestion of pills in a suicide attempt. The girl shared that God spoke with her. Her parents stated that in their religious community it is not uncommon for people to say such things. To seek clarification, the psychiatrist requested permission to speak with the girl's minister. Both the girl and the parents agreed. The pastor supported the family's statements that community members often referred to God speaking with them. The pastor and the congregation were aware of the girl's hospitalization and inquired how to support her on her return home.

When psychiatrists interact with unfamiliar religious or spiritual traditions, they may underdiagnose, attributing perceived pathology to the religion, or overdiagnose. Collaboration with religious leaders may help to clarify the issue (Whitley, 2012). Indeed, many clergy are disappointed by the lack of outreach on the part of mental health professionals. Attempts to collaborate may not always yield consensus regarding a treatment plan. It remains the responsibility of the mental health professional to uphold the role of mandated reporter should neglect or abuse be present.

Some providers feel responsible to counteract the negative legacy that psychiatry has with religion by proactively forming ties with mistrustful religious people. For example, a Holocaust survivor and psychiatrist in Westchester County, New York, who directed a psychiatric hospital, built a relationship with the leaders of an ultra-Orthodox Jewish community. He made inpatient units acceptable to the laws of Torah so that leaders felt comfortable referring members of their community. Ultra-kosher meals were delivered. A girl was kept separate from her peers when they watched secular movies; she watched acceptable Orthodox movies instead. There was a place on the grounds for family members to stay, facilitating visits without use of vehicles on the Sabbath. There was even an *eruv* around the hospital to allow visitors to carry their belongings.

A 10-year-old girl was admitted to a psychiatric facility after calling the police and asking them to kill her. She was obsessed with religious laws and fear of not adhering to them. Her mother was Yiddish-dominant, and the psychiatrist managed to communicate in German. Her Christian psychiatrist explored the meaning of the law with the patient and her mother, wondering whether the law was not a gift from God rather than a tormentor. The psychiatrist relied on the mother, who understood the girl's relationship to the law to be distorted and excessive.

CONCLUSIONS

In summary, it is a provider's responsibility to be aware of his or her own worldview and to explore a patient's religious/spiritual ideology. Provider and patient may cross a boundary as they share religious identities. Providers must be prudent and not violate boundaries by imposing their own beliefs or prescribing religious practices. Should religious beliefs threaten a child's health, these concerns must be addressed with the family. Consultation with clergy can clarify whether such beliefs are consistent with the faith. Faith is not a justification for child abuse or neglect, and the safety of the child is paramount. More frequently, inquiry into a patient's religious world assists in identifying core issues and deepens the healing process.

It may be prudent for mental health providers to be open about their own religious identification and their attitudes toward other religions. In this way, children and their parents can know where their provider stands in the religious realm and whether they feel that there are irreconcilable differences. Parents are then free to seek help elsewhere with the assistance of the provider. A formal process of informed consent makes the spiritual dimension of treatment overt and reciprocally acknowledged.

Religion influences parenting. Young children with behavioral disorders may be labeled as sinners, and corporal punishment may be seen as an acceptable intervention. Consultation with clergy may clarify whether such behavior is normative. However, providers must educate parents about laws against physical abuse and must act to protect the child when indicated, regardless of whether the treatment is religiously endorsed. Exorcisms may be prescribed to children whose hallucinations are labeled demon possession. The nature of the exorcism must be clarified.

A 13-year-old Dominican-American adolescent was diagnosed with depression with psychotic features and had both inpatient and outpatient psychiatric treatment. The Roman Catholic mother was engaged with her daughter in psychotherapy, and both accepted psychopharmacologic intervention. The therapist became concerned she learned that the mother planned to spend part of their vacation in the Dominican Republic seeking a woman's help in performing an exorcism. Further exploration clarified that the exorcism would involve prayer and faith-based counseling. Isabel was looking forward to it and shared after she returned that it had brought her peace.

During adolescence, individuation may lead to discordance between parents' faith-based values and a teen's developing identity. Religions may prohibit masturbation, homosexuality, premarital sex, choice of mate, and substance use. These prohibitions may be protective, with teens involved in certain religious communities being less likely to use substances or to commit suicide. Yet in extreme cases, they may lead to young people being abused or getting expelled from their homes. Indeed, lesbian, gay, bisexual, and transgender (LGBT) youth are often vulnerable to homelessness due to their parents' faith-based intolerance. Other religious institutions have responded by turning their houses of worship into sanctuaries. In New York City, the congregation of Trinity Lutheran Church has created the Trinity Place Shelter, where LGBT youth are welcome 365 days a year (Trinity Place Shelter, 2016).

The Trinity Place Shelter is an example of a resource within a religious community. As mental health providers reach out to religious leaders, resources can be exchanged, and the religiosity gap can be narrowed. Many religious leaders are on the front lines of mental health crises and would value collaboration. Interviews of ministers, rabbis, and imams in the United Kingdom conducted in 2007 found that most had little or no mental health training and lacked confidence in dealing with mental illness in their congregations (Leavey, Loewenthal, & King, 2007). A 2012 survey sent to clergy in North Carolina had a low rate of response yet achieved representation from Christian, Jewish, Hindu, and Muslim religious leaders. Eighty-four percent of respondents saw a need for community mental health services for children and believed that psychiatrists and psychologists had important roles to play in their treatment. Most claimed that they endorsed the use of prescribed psychiatric medication. Yet, 68% indicated a preference to provide counseling rather than refer to mental health providers. As a group, they conveyed lack of confidence in their knowledge of specific disorders and their capacity to identify them. All expressed a desire to collaborate with mental health professionals, yet 48% felt that professionals fail to value their spiritual role in caring for those with mental disorders. They hoped to educate providers regarding their parishioners' beliefs and values. This might ease the clergy's concerns about providers' insensitivity toward spiritual needs. One respondent declared: "Sometimes the clergy and mental health professional ought to collaborate (with the patient's permission) but this is rarely encouraged." Yet, "Attention to religion can aid in the development of culturally competent and accessible services, which in turn may increase engagement and service satisfaction among religious populations" (Blalock & Dew, 2012).

A rapprochement between religion and psychiatry is indicated for the sake of all children and families. Recognition of religion and spirituality enriches our clinical work and calls us to cross over to religious communities to join forces in the struggle for mental health. Mutually shared taboos must be shed to enable cross-disciplinary relationships. On a larger scale, joint efforts of mental health organizations and religious communities have led to such entities as NAMI's FaithNet. This group within the National Alliance on Mental Illness "supports efforts to exchange information, tools, and resources to educate faith communities about mental illness and the vital role spirituality plays in recovery for many" (National Alliance on Mental Illness, 2017). These efforts create a bridge that can enrich children's road to recovery.

REFERENCES

Abernathy, A., & Lancia, J. (1998). Religion and the psychotherapeutic relationship: Transferential and countertransferential dimensions. *Journal of Psychotherapy Practice and Research*, 7, 281–289.

Ahmed, K. (2012). Feeling stressed? A leaflet for Muslims. Royal College of Psychiatrists. Retrieved from http://www.rcpsych.ac.uk/healthadvice/problemsdisorders/leafletformuslimsonstress.aspx.

American Academy of Pediatrics, Committee on Bioethics. (1997). Policy statement: Religious objections to medical care. *Pediatrics*, *99*(2), 279–281.

American Academy of Pediatrics, Committee on Bioethics. (2013). Conflicts between religious or spiritual beliefs and pediatric care: Informed refusal, exemptions, and public funding. *Pediatrics*, *132*(5), 962–965.

American Academy of Pediatrics, Section on Hospice and Palliative Medicine and Committee on Hospital Care. (2013). Pediatric palliative care and hospice care commitments, guidelines and recommendations, *Pediatrics*, *132*(5), 966–972.

Asnaani, A., & Hofmann, S. G. (2012). Collaboration in culturally responsive therapy: Establishing a strong therapeutic alliance across cultural lines. *Journal of Clinical Psychology*, *68*, 187–197.

Black, N. (2004). Hindu and Buddhist children, adolescents and families. *Child and Adolescent Psychiatric Clinics of North America*, *13*(1), 201–220.

Blalock, L., & Dew, R. (2012). A pilot survey of clergy regarding mental health care for children. *Depression Research and Treatment*. doi:10.1155/2012/742410

Breland-Noble, A. M., Wong, M. J., Childrens, T., Jankerson, S., & Sotomayor, J. (2015). Spirituality and religious coping in African American youth with depressive illness. *Mental Health, Religion and Culture*, *18*(5), 330–341.

Ciftci, A., Jones, N., & Corrigan, P. W. (2012). Mental health stigma in the Muslim community. *Journal of Muslim Mental Health*, *7*(1), 17–32. doi:10.3998/jmmh.10381607.0007.102

Comas-Diaz, L., & Jacobsen, F. (1991). Ethnocultural transference and countertransference in the therapeutic dyad. *American Journal of Orthopsychiatry*, *61*, 392–402.

Dein, S. (2004). Working with patients with religious beliefs. *Advances in Psychiatric Treatment*, *10*, 287–294.

Dell, M. L. (2004). Religious professionals and institutions: Untapped resources for clinical care. *Child and Adolescent Psychiatric Clinics of North America*, *13*(1), 85–110.

Freud, S. (1927). *The future of an illusion*. New York, NY: Norton.

Gholipour, B. (2014). Supernatural "jinn" seen as cause of mental illness among Muslims. *Livescience*. Retrieved from www.livescience.com/47394-supernatural-jinn-mental-illness-islam.html.

Hoesli, T. M., & Smith, K. M. (2011). Effects of religious and personal beliefs on medication regimen design. *Orthopedics*, *34*, 292–295.

Josephson, A. (2004). Formulation and treatment: Integrating religion and spirituality in clinical practice. *Child and Adolescent Psychiatric Clinics of North America*, *13*(1), 71–84.

Kelly, J. A., May, C. S., Maurer, S. H. (2016). Assessment of the spiritual needs of primary caregivers of children with life-limiting illnesses is valuable yet inconsistently performed in the hospital. *Journal of Palliative Medicine*, *19*(7), 763–766.

Kleinman, A., & Benson, P. (2006). Anthropology in the clinic: The problem of cultural competency and how to fix it. *PLoS Medicine, 3,* 1673–1676.

Kung, H. (1979). *Freud and the problem of God.* New Haven, CT: Yale University Press.

Leavey, G., Loewenthal, K., & King, M. (2007). Challenges to sanctuary: Clergy as a resource for mental health care in the community. *Social Science and Medicine, 65,* 548–559.

Loewenthal, K. M. (2006). Orthodox Judaism: Features and issues for psychotherapy. *The Psychologies in Religion, 1,* 1–24.

Margolese, H. C. (1998). Engaging in psychotherapy with the Orthodox Jew: A critical review. *American Journal of Psychotherapy, 52*(1), 37–53.

McNeil, B., & Cervantes, J. M. (2008). *Latina/o healing practices: Mestizo and Indigenous perspectives.* New York, NY: Routledge.

McRae, M. B. (1998). Black churches as therapeutic systems: A group process perspective. *Health Education and Behavior, 25,* 778–789.

Mercer, J. A. (2004). The Protestant child, adolescent and family. *Child and Adolescent Psychiatric Clinics of North America, 13*(1), 161–181.

National Alliance on Mental Illness. (2017). NAMI FaithNet [Web page]. Retrieved from http://www.nami.org/faithnet.

Nolan, J. A., & Whetten, K. (2011). Religious, spiritual, and traditional beliefs and practices and the ethics of mental health research in less wealthy countries. *International Journal of Psychiatry in Medicine, 42,* 267–277.

Pridmore, S., & Pasha, M. I. (2004). Psychiatry and Islam. *Australasian Psychiatry, 12,* 380–385.

Rube, D. M., & Kibel, N. (2004). The Jewish child, adolescent and family. *Child and Adolescent Psychiatric Clinics of North America, 13*(1), 137–147.

Sabry, W. M., & Vohra, A. (2013). Role of Islam in the management of psychiatric disorders. *Indian Journal of Psychiatry, 55,* 205–214.

Simpson, A. (2013). *Troubled minds: Mental illness and the church's mission.* Downers Grove, IL: InterVarsity Press.

Sublette, E., & Trappler, B. (2000). Cultural sensitivity training in mental health treatment of Orthodox Jewish inpatients. *International Journal of Social Psychology, 46,* 122–134.

Trinity Place Shelter. (2016). [Web page]. Retrieved from http://trinityplaceshelter.org/.

Whitley, R. (2012). Religious competence as cultural competence. *Transcultural Psychiatry, 49,* 245–260.

Wiener, L., McConnell, D. G., Latella, L., & Ludi, E. (2013). Cultural and religious considerations in pediatric palliative care. *Palliative and Supportive Care, 11*(1), 47–67.

SIXTEEN

Spirituality, Ethics, and People with Intellectual Disabilities

William Gaventa, M.Div., and Mary Lynn Dell, M.D., D.Min.

THERE ARE SIGNIFICANT DISCREPANCIES IN ESTIMATES OF THE NUMBERS of individuals with intellectual disabilities diagnoses. The lack of definitive statistics about these adults may be attributed to a lack of consensus about the definitions of intellectual disability, multiple data sources employing different methodologies, different populations reported (institutionalized or not), and the fact that many are still cared for in homes and settings that are more challenging to include in prevalence estimates (Yang & Tan, 2016). The life expectancy for adults with mild disabilities is approaching that of the general population, and those with more moderate and severe degrees of disability are also living well into their fifties and sixties. Adults with Down syndrome are commonly living into their fifties and beyond (Bittles et al., 2002; Janicki, Dalton, Henderson, & Davidson, 1999; Perkins & Moran, 2010). During the span 2006–2008, one in six children in the United States was estimated to have developmental disabilities, with a wide variety (Boyle et al., 2011). In 2016, the Centers for Disease Control and Prevention estimated that 1 of every 68 children has an autism spectrum disorder (Christensen et al., 2016).

The religious and spiritual lives of people with intellectual disabilities have been recognized and addressed in various ways by psychologists, therapists, social workers, families, other caregivers, and many religious communities for a number of years. Psychiatrists and other medical professionals have served this population through their skills of assessment, diagnosis, and treatment, especially psychopharmacology, and have increasingly recognized the myriad ethical issues associated with their care. However, mental health clinicians typically have had limited opportunities to consider the confluence of religion, spirituality, and ethics when caring for individuals with developmental disabilities, their families, and other caregivers.

This chapter addresses the spirituality of people with intellectual disabilities, with particular focus on those factors that are often critical to understanding their situations and perspectives when ethical topics or dilemmas arise in their mental health care. Basic information on disability and spirituality is provided. Principlism and ethics of care are discussed because these ethical theories are especially well suited to ethical thinking and decision making regarding those with disabilities. Common ways in which spirituality plays out in the lives of the disabled are considered. Throughout the chapter, the importance of family and other caregivers is highlighted. Suggestions for mental health providers are offered, and references for additional reading and study are provided.

AN OPENING STORY

We begin with a true story, adapted in small ways to maintain confidentiality.

Tony was a man who was referred to the student chaplain by the behavior therapist in a community-based agency serving adults with intellectual and developmental disabilities. He was living in one of the group homes, after having come out of a psychiatric center in which he had been placed because of hearing voices. Before that he had lived all his life with his mother, in her home, until she died around Thanksgiving a year earlier. There had been several instances of intense acting-out behavior in the group home and in a day program. The agency was beginning to question their ability to continue their support. Medication changes had not worked. In their initial conversation, the chaplain found out that Tony's mother had died a year before.

Tony had not been able to go to the funeral, nor did he know where she was buried. The chaplain discovered that Tony used to go to Mass with his Mom, that his favorite meal was her macaroni and cheese, and that the behavior therapist had promised they would make a memory box sometime but that had not yet happened. After several other visits—some of which included prayers by the chaplain and by Tony to his mother—and at least one more incident, the chaplain worked with Tony to plan a memorial service for his mother in his group home. They invited staff and a small group of acquaintances. A memory box was made, and the chaplain worked with Tony to prepare refreshments for after the service, including baking macaroni and cheese together. In the subsequent weeks and months, Tony's acting-out behavior diminished significantly, and the agency continued supporting him in their programs. The chaplaincy student continued to meet with Tony until the training program ended. Perhaps most importantly, people began to see Tony and his story, not simply his behavior.

In that short, true story, there are multiple issues related to disability, spirituality, psychiatric supports, systems of support, and the lack of community and relationships often faced by people with intellectual and developmental disabilities who end up in a service system after a double loss (in this case, of his remaining parent and of the home and community in which he had lived). The round robin of transfers between psychiatric and developmental services might have continued had not several people listened intently to Tony's words and behavior and realized that intellectual disability did not mean he was incapable of struggling with a number of spiritual issues including grief and loss. These professionals recognized that one possible course of treatment was to enable Tony to "act out" his grief in culturally sanctioned ways (i.e., through several rituals, in the context of supportive relationships). This enabled Tony to express his feelings in the context of a small caring community who recognized, affirmed, and validated his loss, memories, and transition.

Compared to many other people with intellectual and developmental disabilities, Tony was lucky, strange as it may sound, because he had access to a support network that included spiritual care and practices. No one made the assumption that Tony could not "understand" death because of his intellectual disability. Loss and grief, as well as isolation and disconnection from social connections, friendships, and participation in families and communities, are two of the frequently unnamed oceans in which many people with disabilities swim as people who are so often on the margins of community life. However, those core spiritual and human needs are noteworthy because of the lack of attention and support paid to them by many service providers. Yet the converse is also true: Other people with disabilities have very active and positive spiritual lives, participate in communities of faith, and make significant positive contributions to the lives of their families, others, and communal organizations in which they participate (Carter, Biggs, & Boehm, 2016; Gaventa & Carter, 2012).

Before examining some of these and other core spiritual dimensions of the lives of people with disabilities and their families, we first need to define disability and spirituality. Both are constructs or ways of describing dimensions of human life through different but intimately connected lenses.

DEFINITIONS OF DISABILITY AND SPIRITUALITY

The broad label of disability includes physical, intellectual, psychiatric, and sensory impairments. Disability also includes developmental disabilities originating before birth (e.g., Down syndrome, other genetic conditions), at birth (e.g., cerebral palsy), or in the developmental period (e.g., autism, which first manifests in the developmental period but is thought to include multiple genetic and environmental factors as cause). Disability also includes acquired impairments such as traumatic brain injury, spinal cord injury, and age-related disabilities, including dementia.

The definition has been gradually shifting from what is called a medical model of disability to a bio-socio-ecological model that defines and places disability at the intersection of physical causes interacting with environmental barriers, including physical, communication, attitudinal, and social (including legal) ones. The World Health Organization (WHO) first solidified this change in 1980 by promulgating a threefold definition of disability: It is first a physical *impairment*, which causes lack of capabilities (*disability*) in one or more areas; both of these conditions are heavily impacted by one's social and physical environment, resulting in a disadvantage or *handicap*. In other words, one may have an impairment and lack certain skills, but it is the environment that primarily disables and handicaps (WHO, 1993).

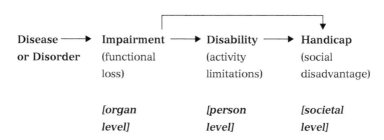

In a more recent model of the definition from the WHO, the International Classification of Functioning, Disability and Health (IFC), the social model became more explicit about the personal and social constructs (attitudes and meanings) of disability and explored environmental disabilities as those that cause a lack of participation (WHO, 2002).

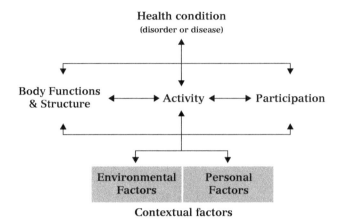

One of the crucial points for the sake of this discussion is that psychiatric conditions can be their own category of disability but they can also be acquired and evident in the lives of people with other forms of disabilities, as illustrated in the story that began the chapter. In the arena of intellectual and developmental disabilities, the label of *dual diagnosis* refers to having both an intellectual disability and emotional/psychiatric conditions, rather than the more typical understanding of dual diagnosis as a combination of psychiatric conditions and drug and/or alcohol addictions or dependencies.

In the context of the social and political movements for disability rights, inclusion, and self-determination, the power of disability as a label is evident in intense discussions and actions related to identity and community (e.g., Davis, 2013). The general rule of thumb is to use person-first language (Snow, 2017), such as, "John is a person with an intellectual disability." However, this is not the case in some circles. For example, the deaf community sees deafness as a culture, so that "John is deaf" or "John is a deaf person" is preferred. It is also not true in some parts of the autism world, in which the label is embraced and affirmed as a positive identity rather than a disabling adjective. Ethical issues and attitudes will be quickly assumed if labels are used without sensitivity, so the second rule of thumb currently is to acknowledge that as a medical or human service professional one has to use a particular term for billing and benefit eligibility, but then ask the person how he or she prefers to have their disability described.

People build their identity in a social context, with attitudes and meanings developed in the context of social expectations, values, assumptions, stereotypes, and traditions (i.e., culture). The question of identity is thus closely related to a second construct that needs definition, spirituality. *Spirituality* and *religion* are often used interchangeably, but there has been significant research and theoretical development leading to a concept of spirituality as a universal dimension of what it means to be human, with religion defined as the most historical and traditional forms in which individuals and cultures have developed and expressed their spirituality (Koenig, 2011; Miller & Thoresen, 2003).

There are many definitions of spirituality arising from different arenas of practice, research, and tradition. For example, famous spiritual figures may be ones known for their skills in prayer, writing, meditation, or other spiritual practices. Other definitions have come from the growing interest in research on spirituality in both acute healthcare and psychiatric/psychological disciplines. There are journals, and associations or parts of associations that explore intersections with spirituality in almost every medical and human service discipline considered to be scientific.

For this discussion on disability, our definition starts from the core values that drive many services and supports related to disability: independence, productivity, inclusion, and self

TABLE 16.1 Spirituality, Values, and Practices

Fundamental Human/ Spiritual Question	Core Spiritual Theme	Policy Value	Practices
Who am I?	Identity/Meaning	Independence	Person-centered language and planning, enhanced growth toward independence
Why am I?	Purpose, calling, vocation	Productivity	Employment, volunteering, making a difference
Whose am I? Who do I belong to? (Also closely related to culture)	Community connection	Integration/ Inclusion	Community inclusion, participation, least restrictive environment, citizenship, friendships
Where have I come from? Who are my people?	Cultural traditions, preferences, ways of understanding	Cultural competence	Person-centered planning, connections, honoring choice and uniqueness
How do I shape my own destiny? Why do bad things happen?	Choice, control, power	Self-determination	Advocacy, rights, empowerment

From Gaventa, W. (2016). Disability and spirituality: Re-membering wholeness. *Journal of Disability & Religion, 20*(4), 307–316.

determination (Gaventa, 2016). Those values are answers, primarily, to core existential questions of what it means to be human (Table 16.1).

Spirituality is understood as a construct that includes three core dimensions:

1. Core values, meaning, and identity, including what is sacred to someone
2. Connections and relationships to self, others, the sacred, time, and place
3. A sense of purpose, call, vocation, or obligation

These dimensions are all related to one's sense of self and the ways that sense of self both shapes and is shaped by the surrounding environment. Identity and relationships, for example, are initially bestowed, but then are further shaped by growth, experiences, preferences, and choices: i.e., they then help shape the surrounding environment.

Most psychiatrists and many other mental health clinicians are familiar with the *principlism school of bioethics,* which is most commonly associated with the work of Tom Beauchamp and James F. Childress (Beauchamp & Childress, 2013). They and other authorities in medical ethics have described four ethical principles that most moral individuals can agree are worthy to consider, abide by, or strive for when wrestling with ethical quandaries. There is general consensus among scholars and clinicians that these principles, perhaps more so than other schemas, form a framework to guide healthcare professionals in their work with patients and families—even when there is no specific ethical dilemma at hand (Ainslie, 2014). These ethical principles are *respect for autonomy, beneficence, non-maleficence,* and *justice* (Beauchamp & Childress, 2013).

According to Beauchamp and Childress (2013), *autonomy* refers to the ability to govern oneself without others attempting to control or limit one's choices. Although some people with intellectual disabilities have severe handicaps that limit their autonomy in the business, legal, and other sectors of our society, their abilities and desires regarding their faith and spiritual beliefs should be respected. Respect for autonomy insists that others in their lives encourage their interest in, and exploration of, spiritual and religious beliefs and practices that enrich, comfort, and facilitate a healthy wholeness of body, mind, and spirit. Respect for autonomy means that psychiatrists and others in their lives may still discuss with the intellectually disabled person and encourage reflection on fundamental human and religious questions. However, since these individuals are autonomous human beings, they must wrestle with these questions just as those who are not disabled in any way. Intellectually disabled individual should be permitted to think about who they are, whose they are, where they have come from, who their people are, how they shape their destiny, and why bad things happen (see Table 16.1).

Beneficence refers to the moral imperative to act so as to benefit others (Beauchamp & Childress, 2013). Of course, the care provided by mental health clinicians and others working with people with intellectual disabilities is offered in the spirit of beneficence, whether the offering consists of psychopharmacology, therapies, psychoeducation, family work, or vocational guidance and training. The Practices column in Table 16.1 reminds clinicians of some of the directions and goals to which their beneficent care contributes. Clinicians must remember that these practices apply to the religious and spiritual realms, not just the secular. A place to live, a job, and even a community of support can be just as hollow for the intellectually disabled as for the nondisabled if longed-for spirituality is lacking or not meeting very personal needs.

Often considered hand in hand with beneficence, *non-maleficence* is the moral imperative not to inflict harm or evil (Beauchamp & Childress, 2013). Psychiatrists try to avoid harming patients by diagnosing accurately, employing the fewest indicated psychopharmacological agents at indicated doses according to evidence-based standards, and referring appropriately to other medical specialists, psychotherapists, social workers, and others. In consideration of Gaventa's table, one can argue convincingly that being dismissive, uninterested, or obstructive with respect to the spirituality of intellectually disabled individuals would constitute maleficence. In some instances, not responding at all or not referring to a religious professional when a patient requests it or when circumstances indicate might also be considered harmful.

Justice means fairness—that which is equitable and does not show favoritism indiscriminately. Bioethics often deals with issues of *distributive justice,* or the application and expression of justice in the allocation of medical goods and services (Beauchamp & Childress, 2013). Certainly, injustices contributed to the rise of disability studies, advocacy groups, special services, and legislation passed to ensure that intellectually disabled people are treated fairly and with respect. Much of what is included in the Policy Value and Practices columns of Gaventa's chart (see Table 16.1) concerns matters of justice. Terms such as independence, productivity, and integration/inclusion describe values that matter to people with disabilities and have driven policies and the passage of new laws designed to "level the playing field" and enable more disabled people to become autonomous or achieve as much as they are able. Many of these values have been pursued through legislation that strengthens the rights of people with disabilities and their families (e.g., the Americans with Disabilities Act). The practices of community inclusion, citizenship, advocacy, rights, and empowerment are definitely issues of justice for people with intellectual disabilities and the medical and other professions that serve them, as well as for spiritual and religious communities and institutions who invite them into their midst to serve and be served.

When collaborating with religious/spiritual professionals or reading literature in the field of disability studies and disability theology, it is important for psychiatrists and non-theologically trained clinicians to be aware that often the religious and theological worlds have expanded the concept of *justice* to include situations, problems, and processes that would not typically be used in medical and psychiatric disciplines. An example is written by sociologist of religion Nancy Eiesland, the author of an early (1994) and seminal book in theology and disability entitled *The Disabled God: Toward a Liberatory Understanding of Disability*. In a 2001 newletter issue focused on faith and people with disabilities, Eiesland observed that the core responsibility of people supporting people with disabilities is to "just listen," by which she meant to listen with an ear for the justice issues in their lives:

> Just listening means attending to the ways in which everyday talk (and sometimes commonly accepted silence) makes claims about justice. They are not theories to be explicated or fully developed agendas to be followed, they are instead calls, pleas, claims upon some people by others. Personal and social reflection on the demands of justice begins in hearing, in heeding a call rather than in asserting and mastering a state of affairs. The call to be just is always situated in concrete social and political practices. Too often temporarily able-bodied people have been eager to devise strategies of response to what they deem as the unhealthy lives of persons with disabilities, before they have just listened. They have attempted to speak for us, deciding how and where we can best serve God, before they have just listened. They have pronounced us sacraments of grace, without listening to our fierce passion to be participants not sacraments. The process of examination of church and society must begin with listening, hearing the calls for justice expressed by people with disabilities who are among us. (Eiesland, 2001)

PEOPLE WITH DISABILITIES AND SPIRITUALITY

People with various forms of disability are quite "normal" in that they can have emotional and psychiatric issues just as anyone else can. The same applies to their experience, expression, and commitments in the realms of spirituality and faith or religion. Their spirituality, like anyone else's, is impacted by their personal experiences and quests, family environment, social context, culture, and religious interests.

However, returning to the interplay in the chart of spiritual questions, themes, social values, and practices, there are many ways by which the spiritual dimensions of disability are heightened or impacted by the lived experience of disability. Three of them are discussed in this section.

Identity

Social context makes assumptions about the meaning of disability and identity of people with disabilities. People with disabilities have been historically treated as outcasts, sinners, diseases, freaks, saints, objects of pity, beggars, advocates, and citizens (Bogdan, Elks, & Knoll, 2012; Kunc, 1996). They are thus swimming in a sea of interpretations and projections about their spirituality that shape their identities in negative or positive ways. For example, they can be seen as heroic overcomers of disability, or as sinners who are responsible for their own disability, or still in some parts of the world, as inhabited by demons or evil spirits.

For people with intellectual and developmental disabilities, the older scientific labels are now pejorative, including moron, feeble-minded, imbecile, and retarded. Whatever label is used, there are assumptions about their capacity to reason and make choices. It is clear, however, that people with even minimal intellectual ability can express preferences that are easily known by people who are close to them. One of the most promising legal developments in the last decade has been the development of "supported decision making" as a substitute for "legal consent." (See the Web site of the National Center for Supported Decision Making, http://supporteddecisionmaking. org.) These approaches start from opposite foundations. Legal consent and guardianship assume that someone is not capable of making decisions, which frequently leads to multiple decisions being made for them by others without their involvement or participation (i.e., they have no voice). Supported decision making assumes that a close circle of caregivers around a person can help determine the choices that person would prefer because of their intimate knowledge of the individual and their ability to involve him or her to the fullest extent possible.

Community

Understanding a dimension and outcome of disability as lack of participation also means that many people with disabilities are isolated and have limited circles of friends, companions, and co-workers. Loneliness and isolation influence quality of life and also have physical and emotional side effects. There is an exercise in person-centered planning strategies in the world of intellectual and developmental disabilities called the relationship map:

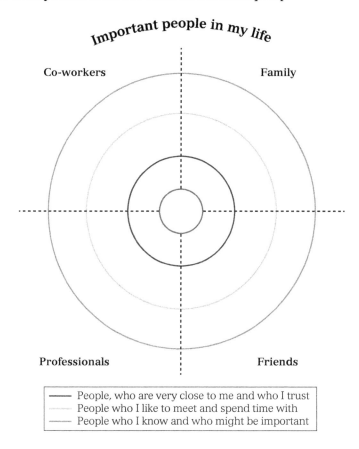

Frequently, people with disabilities have a few family members and fewer friends, especially in the circles closest to them, but multiple co-workers and professionals, who are usually more distant in terms of intimacy and closeness. This is often a stark and graphic illustration of the lack of positive friendships and involvement in community organizations other than service systems in which they are a consumer, client, or patient. So the question of "Who do I belong to?" often has limited answers. Lack of friendships is increasingly recognized as a core indicator of quality of life (Reinders, 2008). It can also be a matter of life or death. The person with multiple disabilities who is in the hospital for an acute care condition or illness is assumed to be lacking in quality of life because of value judgments made about the disability or assumptions about the lack of connections and community around that person. However, in an era of community inclusion, it is increasingly true that a wide network may be invested in the support and care of these individuals through family relationships, schools, Special Olympics, faith communities, and more. Beyond inclusion is a sense of belonging, with multiple dimensions (Carter, 2016).

Purpose

As for Identity, assumptions about the purpose of life for people with disabilities, particularly by others, have a profound impact on their spiritual lives and, indeed, on ethical issues that arise in their care and support. In a social context, others may assume that disability means life has little or no purpose or that a person with a disability is either a "consumer" of public goods and services or a "super-crip," an overcomer and achiever in spite of disability. That context makes it very difficult for people with disabilities to find opportunity and supports to discover their own sense of purpose, vocation, and call. People may say that the purpose of individuals with disabilities is to teach the rest of us important lessons about our own assumptions and the illusions that cover our own awareness of weakness, vulnerability and limitation. People with disabilities can also resent that role, as did the advocate and comedian Stella Young, who railed against "inspiration porn" (Young, 2014)—or a disability advocate who once told one of us, "Don't use me to work out your crap!"—especially if typical people are not willing to confer on them the value and worth attributed to teachers.

That "why" question of individual purpose for people with disabilities is often completely overshadowed by theistic questions about the purpose of assumed suffering coming toward them: "Why do I/you have this disability?" (Paterson, 1970, p. 41, quoted in Gaventa, 2016), "Why, God?" or "Why me/our child?" Questions from individuals who acquire a disability or from parents after receiving a diagnosis for their child are part of a profound personal emotional and spiritual journey of loss, grief, lamentation, and adaptation toward coping with what is sometimes called a "new normal" (Frank, 1997; Paterson, 1970; Reinders, 2014). In George Paterson's model of the question, disability or another event assumed to involve suffering can be caused by God for redemptive or retributive purposes, or not caused by God and thus either absurd or providential (i.e., God did not cause it, but God's presence and assistance were found in the journey).

IMPLICATIONS IN EXPERIENCE AND PRACTICE

If you ask a person with a disability and/or their family to tell you about their spiritual journey as part of your care and support, you will usually get a long story, either about the importance of their faith or spiritual community on the one hand or, on the other their experiences of feeling neglected, unwelcome, and/or hurt by things people say, even including outright requests from clergy and congregations for the family to leave or take their child out of a religious education program. One of the immediate ethical implications for psychiatrists and service providers is self-understanding of their role as professionals, their willingness to explore the arenas of spirituality and faith, and their willingness and ability to follow up on those issues in collaboration with the family. One of the more positive developments in psychiatry and psychology is that spirituality is not so quickly equated with symptoms of illness as was once the case. One of us heard a woman in New Jersey tell the story of her journey from mental illness through seminary to a role as chaplain. She noted than in her extensive psychiatric care, her interest in spirituality and faith was interpreted by psychiatrists and therapists as a symptom, while in her faith community, her mental illness made her an outcast.

A recent study by Erik Carter and colleagues involving 500 families in Tennessee found that the families placed significant importance on the role of spirituality in their family life and for their children (Liu, Carter, Boehm, Annandale, & Taylor, 2014), but that its interest and importance was not discussed or honored by the disability and health systems with which they dealt, nor by their faith community (Carter, 2013). One of the widely used models of spiritual assessment, the FICA process developed by Christina Puchalski at the George Washington Institute on Spirituality and Health (http://smhs.gwu.edu/gwish/clinical/fica/spiritual-history-tool), provides a simple yet comprehensive process for addressing spiritual questions and concerns (Puchalski & Romer, 2000). The FICA tool has four areas of questions that can be explored either quickly or in depth:

> _Faith:_ Preference, choice, tradition, identity. Do you consider yourself a person of faith, or are you religious?
> _Influence and Importance:_ How important is it to you? How does it influence your daily life?
> _Communal Expression:_ What form does it take, if any? Would you like it to?
> _Assistance:_ How can I/we assist you to address this part of your identity as part of your treatment or supports?

This is but one way in which issues related to spirituality and its power for healing and support as well as their opposites might be explored.

The following discussion is not exhaustive but is meant to present some of the variety of possible ways in which issues in spirituality are played out in the lives of people with disabilities.

Equating Faith or Spirituality with Reason and Capacity to Understand

People often assume that individuals with intellectual and developmental disabilities cannot understand matters of faith or spirituality—or, if they do understand, that they experience them only as "eternal children." Clergy and congregations do not make the same assumption about children because there are multiple ways in which faith communities provide opportunities for learning and growth. Anyone involved in inclusive spiritual supports can tell stories of profound questions or insights voiced by people who do not have high IQs. It becomes an issue for the whole family when a child with a disability is refused rites of transition such as first Communion, baptism, confirmation, or bar/bat mitzvahs. A Roman Catholic mother once told a nun visiting a worship service at a residential facility after her son had received first Communion in his late twenties, that "when the priest rejected my son as a child, they rejected me." At an inclusion workshop, one of us heard two parents talk about their faith experiences. One mother had a child on the autism spectrum, and the other a child with mental health issues. The first mother had been asked to leave 13 congregations, the second, 17. That is an extreme, but the amazing part was that both had eventually found welcoming and inclusive faith communities. The young man with mental illness in fact found a community for himself, and then invited his parents to join him, after they had given up trying. There are now multiple resources and examples of ways that children and adults with many forms of disability are being given the opportunity to learn and grow in their spiritual lives in the context of faith communities.

A second and similar manifestation of this false equation of spiritual issues and needs with reason concerns assumptions about the capacity of individuals with intellectual and developmental disabilities, including those on the autism spectrum, to understand death or experience grief and loss, as was illustrated earlier in this chapter. The loss of close relationships with family, friends, or staff can have a profound impact on individuals with disabilities; if not recognized and honored, this becomes "disenfranchised grief" and can lead to behavioral acting out in ways that are injurious to oneself or others. Again, there is a growing body of research about grief and loss for individuals with intellectual and developmental disabilities. Adapted materials for helping them understand at the level of their ability are available. There is increased focus on the importance of their being included in culturally normative ways of expressing and responding to grief and loss, such as attending wakes and funerals, sending sympathy cards, making memorials, visiting gravesides, praying, and taking opportunities to share and express one's feelings. As this is being written, there is an online conversation among people who are searching for resources online to help a teenager with autism who found a parent who had committed suicide. One of the clear ethical implications for psychiatrists and others who may be consulted to deal with acting out behaviors is the need to explore the causes of the behavior and see if there are potential connections to grief and loss. Approaches such as positive behavior supports are much more humane and ethical than a quick resort to medication.

Finally, a third manifestation is expressed in behavior in congregational settings not related to grief or loss. Young people and adults with intellectual and developmental disabilities, especially those on the autism spectrum, often grow up without the opportunity to participate regularly with their families in their faith tradition. Later, if the doors open and people seek to include them, their lack of appropriate behavior is often blamed on their disability (e.g., "They don't know better," "They act that way because they are [you name the disability"]). The real issue is that they have not had the chance to grow up and absorb (i.e., practice) the traditions and expectations of that faith community or any other. In the language framework of autism supports, every faith community has a hidden curriculum of rules, expectations, and behaviors that one may step right over or violate because they are not explicit and because individuals have not had time to learn through practice and repetition. As in many areas of adaptive supports, when faith communities realize the problem and implement ways of helping people learn and practice, the resulting changes can be appreciated by any stranger who comes to that congregation.

Judgments by Others About the Connection Between Disability, Sin, and Faith

Individuals with disabilities of many varieties tell stories about experiences of being asked by others (religious or not) what they did that caused their disability. It is a common question or assumption. Had they been cursed by God or others? Are they now, in one sense or another, "unclean?" The assumption is that there must be a reason or cause which could have been avoided. Often there is not, but that does not stop the questions. The psychological and spiritual implications of guilt, rejection, and stigma are clear.

There is a second dimension of this connection that is just as problematic: the assumption or belief that stronger faith will lead to a cure. It is a connection that is rejected in the Christian tradition in the Gospel of John, Chapter 9, when the disciples asked why a man was born blind: "Was it his fault or his parents?" The reply was neither. The answer, "so that the grace of God might be manifest," is often misinterpreted to mean that he was created this way so that Jesus could heal him through a miracle. A more accurate interpretation is that this is an opportunity for others to respond, out of their sense of the grace of God, and extend that grace to the blind man as well. Many people who use wheelchairs or who have other obvious physical disabilities can recount stories about strangers who have come to them and asked if they could "pray over them." People with disabilities have to develop their own ways of responding to those invasions of spiritual space and meaning. One man with a physical disability had his own answer that reversed the question. Told by a stranger on the street that if he had enough faith, he could be cured, his response was, "If you had enough faith, you could heal me."

To be fair, secular practices have also put this kind of spiritual pressure and judgment on people with disabilities. Some treatment regimens for children with multiple disabilities, such as the once popular "patterning" and others for autism, often imply, implicitly or explicitly, that if someone does not make progress, it is because they or their parents are not following the regimen tightly enough. Mental health professionals know that people with mental illness often face prescriptions from others that if they would just get their act together, they would be all right. One of the clear ethical issues in all of these diagnoses or prescriptions is that people would never make the same connection regarding a person with an acute medical illness or disease for which there is an assumed cure.

Issues of Hospitality: Access, Accommodation, Participation, and Welcome

People with disabilities and their families have far too many experiences of not being able to get into a community building, such as a church or synagogue, but they may report that the attitudinal barriers are even worse. Those are the ones that impact their sense of welcome and their ability to participate and belong. The clear connection between spirituality, ethics, and these social constructs of disability is not simply related to rights to participate as citizens but to the fact that lack of welcome or rejection violates in fact what the faith community or other organization preaches. For example, most churches have on their signs or Web pages the invitation that "Everyone is welcome." That may not turn out to be the case, and even if a person with a disability is welcome, issues of access and accommodation may make participation impossible. The deeper ethical issue for communities of faith is that all of the major faith traditions have two core injunctions: first, something like the Golden Rule of "doing unto others as you would have them do unto you" and, second, a version of "love your neighbor as yourself," or "show hospitality to strangers."

The spiritual and psychological impact of failed hospitality can be profound. A favorite story is of the parents who, when asked in private to "Tell me your church story," said their experience was still too hard to talk about in public. Where they previously lived, their daughter, labeled as microcephalic and moderately retarded, had been a supported employee at McDonald's. When they moved to a different state, their new community did not have a supported employment program, and the daughter returned to a sheltered workshop, where she began to lose some of the social skills she had acquired as an employee. They began to "church shop," and after yet another bad experience in a young adult program, they came home to hear the daughter say, "No more church, Mom." The mother tried to convince her that the church was God's house and that they needed to belong, whereupon the daughter cut to the quick with the simple statement: "Well, it may be God's house, but He is not home." This is just one example of the ways in which spirituality and faith may be used to make barriers of access and welcome even worse by assumptions and practices that are justified in God's name. It is also an example of the kind of profound insight that can come from people whose capacity for spirituality is often questioned.

For practitioners, this dimension of spirituality raises at least three important questions. First, how much attention should be paid to the importance of friendships and relationships that are reported by patients or clients and to the importance of a supportive community? A practitioner may not agree with the tenets or beliefs of an individual's or family's faith community, but can the practitioner understand the value and support provided by that community? Likewise, can expressions of stress be seen as reflecting a lack of supportive community rather than an individual psychological issue? A mother once said, "I went to my pastoral counselor because of the stress in our family around care for our disabled child. All he wanted to do was talk about my relationship with my mother, and what I most needed was some respite care." Thankfully, respite care is becoming a known concept in faith communities as a way of supporting 24/7 caregivers and those caregivers who are "sandwiched" between children and parents. It is but one of many ways that faith communities can provide emotional, material, and practical supports.

Second, what is a clinician's professional responsibility toward people who share stories related to a lack of welcome? Does their role include advocacy, such as using the FICA model of spiritual supports and asking whether a person or family might like assistance in addressing these issues or talking with a pastor of their congregation? In the area of mental illness, a promising development is the partnership between the American Psychiatric Association and a number of faith-based organizations who are working on this issue to build more effective collaborative practices between psychiatrists and clergy (www.psychiatry.org/faith).

Third, what clinical settings and practices are hospitable and welcoming to people with disabilities? Many human service offices and agencies communicate an inhospitable welcome. (For an excellent team study guide, see the Bruce Anderson CD, "Our Door is Open: Creating Welcome in Helping Organizations," available at http://www.communityactivators.com.) Environments can be very stressful to some people with mental health issues and to others on the autism spectrum.

Gifts and Weaknesses, Strengths and Deficits, Givers and Receivers

Of equal importance to the previous three areas is the question of whether spiritual communities and human service practitioners can focus as intentionally on someone's gifts and strengths as they do on deficits, needs, and assumed weaknesses. Coping with disability of any kind is a lifelong journey. If we believe, as we say we do, that everyone has gifts and strengths, then how can we help someone to build on those? Spiritual traditions may express this in terms of everyone being created in the image of God, everyone having value and worth, and everyone having both a vocation and a call. This attitude is manifest in the recovery movements in mental health (Pagano, Post, & Johnson, 2011; Post, Pagano, Lee, & Johnson, 2016), just as it is in person-centered planning processes (O'Brien & O'Brien, 1998; Smull & Sanderson, 2005) in the worlds of intellectual and developmental disabilities and other forms of disability (see also http://www.learningcommunity.us). It may be both a matter of perspective and a matter of time: Are we willing to get to know people with disabilities in the fullness of their lives, and perhaps help them to discover, see, and claim their own strengths and gifts? Those may be passions, interests, and skills that have nothing to do with one's disability, or they may be gifts and strengths that have arisen from having to cope with the issues they have encountered because of the disability.

The naming and recognition of gifts and strengths is but the first step. The second is helping people find ways to express and use them. Perhaps stated most simply, people like to be givers and contributors as well as receivers. In the Christian tradition, there is a familiar saying, "It is more blessed to give than to receive." The truth of the matter is that it is also a whole lot easier. One of the real issues for typical people (and even more so for professional caregivers) is that it is hard to recognize and affirm one's own needs by asking for support from others or by learning effective skills in self-care. The social and cultural roles of people with disabilities often lead to their being seen simply for their needs. They become seen as receivers, consumers, clients, patients, or, more dangerously, as "takers."

At an early inclusive faith supports conference in the late 1970s, a woman named Kathy, who had fairly significant cerebral palsy, told her story of being sent to an institution out in the country as a child, being "repatriated" to a smaller institution in the city where the workshop was taking place, then moving to a supported living arrangement for people with disabilities and finally to her own apartment. Her qualities of perseverance and determination were evident in her story. In her halting voice, she closed with this simple injunction: "It is really important for you to be nice to handicapped people, but it is more important for you to let them be nice to you."

In a small book called *Flourish: People with Disabilities Living Life with Passion*, Karin Meiberg-Schwier (2012) outlined key strategies that have helped people flourish and told the stories of a number of people with various forms of disability. All of them found ways to use their gifts and strengths in service with and to others and their communities. These included volunteer roles, jobs, microbusiness entrepreneurship, and more. One story of a young man named Jason highlighted the variety of ways in which he was active in his faith community. Congregations working on inclusive supports are finding many ways to recognize gifts and help them be used in what Wolf Wolfensberger (1983) called socially valued roles (also see http://www.socialrolevalorization.com/en/).The outcomes for identity, connection, and sense of purpose are clear. One of the statements frequently made by faith communities is that they began by "ministering to" people with disabilities, then including them along with themselves, and finally recognizing that the congregation was receiving just as much as it was giving. One of the core commitments of a congregation or community is recognizing that if they cannot find a way to use someone's gifts, it says more about their lack of imagination than it does the ability of the individuals involved.

These are spiritual dimensions of life and support that do not have to be expressed or experienced only in communities of faith. They can be experienced anywhere. But one of the implications, and indeed one of the ethical questions, is whether professional caregivers can recognize and acknowledge the contributions to their own lives of people with disabilities whom they support. An honest discussion would reveal ways in which the people they support are central to their understanding of vocation and meaningful purpose. For people with disabilities, who so rarely hear about the ways in which make a contribution to others, a final ethical implication, perhaps related to justice, is whether we as professionals are able to find ways to tell them so and to affirm the mutuality of the relationships in which we are involved.

ETHICS OF CARE

Earlier in this chapter, principlism ethics was reviewed as it applies to intellectual disability and set in conversation with Gaventa's four key elements: the fundamental human/spiritual question, the core spiritual theme, the policy value, and practices (see Table 16.1; Gaventa, 2016). As this chapter has unfolded, the roles of patient and caregiver experience, gifts and graces, relative strengths and weaknesses, and givers and receivers have been discussed. Clearly, relationships are of prime importance, as is the need for psychiatrists and other mental health professionals to understand and *work* to form helpful and enduring relationships with patients, their families, and other care providers. In many ways, the ethics of working with the spirituality of people with intellectual disabilities agrees with several of the key premises of the ethics of care and caring.

The ethics of care originated in feminist ethics, a paradigm that grew to address what many viewed as a very male-dominated approach to ethics that existed at least until the 1970s. Feminists and others struggled with many aspects of deontology, principlism, and utilitarianism. Carol Gilligan, in particular, is credited with the observation that men tend to be rule-focused in their moral development and in reasoning, behaviors, and interpersonal relationships (Gilligan, 1982). This affects the way in which they analyze and tackle problem solving and ethical dilemmas. Alternatively, women address ethical problems while valuing and prioritizing interpersonal relationships and caring for others (Gilligan, 1982; Gordon, 2015; Tronto, 2014).

Burnor and Raley (2011), informed by the feminist philosophers Nel Noddings (2003) and Virginia Held (2007), summarized the key points of care ethics as follows:

1. The fundamental moral obligation is to interact with others from the perspective of caring, and that happens in relationship.
2. These caring relationships involve more than one person and therefore involve varying degrees of mutuality.
3. Caring relationships affect those involved and hence can be transforming in nature.
4. Authentic caring leads to doing.

Although the ethics of care has been criticized for not providing a consistent method or roadmap for ethical analysis, its application to people with intellectual disabilities and their families and caregivers is obvious. The ethics of care is a helpful vehicle for identifying and discussing the needs of vulnerable populations in general, and it also provides a basic structure or set of priorities for the consideration of the lives of those with disabilities in families, religious communities, and other social groups to which they belong (Gordon, 2015; Lo, 2013).

ADDITIONAL PARENTAL
AND FAMILY CONSIDERATIONS

As mentioned several times in this chapter, families and other groups who know and care for the intellectually disabled are extremely important. Although this is certainly true for disabled children, the importance of families and nonmedical caregivers is often greater for disabled adults than in non-disabled adult populations.

Regardless of the specific disability, the challenges parents face unfold as their child grows into adolescence and into adulthood (Wang, 2012). Parents of babies and young children face delays in feeding and eating skills, toilet training, speech, and language. In addition to a never-ending string of physicians' appointments, there are often occupational, physical, speech and language, behavioral training, and other therapy appointments on a regular basis. As the child grows older, there are many more meetings with schools for educational planning than for typical children. Haircuts, buying shoes, and teeth brushing can be struggles for years. Many children are taking multiple medications prescribed by several physicians, so parents must keep track of refills and insurance issues, not to mention frequent runs to the pharmacy. Even if there are no or only mild physical disabilities, intellectual limitations can make the child prone to dangerous behaviors, such as leaving the house unnoticed, wandering, climbing through windows onto the roof, or locking themselves in bathrooms or other spaces where adults unable to get them out from the outside. Many parents need to spend extra time and money modifying their homes to keep their children safe. As the disabled adolescent transitions to adulthood, parents often feel strained by financial, legal, and other care burdens. Parents find that they do not have enough time or energy to attend to their marriage, their careers, and their other children. The health of the caregiver may suffer because there is extremely limited time for attending to their own healthcare, diet, and exercise. Incomes and careers are limited, and saving money for the child's present and future care undermines retirement plans. Over time, the parents lose touch with old friends and sacrifice hobbies and recreational pursuits; their worlds can contract and be limited by their burden of care. In addition, they may be and/or feel ostracized or neglected by their religious communities due to their child's behaviors and needs.

Siblings of intellectually disabled individuals also require special consideration by both mental health clinicians and religious/spiritual care providers (Autism Society of America, 2017). Some adult siblings look back on their experiences of growing up with a disabled brother or sister positively, stating that they learned virtues of tolerance and patience and developed helping skills that they value and that have even given them advantages over others after they left their family of origin. Others carry resentment of the time, energy, and money required by their sibling that subtracted from their own lives; they remember the embarrassment and frustration they experienced and attributed to the affected sibling. Still others are able to process both the blessings and the burdens of their experiences.

As mentioned earlier, given the unifying theme of relationships, the ethics of care can be helpful in sorting through the ethical issues with both psychiatric and religious/spiritual considerations. In addition, Jonsen, Siegler, and Winslade's Four Topics Model (see Chapter 1), especially the section on contextual features, is a very relevant guide for obtaining information about family, religious, financial, and legal factors that are important to the analysis of ethical quandaries (Jonsen, Siegler, & Winslade, 2015).

TRENDS IN SPIRITUAL CARE AND BELONGING FOR PEOPLE WITH INTELLECTUAL DISABILITIES AND THEIR FAMILIES

In the last two decades, many faith traditions and local faith communities have realized the need to provide spiritual care to people with all types of disabilities and their families. This trend has gone beyond mandated wheelchair access to houses of worship to include adapted religious education courses to meet the needs of various disabilities and special worship services that accept and accommodate those with movement disorders, short attention spans, impulsiveness, medical equipment, or vocalizations that might distract able-bodied worshipers, who may view these as disruptions to their own worship and religious/spiritual practices. People with disabilities are encouraged not only to attend but to share in planning and participation in the worship services and other activities of the faith community. In addition to or instead of special services for people with disabilities only, many congregations intentionally have educated themselves about intellectual disabilities and include people with disabilities and their families in all programming and events of the community.

Psychiatrists and other mental health clinicians caring for people with intellectual disabilities and their families are well advised to be aware of faith communities of all traditions in the areas in which they practice that provide these opportunities for inclusion and service. People with developmental disabilities benefit from being connected to churches, synagogues, mosques, and other places of worship, especially from the relationships they develop with other people who belong there and with the religious/spiritual leaders who lead and serve these groups. These communities and their leaders may also be of assistance to psychiatrists and others in the medical field, helping clinicians to understand their patients better and providing insights in the event of ethical dilemmas.

CONCLUSION

As illustrated in this chapter, the spiritual and religious needs of people with intellectual disabilities and their caregivers are broad and significant. So too are the gifts and insights they offer to faith communities and to the psychiatrists and mental health providers with whom they interact. In situations involving ethical questions and quandaries, spiritual and religious considerations may be as prominent—if not more so—than medical and psychiatric elements. Spiritually and culturally informed clinicians should be able to recognize and assist their intellectually disabled patients as they navigate these matters of psychiatric, ethical, and religious/spiritual importance.

RELATED BOOKS AND WEB SITES OF INTEREST

Abrams, J. Z. (1998). *Judaism and disability: Portrayals in ancient texts from the Tanuch through the Bavli*. Washington, DC: Gallaudet University Press.

Brock, B., & Swinton, J. (Eds.). (2012). *Disability in the Christian tradition.* Grand Rapids, MI: Eerdmans.

Collaborative on Faith and Disability. http://faithanddisability.org. Resources, references and plenary presentations from the Summer Institute on Theology and Disability.

Gaventa, W. C., & Coulter, D. L. (Eds.). (2014). *Spirituality and intellectual disability: International perspectives on the effect of culture and religion on healing body, mind, and soul.* New York, NY: The Haworth Pastoral Press.

Meyer, D. (2017). What siblings would like parents and service providers to know. Retrieved from https://www.siblingsupport.org/documents-for-site/WhatSiblingsWouldLikeParentsand ServiceProviderstoKnow.pdf

Newman, B. J. (2011). *Autism and your church: Nurturing the spiritual growth of people with autism spectrum disorders* (2nd ed.). Grand Rapids, MI: CRC Publications.

Picard, A., & Habets, M. (Eds.). (2016). *Theology and the experience of disability.* New York, NY: Routledge.

Pinsky, M. E. (2012). Amazing gifts. Herndon, VA: The Alban Press.

Scully, J. L. (2008). *Disability bioethics: Moral bodies, moral difference.* New York, NY: Rowman & Littlefield.

Schumm, D., & Stoltzfus, M. (Eds.). (2011). *Disability and religious diversity: Cross-cultural and interreligious perspectives.* New York, NY: Palgrave Macmillan.

Schumm, D., & Stoltzfus, M. (Eds.). (2011). *Disability in Judaism, Christianity, and Islam.* New York, NY: Palgrave Macmillan.

Sibling and Leadership Network. Online resources for adult sibs. http://siblingleadership.org. Focused on adult sibling.

Sibling Support Network. https://www.siblingsupport.org. Focused on children and youth siblings.

Webb-Mitchell, B. (1996). *Dancing with disabilities: Opening the church to all God's children.* Cleveland, OH: United Church Press.

Yong, A. (2011). *The Bible, disability, and the church: A new vision of the people of God.* Grand Rapids, MI: Eerdmans.

Yong, A. (2007). *Theology and Down syndrome.* Waco, TX: Baylor University Press.

REFERENCES

Ainslee, D. C. (2014). Principlism. In B. Jennings, B. (Ed.). *Bioethics* (4th ed., pp. 2485–2489). Farmington Hills, MI: Gale Resources, Cengage.

Autism Society of America. (2017). Web site. Retrieved from http://www.autism-society.org.

Beauchamp, T. L., & Childress, J. F. (2013). *Principles of biomedical ethics* (7th ed.). Oxford, England: Oxford University Press.

Bittles, A. H., Petterson, B. A., Sullivan, S. G., Hussain, R., Glasson, E. J., & Montgomery, P. D. (2002). The influence of intellectual disability on life expectancy. *Journal of Gerontology: Series A, Biological Sciences and Medical Sciences, 57*(7), M470–M472.

Bogdan, R., Elks, M., & Knoll, J. (2012). *Picturing disability: Beggar, freak, citizen, and other photographic rhetoric.* Syracuse, NY: Syracuse University Press.

Boyle, C. A., Boulet, S., Schieve, L. A., Cohen R. A., Blumberg, S. J., Yeargin-Allsopp, M., . . . Kogan, M. D. (2011). Trends in the prevalence of developmental disabilities in U.S. children, 1997–2008. *Pediatrics, 127*(6), 1034–1042.

Burnor, R., & Raley, Y. (2011). *Ethical choices: An introduction to moral philosophy with cases.* New York, NY: Oxford University Press.

Carter, E. W. (2013). Supporting inclusion and flourishing in the religious and spiritual lives of people with intellectual and developmental disabilities. *Inclusion, 1*, 64–75. doi:10.1352/2326-6988-1.1.064

Carter, E. W. (2016). A place of belonging: Research at the intersection of faith and disability. *Baptist Review and Expositor*(2).

Carter, E. W., Biggs, E. E., & Boehm, T. L. (2016). Being present versus having a presence: Dimensions of belonging for young people with disabilities and their families. *Christian Education Journal 13*(1), 127.

Carter, E. W., Boehm, T. L., Annandale, N. H., & Taylor, C. (2016). Supporting congregational inclusion for children and youth with disabilities and their families. *Exceptional Children, 82*(3), 372–389.

Christensen, D. L., Baio, J., Braun, K. V. N., Bilder, D., Charles, J., Constantino, J. N., . . . Yeargin-Allsopp, M. (2016). Prevalence and characteristics of autism spectrum disorder among children aged 8 years: Autism and Developmental Disabilities Monitoring Network, 11 sites, United States, 2012. *MMWR Surveillance Summaries, 65*(SS-3), 1–23.

Davis, L. J. (2013). *The end of normal: Identity in a biocultural era.* Ann Arbor, MI: University of Michigan Press.

Eiesland, N. L. (1994). *The disabled God: Toward a liberatory theology of disability.* Nashville, TN: Abingdon Press.

Eiesland, N. L. (2001). Liberation, inclusion, and justice: A faith response to persons with disabilities. *Impact: Feature Issue on Faith Communities and Persons with Disabilities, 14*(3) [online]. Minneapolis, MN: University of Minnesota, Institute on Community Integration. Retrieved from https://ici.umn.edu/products/impact/143/default.html.

Frank, A. (1997). *The wounded storyteller: Body, illness, ethics.* Chicago, IL: University of Chicago Press.

Gaventa, W. (2016). Disability and spirituality: Re-membering wholeness. *Journal of Disability & Religion, 20*(4), 307–316.

Gaventa, W., & Carter, E. W. (Eds.). (2012). Spirituality: From rights to relationships [Special issue]. *TASH Connections, 38*(1).

Gilligan, C. (1982). *In a different voice: Psychological theory and women's development.* Cambridge, MA: Harvard University Press.

Gordon, J.-S. (2015). *Bioethics.* Internet Encyclopedia of Philosophy. Retrieved from www.iep.utm.edu/bioethic.

Held, V. (2007). *The ethics of care: Personal, political, and global.* New York, NY: Oxford University Press.

Janicki, M. P., Dalton, A. J., Henderson, C. M., & Davidson, P. W. (1999). Mortality and morbidity among older adults with intellectual disability: Health services considerations. *Disability and Rehabilitation, 21*(5–6), 284–294.

Jonsen, A. R., Siegler, M., & Winslade, W. J. (2015). *Clinical ethics: A practical approach to ethical decisions in clinical medicine* (8th ed.). New York, NY: McGraw-Hill Education.

Koenig, H. (2011). *Spirituality and health research: Methods, measurements, statistics, and resources.* Conshohocken, PA: Templeton Press.

Kunc, N. (1996). *A credo for support.* Written version with music retrieved from https://www.youtube.com/watch?v=21uHYEqKOOw; spoken version by People First retrieved from https://www.youtube.com/watch?v=wunHDfZFxXw.

Liu, E. X., Carter, E. W., Boehm, T. L., Annandale, N., & Taylor, C. (2014). In their own words: The place of faith in the lives of young people with intellectual disability and autism. *Intellectual and Developmental Disabilities, 52*, 388–404. doi:10.1352/1934-9556-52.5.388

Lo, B. (2013). *Resolving ethical dilemmas: A guide for clinicians* (5th ed., pp. 3–65, 263–270). Philadelphia, PA: Lippincott, Williams, & Wilkins.

Meiberg-Schwier, K. (2012). *Flourish: People with disabilities living life with passion.* Saskatoon, Canada: Copestone.

Miller, W., & Thoresen, C. (2003). Spirituality, religion, and health: An emerging research field. *American Psychologist*, *58*(1), 24–35.

Noddings, N. (2003). *Caring: A feminine approach to ethics and moral education* (2nd ed.). Berkeley, CA University of California Press.

O'Brien, J., & O'Brien, C. (Eds.). (1998). *A little book about person centered planning*. Toronto, Canada: Inclusion Press.

Paterson, G. W. (1975). *Helping your handicapped child*. Minneapolis, MN: Augsburg Publishing House.

Perkins, E. A., & Moran, J. A. (2010). Aging adults with intellectual disabilities. *JAMA*, *304*(1), 91–92.

Pagano, M. E., Post S. G., & Johnson, S. M. (2011). Alcoholics Anonymous-related helping and the helper therapy principle. *Alcohol Treatment Quarterly*, *29*(1), 23–34.

Post, S. G., Pagano, M. E., Lee, M. T., & Johnson, B. R. (2016). Humility and 12-step recovery: A prolegomenon for the empirical investigation of a cardinal virtue in Alcoholics Anonymous. *Alcoholism Treatment Quarterly*, *34*(3), 262–273.

Puchalski, C. M., & Romer, A. L. (2000). Taking a spiritual history allows clinicians to understand patients more fully. *Journal of Palliative Medicine*, *3*(1), 129–137.

Reinders, H. (2008). *Receiving the gift of friendship: Profound disability, theological anthropology, and ethics*. Grand Rapids, MI: Eerdmans.

Reinders, H. (2014). *Disability, providence and ethics: Bridging gaps, transforming lives*. Waco, TX: Baylor University Press.

Smull, M., & Sanderson, H. (2005). *Essential lifestyle planning for everyone*. Annapolis, MD: The Learning Community.

Snow, K. (2017). Disability is natural! [Web site]. Retrieved from https://www.disabilityisnatural.com).

Tronto, J. C. (2014). Care ethics. In B. Jennings (Ed.). *Bioethics* (4th ed., pp. 495–504). Farmington Hills, MI: Gale Resources, Cengage.

Wang, K. Y. (2012). The care burden of families with members having intellectual and developmental disorder: A review of the recent literature. *Current Opinion in Psychiatry*, *25*, 348–352.

Wolfensberger, W. (1983). Social role valorization: A proposed new term for the principle of normalization. *Mental Retardation, 21*(6), 234–239.

World Health Organization. (1993). *International classification of impairments, disabilities and handicaps: A manual of classification relating to the consequences of disease*. Published in accordance with resolution WHA29.35 of the Twenty-ninth World Health Assembly, May 1976 [reprinted with foreword]. Geneva, Switzerland: World Health Organization.

World Health Organization. (2002). *Toward a Common Language of Disability, Functioning and Health*. http://www.who.int/classifications/icf/training/icfbeginnersguide.pdf

Yang, K. L., & Tan, H. E. (2016). Disability statistics. Cornell University Institute on Employment and Disability. Retrieved from http://www.yti.cornell.edu.

Young, S. (2014). "I'm not your inspiration, thank you very much." TED talk. Sydney, Australia. Retrieved from https://www.ted.com/talks/stella_young_i_m_not_your_inspiration_thank_you_very_much?language=en.

SEVENTEEN

Mental Disorder and Transformation

Perspectives from Community Psychiatry

Tony Benning, M.D.

> *Psychopathology is a means rather than an end—the less idealized part of the romantic journey*
>
> (Mcdaniel, 1989)

INTRODUCTION

In recent decades, psychiatry and associated mental health disciplines have struggled to balance their historical professional identities of compassion and focused attention to complementary, integrated elements of the biopsychosocial model of assessment and treatment with the explosion of new information and tools from basic neuroscience and advanced social sciences. Certainly these scientific advances have saved lives and improved the quality of life for countless individuals and societies at large. As other medical specialties have done, psychiatry has developed both formal, organized subspecialties and focused areas of research and education as knowledge has increased. These specialized areas of expertise include psychopharmacology, geriatrics, consultation liaison (psychosomatics), forensics, new evidence-based forms of psychotherapies, addictions, child and adolescent psychiatry, and complex neuroimaging and treatments such as electroconvulsive therapy, vagal nerve stimulation, and transcranial magnetic stimulation.

In this time of 21st century specializations and neuroscience advances, our mental health and theological professionals, guilds, and religious communities must also remember that, all over the globe, still exist vast areas—rural, suburban, and urban—of very limited access to mental health care. Similarly, even in areas where adequate numbers of providers practice their professions, access to preferred services may not be available for financial and other reasons. In these instances, it is the community psychiatrist and community mental health systems who step up and who must have a constant, up-to-date repertoire of assessment and treatment tools to employ competently and swiftly for any individual, family, psychodynamic, and/or medical issues that present unannounced.

This chapter presents reflections from one community psychiatrist's practice regarding the intersection of psychiatry, ethics, and religion and spirituality in his daily work.

R. D. Laing famously wrote, "Madness need not be all breakdown. It may also be breakthrough. It may be liberation and renewal as well as enslavement and existential death" (Laing, 1967). That the personal meanings in psychosis could have transformational significance was a major contention for Laing, especially in his later thought (Bentall, 2005). Recent decades have seen a steadily growing interest in the relationship between mental illness—especially psychosis—and transformation.

In *Trials of the Visionary Mind*, John Weir Perry, a psychiatrist based in the San Francisco area, brought a neo-Jungian perspective to his analysis of the contents of psychotic experiences—or visionary states, as he preferred to call them (Perry, 1999). Perry found that the commonly occurring themes in psychosis (such as kingship and cultural disintegration followed by renewal) resembled those found in the great universal myths. Lukoff and Everest (1985) also interpreted the psychotic process as an encounter with mythical realities by drawing heavily on the concept of the hero's journey as elaborated by Joseph Campbell (1972). They suggested that the psychotic journey, as a mental odyssey of sorts, recapitulates the sequential stages of separation, initiation, and return seen in the mythical hero's odyssey.

More recently, Nixon, Hagen, and Peters (2010) undertook a phenomenological inquiry of six individuals who had experienced psychosis as having spiritual or otherwise positive significance. Four major themes emerged with respect to participants' experiences of transformation:

1. Detachment and mindfulness
2. Accepting the dissolution of time into now
3. Embracing a spiritual pathway
4. Realignment of career path

Several authors have alluded to the fact that there may be significant overlap with regard to the way in which spiritual experience and psychiatric disorder present. Fulford and Jackson (1997), for example, suggested that pathological and spiritual psychotic phenomena cannot be distinguished on the basis of either form or content, nor from the relationship with other symptoms, nor by reference to descriptive criteria of mental illness. They showed that a distinction can be drawn only by considering the significance of the experience and examining the way in which it is embedded within the value system and set of beliefs of the individual. Moreira-Almeida and Cardena (2011) arrived at a similar conclusion on the basis of a Brazilian study showing that, from a phenomenological perspective, there is little to distinguish between those psychotic symptoms that are associated with a disorder and those that occur in otherwise healthy and well-functioning members of the general population. They emphasized the role of society's frame of reference in influencing the trajectory of the symptoms such that they can become either illness or a stimulus for personal growth.

Underrepresented in the literature is an exploration of the sorts of ethical, clinical, and pragmatic dilemmas that are faced by clinicians as they try to assist clients in a manner that honors the transformational dimension of mental illness. This chapter attempts to address that gap in the literature by describing the presentation and management of three clinical cases from the author's community psychiatric practice. The hope is that doing so will assist other clinicians facing similar dilemmas at the intersection of psychiatry, ethics, and religion.

THREE CLINICAL CASES FROM A COMMUNITY SETTING

Charlie

The first case to be discussed here is that of Charlie, a 60-year-old man from a British Columbia First Nations background. Charlie had no past psychiatric history until he experienced psychotic symptoms 2 months before he first presented to the clinic. His symptoms included a fairly sudden onset of sleep disturbance and auditory hallucinations in which he heard distressing screams of children and other family members. There appeared to be some delusional elaboration too, as he had called the police on several occasions to report that his family members were being tortured. He had become mistrustful in recent months and had developed the belief that others, including his sons, were communicating with him over long distances by inserting thoughts into his mind. Charlie was reluctant to seek medical help, convinced that what he was going through—as distressing as it was—amounted to a normal spiritual experience. Specifically, he believed that his experience was a spiritual song, although he was reluctant to elaborate further on this. The first time Charlie came to see the psychiatrist, he was extremely ambivalent, so much so that he terminated the interview prematurely, after about 10 minutes.

The psychiatrist's dilemma arose from a wish to navigate through a range of potentially contradictory ethical imperatives. Using Jonsen, Siegler, and Winslade's Four Quadrant Model (2006), the first of those ethical imperatives was in keeping with the upper left quadrant, Medical Indications (see Chapter 1). According to Jonsen et al., that quadrant encompasses such questions as *What is the patient's medical problem? What is the History? What is the diagnosis?* and *What are the goals of treatment?* Such questions obligated the psychiatrist to prioritize arranging appropriate investigations (namely a computed tomographic [CT] scan of the head) to rule out serious intracerebral pathology and to consider initiating antipsychotic medication. Evidence-based psychiatric practice dictated that priority be given to screening for organic pathology in anyone in such a relatively late age group who presents with a first onset of psychosis. Such undertakings would be in keeping with the very fundamental medical ethical principles of beneficence and non-maleficence, both ethical imperatives emphasized by Jonsen et al. as being relevant to the Medical Indications quadrant. Wanting to take all relevant factors into consideration before proceeding any further with this clinical quandary, the psychiatrist was interested in conceptualizing this case in a way that was inclusive of the remaining quadrants: Patient Preferences, Quality of Life, and Contextual Features.

Jonsen et al.'s Patient Preferences quadrant places emphasis on the ethical imperative of patient autonomy. Questions that inform the exploration of autonomy include, *Is the patient mentally capable and legally competent?* and *What is the patient's stated preference for treatment?* There was acknowledgment of the fact that Charlie expressed a preference not to be evaluated or treated along conventional, Western-style lines and that his explanatory model for his experience was a "spiritual song." However, Charlie's competence to make such a decision was highly questionable. He did not convey appreciation of the potential consequences of not undergoing those investigations and treatments. The patient's mistrust affected his ability to believe that the psychiatrist's management was motivated by an ethic of beneficence.

The Contextual Features quadrant behooves clinicians to be mindful about such issues as religion and culture, as well as the family's views on treatment decisions. Therefore, the psychiatrist asked Charlie to invite his daughter to a meeting. The psychiatrist was interested in her views about spiritual songs as understood by the local First Nation community or whether, in fact, she thought that the problem lent itself to a more Western-style explanation and intervention. The psychiatrist's intention was that, with Charlie's permission, his daughter would be asked to play the role of cultural broker.

The psychiatrist met Charlie a few weeks after the initial meeting in the company of his daughter, an occupational therapist. Her opinion was quite clear; this was a psychosis, and her father should have a CT scan and be started on antipsychotic medication. Visibly distressed, the daughter implored the psychiatrist: "All I want is to have my dad back." Further, the daughter acknowledged the legitimacy of the concept of a spiritual song but was not of the view that her father's presentation could be explained by such a phenomenon. She stated that the family had consulted an elder in the community who had advised that spiritual songs do not usually persist more than a few days at most.

Hearing these facts stated in Charlie's presence, as well as witnessing the daughter's clear emotional distress, facilitated a shift in Charlie. He became more agreeable to undergoing a CT scan and a trial of antipsychotic medication. Charlie's resistance to thinking of his experience as an illness had softened significantly. The psychiatrist avoided using the term "psychosis" out of a concern that Charlie would perceive this as the imposition of a Western worldview, thus alienating him and leading to unnecessary harm. The psychiatrist did, however, use such words as "breakdown" and acknowledged that the experiences Charlie was having were causing much "distress" for him and his family. On the basis of the new information offered by the daughter, the psychiatrist avoided using the term "spiritual song," but it was suggested to Charlie that when he became "better" and reflected on his experiences, he might come to see that it was of some value. The psychiatrist talked about the fact that recovery from breakdown may well be associated by some persons with a feeling of having undergone a transformation or alteration of one's priorities, commitments, or worldview. A valuable therapeutic bond was forged in this meeting. The terms psychosis and spiritual song had both been avoided, while at the same time the idea was embraced that what Charlie was going through was distressing and undesirable but could have meaningful or transformational significance. The psychiatrist found it profitable to deploy Jonsen's Four Quadrant Model. The model served as a safeguard against the strictly medical approach to clinical cases, one that risks riding roughshod over cultural explanatory models and such imperatives as patient self-determination. The improved therapeutic relationship constituted powerful evidence of the model's usefulness.

Alice

The second case concerns Alice, a 58-year-old woman who presented with a 4-week history of signs and symptoms that were in keeping with a manic episode with psychotic features. There was neither a personal nor a family history of mood disorder. The only significant history was that of alcohol dependency, which had been in remission for almost 2 years. Alice had been brought into hospital by her concerned family. Given the florid nature of her psychiatric presentation, as well as lack of insight, she was detained in hospital involuntarily under Canada's Mental Health Act.

Alice's manic symptoms included hyperactivity, rapid speech, overfamiliarity, increased energy levels, and reduced need for sleep. The psychotic aspect of Alice's presentation took the form of a feverish religious preoccupation. She spoke about being constantly watched by her personal angel and emphatically expressed her belief that she was on a special religious mission and that sermons in the church were being prepared especially for her. There were clear grandiose delusions, revealed, for example, by her claim that she had the ability to make stars dance. She was vocal regarding her belief that the rapture was imminent. (By this, she was referencing the Christian eschatological belief that either before or at the time of the second coming of Christ, believers, both dead and alive, will be raised). There was no hostility or aggression. Although she lacked insight, she did agree to take medication. After a week or so, she was permitted to have passes to visit the immediate vicinity of the hospital. During the passes, she started attending services at the local church, where she sought the counsel of the minister.

Alice met the criteria for a manic episode with psychotic features. The psychiatrist was obliged to keep her safe, to initiate standard medication, to provide psychoeducation, and to discuss the diagnosis and prognosis with her and her family. The relatively late age at apparent first onset of a psychotic disorder behooved a thorough screening for undisclosed organic disease.

One day when Alice was still in the hospital and still experiencing psychotic as well as manic symptoms, she shared with the psychiatrist the fact that she wanted to consecrate her newly found Christian convictions by undergoing a baptism. This presented the treating psychiatrist with an ethical dilemma. No one wanted to see Alice inadvertently harm herself by making a religious commitment in the context of an acute psychiatric episode that she might regret or at least have a change of heart about when recovered. In this respect, an imperative of beneficence was clearly at play. On the other hand, many psychiatric patients express their religious convictions in various ways without the involvement of mental health professionals and are not harmed in doing so. Different historical epochs and cultural settings have had a large determining influence in such matters. On reflection, the psychiatrist's discomfort about preventing Alice from undergoing baptism stemmed from a desire to respect her autonomy. The psychiatrist proceeded to arrange a meeting attended by himself, Alice, and the minister.

This meeting proved to be very productive. The minister and the psychiatrist were able to establish common ground, and this was evident to Alice. It was agreed that Alice was psychiatrically unwell and that, for now, she required hospital care. It was also agreed that there was something very meaningful and legitimate about her religious fervor. As such, there would be no reason for Alice not to continue with her voracious bible reading and church attendance. Those activities certainly spoke to the Quality of Life imperatives of Jonsen's model. The minister advised Alice that it might be best to hold off from committing to a baptism until she was further along in her recovery and, ideally, discharged from hospital. The minister emphasized that a decision to undergo baptism should not be made without due thought and prior reflection: "It is not a decision to be taken lightly." Despite some initial resistance, Alice agreed to follow the minister's advice and postponed her baptism.

When facing real-life ethical dilemmas at the interface of psychiatry and spirituality, the foregoing two cases demonstrate the usefulness of bringing a third person, a broker, into the dialogue. In both cases, a positive relationship was maintained between psychiatrist and patient, and neither the conceptualization of the phenomenon in question as "illness" nor the idea that it might be "meaningful" had to be jettisoned. It was possible to retain a sense of both through the avoidance of a dogmatic insistence that any given phenomenon must be understood as *either* one thing *or* another. In this way, a balance was struck between the ethical principles of beneficence, non-maleficence, and patient autonomy, without any one principle having to be overridden by another. Another helpful factor was that the broker, in both cases, was as interested as the psychiatrist in approaching the situation from the sort of broad-based, inclusive ethical standpoint that Jonsen's model represents.

Samantha

The third case is that of Samantha, a 25-year-old Canadian immigrant of Vietnamese origin who was referred for ongoing psychiatric care at the community mental health center. In recent years, in a different community, she had had three psychiatric hospitalizations for psychosis, including persecutory delusions and threatening auditory hallucinations, and had been diagnosed with paranoid schizophrenia. Nonadherence to medication had been a major issue and was thought to have contributed to her second and third psychotic episodes.

In an early interview with Samantha and her mother, assisted by a Vietnamese interpreter, the psychiatrist asked Samantha's mother about her understanding of those problems that had been afflicting her daughter and what she considered to have caused them. She replied that the family were Buddhists, and they believed that her daughter's illness was caused by her having been possessed by malevolent ancestral spirits who were upset about having been forgotten by their descendants. The mother went on to describe the sorts of help-seeking that the family had pursued in the light of their understanding of the causes of illness. Several members of Samantha's extended family had visited the cemetery in Vietnam to offer gifts and prayers to ancestral spirits in an attempt to win their good favor and earn their forgiveness. After Samantha became sick, it also had become regular practice for the family to visit a local Canadian Buddhist temple.

The nature of the help-seeking was very heavily influenced by the family's cultural explanatory model, which was laden with a syncretic mix of Buddhist and indigenous Vietnamese illness concepts. In keeping with the Patient Preferences and Contextual Features quadrants of Jonsen's model, the psychiatrist respected the family's beliefs about the origins of Samantha's illness but was concerned that doing so would be perceived as a green light for Samantha to discontinue her medication, which both she and her mother wanted to do. The psychiatrist proceeded by trying to reconcile the family's explanatory model with a Western one, reinforcing the fact that antipsychotic medication had been a major contributory factor to Samantha's recovery after each of her previous episodes of illness. Reinforced too was the prediction that coming off medication would likely result in her becoming sick again very quickly.

Unfortunately, the psychiatrist did not feel that he had been successful so far, despite much effort, in engendering in Samantha or her family a willingness to hold together in a reconciliatory embrace both Western and Eastern conceptualizations of illness. Samantha adhered to antipsychotic medication only because it was administered in the form of a monthly injection and because she was subject to the powers of the Mental Health Act. The psychiatrist was not entirely free of conflict, for there remained a worry about imposing on Samantha and her family a Western secular worldview. This is a worldview that prizes scientific truths above all else; it privileges biomedical disease causation models at the expense of all others, and it is a worldview that Samantha and his family considered incongruent and incompatible with theirs. The term "schizophrenia," the ensemble of meanings that attend it, and the assumptions about causality that are implicit to it—as the psychiatrist was learning quickly—fell well outside the worldview subscribed to by Samantha and her family. They were not at all signed up to any of that! Yet, the physician was permitted by the conventions of Western psychiatric practice to deliver a diagnosis of schizophrenia, with or without their consent, even if it meant overriding the patient's right to self-determination (Bradfield, 2002). The medication was administered to Samantha on a monthly basis, contrary to her wishes, on the basis of the well-rehearsed path of ethical reasoning in such situations that holds the preservation of autonomy to be a subordinate principle to the principle of beneficence. Furthermore, the psychiatrist's practice was taking place under the canopy of a legislative system that permits the enactment of decisions that override the autonomy of individuals such as Samantha and their families. Jonsen's model informs our conceptualization of the ethical factors that are of relevance to cases such as these because context encompasses the ways in which the law impacts clinical decision making.

The psychiatrist has often wondered how the family's experience would have been different had Samantha developed psychosis in rural Vietnam, their country of origin. There, Samantha and her family likely would have been freer than they were in Canada to venture along the spiritual path upon which Samantha's sickness appears to have catapulted them. Had Samantha fallen sick in Vietnam, the family would likely have been more successful than they were ever likely to be in Canada in escaping the reach of the long and very strong arm of mental health law.

CONCLUSION

Contending that the "first attempt to assert meaning in psychopathology" is likely to have come from Plato, Littlewood (1988) brought attention to Plato's greater interest in "meaning" than in "etiology." Littlewood went on to speculate that the shift in the early modern period from the authority of clergy to that of medicine all but stamped out any discourse around psychopathology that was not concerned with etiology and disease causation. At the beginning of the 20th century, William James, in his magisterial *The Varieties of Religious Experience*, also engaged with such issues, demonstrating an acute sensitivity to the perils of what he referred to as "medical materialism" (James, 1958). This medical materialism (or medical reductionism) reveals itself in what James called "nothing but" explanations, ones that view St. Paul's visions on the road to Damascus, for example, as nothing but epilepsy and the mystical experiences of St. Teresa of Avila as nothing but hysteria (James, 1958). In this respect, as in others, James demonstrated his grasp of issues that remain highly relevant in the contemporary era, an era in which neuroscientific discourse asserts a greater hold on a wider range of human experience than was the case at the turn of the 20th century.

The backbone upon which this chapter rests is the contention that considerations of meaning and transformation ought to be afforded a space within psychiatrists' conceptual purview, in the interests of a shift toward epistemological pluralism and away from medical reductionism. Envisioned here is a sort of holy marriage between the *objective* fact-based concerns with etiology and disease causation on one hand and the *subjective* value-based concerns with meaning, purpose, and transformation on the other. As a clinical tool, Jonsen's Four Quadrant Model of ethical case analysis very much reflects that pluralistic ethos, and further, as has been shown in this chapter, constitutes an effective and pragmatic tool for use in clinical practice.

On a practical and organizational level, the case vignettes discussed in this chapter speak to the potential value of effective collaboration between community psychiatrists and religious leaders. Even though the specific cultural and demographic context affects whether and to what extent community psychiatrists in any given community will forge collaborative relationships with traditional healers, clergy, or other religious/spiritual professionals, the guiding principle still applies: The needs of patients who invoke a spiritually-informed explanation of their psychological distress are likely to be better served if there are greater working relationships between psychiatrists and representatives of particular religious/spiritual traditions. Several authors have raised the need to forge greater collaborative connections of this sort (e.g., Farrell & Goebert, 2008; John & Williams, 2013), and this chapter very much upholds and reinforces that view.

It might also be noted that the general thrust of this chapter is entirely in keeping with the values and principles that are coming to be associated with the so-called recovery movement (Whitley & Drake, 2010) in mental health, a key aspect of which is to include the spiritual and existential dimensions of human experience. Moreover, the subject matter of this chapter is likely to be done justice only when based on an effective interweaving of theory and praxis. Therefore, in addition to theoretical reflection, clinicians working at the interface of psychiatry and religion/spirituality are likely to profit from discussion of the sorts of ethical and pragmatic issues that arise there, as well as from dissemination of strategies that have been found to be helpful. Hopefully, this chapter has contributed in a small way to both of those.

REFERENCES

Bentall, R. (2005). R. D. Laing: An appraisal in the light of recent research. In S. Raschid (Ed.). *R. D. Laing: Contemporary perspectives* (pp. 221–245). London, England: Free Association Books.

Bradfield, B. (2002). Mental illness and the consciousness of freedom: The phenomenology of psychiatric labelling. *Indo-Pacific Journal of Phenomenology, 2*(1), 1–14.

Campbell, J. (1972). *The hero with a thousand faces.* Princeton, NJ: Princeton University Press.

Farrell, J. L., & Goebert, D. A. (2008). Collaboration between psychiatrists and clergy in recognizing and treating serious mental illness. *Psychiatric Services, 59*(4), 437–440.

Fulford, K. W. M. & Jackson. M. (1997). Spiritual experience and psychopathology. *Philosophy, Psychiatry and Psychology, 4*(1), 41–65.

James, W. (1958). *The varieties of religious experience.* New York, NY: Mentor Books.

John, D. A. & Williams, D. R. (2013). Mental health service use from a religious or spiritual advisor among Asian Americans. *Asian Journal of Psychiatry, 6*(6), 599–605.

Jonsen, A. R., Siegler, M., & Winslade, W. J. (2006). *Clinical ethics: A practical approach to ethical decisions in clinical medicine.* New York, NY: McGraw-Hill.

Laing R. D. (1967). *The politics of experience and the bird of paradise.* Harmondsworth, UK: Penguin.

Littlewood, R. (1988). The imitation of madness: The influence of psychopathology on culture. In R. Littlewood, *The butterfly and the serpent: Essays in psychiatry, race, and religion* (pp. 123–146). London, England: Free Association Books.

Lukoff, D., & Everest, H. (1985). The myths in mental illness. *Journal of Transpersonal Psychology, 17*(2), 123–153.

Mcdaniel, J. (1989). *The madness of the saints: Ecstatic religion in Bengal.* Chicago, IL: University of Chicago Press.

Moreira-Almeida, A., & Cardena, E. (2011). Differential diagnosis between non-pathological psychotic and spiritual experiences and mental disorders: A contribution from Latin American studies to the ICD-11. *Revista Brasileria de Psiquiatria, 33*(1), 29–36.

Nixon, G., Hagen, B., & Peters, T. (2010). Psychosis and transformation: A phenomenological inquiry. *International Journal of Mental Health and Addiction, 8*(4), 527–544.

Perry. J. W. (1999). *Trials of the visionary mind: Spiritual emergency and the renewal process.* New York, NY: SUNY Press.

Whitley, R. & Drake, R. E. (2010). Recovery: A dimensional approach. *Psychiatric Services, 61*(12), 1248–1250.

EIGHTEEN

International Perspectives on Ethical Issues in Religion and Psychiatry

Walid Sarhan, M.B., B.S., FRCPsych,
and Wai Lun Alan Fung, M.D., Sc.D., FRCPC

GLOBALLY, DISCUSSION OF THE PLACE OF SPIRITUALITY AND RELIGION within psychiatry has become particularly timely, both because of a resurgence of interest in religious belief and practice in many parts of the world and because of the increased movement of the world's populations, with the subsequent assimilation of a variety of belief systems and practices (Boehnlein, 2006). Because mental health providers everywhere are increasingly treating immigrants and refugees whose backgrounds are much different from their own, it is important for them to understand cultural factors, including religious thought and practices, that relate to mental health and illness.

Acculturation can bring about change in religious traditions, just as it can dynamically influence other areas of life for individuals and groups. Increased religiousness in contemporary societies has both positive and negative aspects (Boehnlein, 2006). One benefit is that religious belief systems may provide meaning for individuals or groups who have survived war, civil violence, torture, and/or natural disasters. Furthermore, a broad spectrum of religious organizations have historically funded and operated mental health services in various countries; clinicians need to be knowledgeable about the beliefs and political structures of these organizations so that the effectiveness of their services can be enhanced.

On the negative side, any religious fundamentalism can be damaging not only to individuals' mental health and social adjustment but also to peaceful coexistence among cultures. Religious fundamentalism is commonly seen by the public to be some sort of psychological imbalance, and mental health professionals may be asked to comment on behaviors that are seen as strange by the majority in society. This raises critical ethical questions about how psychiatric diagnoses and labels should be used to describe the individual who is acting upon a religious ideology. Should a religious ideology be described as a set of overvalued ideas or as a force contributing to terrorism?

INTERNATIONAL PATTERNS
OF SPIRITUALITY AND RELIGION

Worldwide, more than 8 in 10 people identify with a religious group. A comprehensive demographic study of more than 230 countries and territories conducted by the Pew Research Center's Forum on Religion & Public Life (Hackett & Grim, 2012) estimated that there are 5.8 billion religiously affiliated adults and children around the globe, representing 84% of the 2010 world population of 6.9 billion.

The demographic study—based on analysis of more than 2500 censuses, surveys and population registers—found 2.2 billion Christians (32% of the world's population), 1.6 billion Muslims (23%), 1 billion Hindus (15%), almost 500 million Buddhists (7%), and 14 million Jews (0.2%) around the world as of 2010 (Hackett & Grim, 2012). In addition, more than 400 million people (6%) practiced various folk or traditional religions, including African traditional religions, Chinese folk religions, Native American religions, and Australian aboriginal religions. An estimated 58 million people—slightly less than 1% of the global population—belonged to other religions, including the Baha'i faith, Jainism, Sikhism, Shintoism, Taoism, Tenrikyo, Wicca, and Zoroastrianism. Whereas roughly one in six people around the globe (1.1 billion, or 16%) had no religious affiliation, surveys indicated that many of the unaffiliated hold some religious or spiritual beliefs (such as belief in God or a universal spirit) even though they do not identify with a particular faith (Hackett & Grim, 2012).

For adolescents and young adults, Lippman and McIntosh (2010) reviewed the findings from four international surveys—the World Values Survey, the Civic Education study by the International Association for the Evaluation of Educational Achievement (IEA), the Young Europeans survey, and the Religion Monitor survey—which provide useful information on the patterns of spirituality and religiosity in many regions around the globe. Although the different measures and samples used did not permit direct comparison, these nationally representative surveys revealed consistent patterns that help explain the demographics of selected aspects of spirituality and religiosity (Lippman & McIntosh, 2010). One is the relationship between a country's level of economic development and the spirituality and religiosity of its population. As countries develop economically, less emphasis is placed on dominant religious traditions and values and more on secular institutions, as well as educational and economic accomplishment, powered by the need for trained workforces in industrialized societies (Inglehart, Basañez, Díez-Medrano, Halman, & Luijkx, 2004). Another pattern is the clear imprint of religion on beliefs in countries with a history of an influential religious tradition, such as Islam or Catholicism, such that young adults from these countries score relatively high on questions of spirituality and religiosity. Likewise, there is an imprint of the secular traditions of communist, socialist, and welfare states, reflected in the low importance given to religion and God in countries of the former Soviet Union, where religion was suppressed for so long and atheism was espoused by the state and widely adopted by citizens, and in the Nordic welfare states. In addition, formerly Confucian societies (i.e., Japan and China) have a tradition of secular bureaucratic authority that is reflected in the low importance attached to God and religion in those countries (Inglehart et al., 2004). It should nonetheless be noted that these survey items do not adequately capture the diversity of how young people experience and shape their spiritual identities across different cultures, contexts, and religious traditions (Lippman & McIntosh, 2010).

INTERNATIONAL PERSPECTIVES
ON PROFESSIONAL ETHICS IN PSYCHIATRY
AND THE INTERSECTIONS BETWEEN
SPIRITUALITY/RELIGION AND PSYCHIATRY

Triggered by the political misuse of psychiatric concepts, knowledge, and techniques in countries such as the former Soviet Union, Romania, and South Africa that came to public awareness during the early 1970s, the Declaration of Hawaii—prepared by Dr. Clarence Blomquist as the first positional statement of the psychiatric profession concerning ethical questions—was adopted by the General Assembly of the World Psychiatric Association (WPA) in Hawaii in 1977 to help psychiatrists in conflicts of psychiatric decision making (Helmchen & Okasha, 2000). Growing needs and new ethical dilemmas of the 1990s led the WPA to develop new recommendations regarding the duties of psychiatrists, which resulted in the Declaration of Madrid, adopted by the WPA in 1996 and subsequently enhanced by the WPA General Assemblies in 1999, 2002, 2005 and 2011.

The Declaration of Madrid outlines the ethical boundaries for psychiatric work. It states that as practitioners of medicine, psychiatrists must be aware of the ethical implications of being a physician and of the specific ethical demands of the specialty of psychiatry. As members of society, psychiatrists must also advocate for fair and equal treatment of the mentally ill and for social justice and equity for all. It formulates seven general guidelines with an increased emphasis on research and resource allocation and gives five specific guidelines on euthanasia, torture, the death penalty, selection of sex, and organ transplantation (Helmchen & Okasha, 2000). The Declaration affirms that ethical practice is based on the psychiatrist's individual sense of responsibility to the patient and judgment in determining what is correct and appropriate conduct. External standards and influences such as professional codes of conduct, the study of ethics, or the rule of law by themselves will not guarantee the ethical practice of medicine. Psychiatrists should keep in mind at all times the boundaries of the psychiatrist–patient relationship and should be guided primarily by respect for patients and concern for their welfare and integrity.

The WPA Ethics Committee recognized the need to develop a number of specific guidelines regarding 16 specific situations including the following two. First, psychiatrists shall not take part in any process of mental or physical torture, even when authorities attempt to force their involvement in such acts. On several occasions, psychiatrists have reportedly been involved in such acts of torture. Second, psychiatrists shall not make pronouncements to the media about the presumed psychopathology of any individuals. This ethical principle is repeatedly violated when psychiatrists talking to the media claim that a certain terrorist or criminal is or is not suffering from mental illness. If the psychiatrist knows the person professionally, he is breaking confidentiality, and if not, he is violating this article from the Declaration of Madrid (WPA, 1996).

In addition to the WPA and the various national psychiatric professional organizations, the United Nations (UN) has also been involved in setting international standards of law and ethics in the general area of mental healthcare and psychiatry. The preeminent or overarching relevant provisions—namely, that people everywhere enjoy equal rights to freedom of the person, freedom of political and religious belief, freedom of expression, the right to a fair trial, and so forth—are comprehensively set forth in the Universal Declaration of Human Rights and the International Covenant on Civil and Political Rights (ICCPR) (Human Rights Watch & Geneva Initiative on Psychiatry, 2002). In the early 1980s, the UN undertook a major investigative review of mental healthcare provision around the world in response to growing international concern over the political misuse of psychiatry in countries such as the former Soviet Union and South Africa. This review focused on the rules, procedures, and practices pursued by various countries in the area of involuntary psychiatric commitment and treatment. In 1983, Special Rapporteur Erica-Irene Daes presented the results of the investigative review and recommended that the UN Commission on Human Rights should, among other things, urge all member States "[to] prohibit the expression of verbal psychological and psychiatric abuses, in particular for political or other non-medical grounds." After several years of discussion and drafting work within the UN, this initiative bore legislative fruit in December 1991, when the world body's General Assembly adopted a wide-ranging set of provisions entitled *Principles for the Protection of Persons with Mental Illness and for the Improvement of Mental Health Care*. Taken together, the UN's 1991 Principles and the WPA's Declarations of Hawaii and Madrid provide the core set of international standards upon which the ethical and legal practices of psychiatrists around the world should properly be evaluated (Human Rights Watch & Geneva Initiative on Psychiatry, 2002).

In addition to the WPA and UN, grassroots initiatives have also played a prominent role in the field of ethics and psychiatry. For instance, Geneva Initiative on Psychiatry, an international foundation, was formed in 1980 to combat the political abuse of psychiatry, which at that moment was widely used as a tool of repression in the Soviet Union and in a number of Eastern European countries (Human Rights Watch & Geneva Initiative on Psychiatry, 2002). It has been the main development agency working in mental health care in Central and Eastern Europe and the new independent states of the former USSR, focusing its efforts on the principle of empowerment of local mental health reformers and their organizations. It has collaborated with international organizations such as the WPA and the World Health Organization, and strives, at the local level, to promote and deepen cooperation between mental healthcare facilities and their users, family members, and user organizations. It aims at monitoring the human rights situation in mental health in all countries where it operates, and it combats the political abuse of psychiatry wherever it is found to occur (Human Rights Watch & Geneva Initiative on Psychiatry, 2002). In 2005, the organization was renamed the Global Initiative on Psychiatry.

The importance of ethical implications of spiritual and religious considerations for the clinical practice of psychiatry has been addressed by various national and international psychiatric organizations in the form of guidelines and position statements.

In 1990, the American Psychiatric Association (APA) published *Guidelines Regarding Possible Conflict Between Psychiatrists' Religious Commitments and Psychiatric Practice*, which emphasized the need for psychiatrists to respect their patients' beliefs and warned against imposition of psychiatrists' beliefs on their patients (APA, 1990). These guidelines provide ethical and professional boundaries within which matters of religion and belief may properly be attended to by psychiatrists, for the benefit of their patients, while ensuring that potential conflicts between the beliefs of psychiatrists and patients are handled appropriately and that potential abuses are avoided. These guidelines were updated in 2006 as the *APA Resource Document on Religious/ Spiritual Commitments and Psychiatric Practice* (Peteet et al., 2006).

In the United Kingdom, the Royal College of Psychiatrists published a Position Statement titled *Recommendations for Psychiatrists on Spirituality and Religion* in 2011, which was subsequently updated in 2013 (Cook, 2013). This document acknowledges that both the evidence base and patient opinions indicate that spirituality and religion are significant in clinical practice and research. Good clinical practice requires both an awareness of the ethical and professional boundaries associated with spirituality and religion in psychiatry and competence in managing them appropriately, respectfully, and sensitively (Cook, 2013). The full text of the Position

Statement is available from <http://www.rcpsych.ac.uk/pdf/PS03_2013.pdf>. Some of its seven recommendations are the following:

- A tactful and sensitive exploration of patients' religious beliefs and spirituality should routinely be considered and will sometimes be an essential component of clinical assessment.
- Psychiatrists should be expected always to respect and be sensitive to the spiritual/religious beliefs and practices of their patients or to the lack of them, and of the families and caregivers of their patients.
- Psychiatrists should not use their professional position for proselytizing or undermining faith and should maintain appropriate professional boundaries in relation to self-disclosure of their own spirituality/religion.
- Psychiatrists, whatever their personal beliefs, should be willing to work with leaders/members of faith communities, chaplains and pastoral workers in support of the well-being of their patients, and should encourage all colleagues in mental health work to do likewise.

In 2016, the WPA published the *Position Statement on Spirituality and Religion in Psychiatry* (Moreira-Almeida, Sharma, Janse van Rensburg, Verhagen, & Cook, 2016), the full text of which is available from http://onlinelibrary.wiley.com/doi/10.1002/wps.20304/full. This statement essentially reaffirms the recommendations by the Royal College of Psychiatrists. In addition, it recommends that "psychiatrists should be knowledgeable concerning the potential for both benefit and harm of religious, spiritual and secular worldviews and practices and be willing to share this information in a critical but impartial way with the wider community in support of the promotion of health and well-being." Overall, it emphasizes that "the approach to religion and spirituality should be person-centered." The concept of person-centered care is closely related to the ethical principles of autonomy and beneficence.

Case Study 1: Terrorism

There is neither an academic nor a legal consensus regarding the definition of terrorism (Schmid, 2011; Williamson, 2009). Various legal systems and government agencies use different definitions. Moreover, governments have been reluctant to formulate an agreed upon, legally binding definition. These difficulties arise from the fact that the term is politically and emotionally charged (Hoffman, 1998).

A 2003 study by Jeffrey Record for the US Army quoted a source (Schmid & Jongman, 1988) that counted 109 definitions of terrorism covering 22 different definitional elements. Record continued, "Terrorism expert Walter Laqueur also has counted over 100 definitions and concludes that the 'only general characteristic generally agreed upon is that terrorism involves violence and the threat of violence.' Yet terrorism is hardly the only enterprise involving violence and the threat of violence. So does war, coercive diplomacy, and bar room brawls" (Laqueur, 1999).

The American Psychological Association has stated clearly on several occasions the difficulty of giving simplistic answers to questions about the psychological aspects of terrorism (DeAngelis, 2009).

Unfortunately, in recent decades, many areas of the globe—such as Northern Ireland, the Balkans, Africa, and the Middle East—have seen the politicization of religious beliefs resulting in the destruction of lives and cultures. This is a very important realm for psychiatry because survivors of regional war trauma and violence frequently migrate to other countries, where they subsequently attempt not only to acculturate but also to place their traumatic experiences into a meaningful context. Another source of tension in the current era is the resurgence of religion in many parts of the world in response to the increasing secularization of developing societies. This tension frequently leads to a polarization of beliefs and perspectives and a hardening of attitudes and opinions when, in fact, religious and secular perspectives may be complementary in understanding the human condition and human behavior.

Suicide Terrorism

Suicide terrorism is the most lethal form of terrorism, and it is on the increase. In 2013 alone, some 384 suicide terrorist acts were carried out in 18 countries causing 3743 deaths—representing a 46% growth over the number of attacks in 2012 and a 66% increase in the number of lethal casualties (Sheehan, 2014).

Most of the research on suicide terrorism has been conducted in the fields of political science and international relations. The prevailing wisdom within this literature is that suicide terrorists are not suicidal. But how good is the evidence for this assumption? Knowing whether suicide terrorists are suicidal has implications for prevention, rehabilitation, and the "softer" side of counterterrorism designed to win minds and hearts. In addition, it may deepen our understanding of suicide itself. Much of the evidence against the possibility that suicide terrorists are suicidal is based on anecdotes or faulty assumptions about suicide. Relatively few formal systematic studies of suicidality in suicide terrorists have been conducted. Nonetheless, there is emerging evidence that suicidality may play a role in a significant number of cases. The field needs a more multidimensional approach, more systematic data at the individual level, and greater international cross-disciplinary collaboration. Would-be suicide terrorists (intercepted and arrested on their way to an attack) should be routinely interviewed using standard internationally accepted psychiatric diagnostic interviews as well as suicidality and homicidality rating scales. Psychological autopsies should also be routinely conducted worldwide. Because no one research site can collect all of the information that is needed, the creation of an internationally shared database that focuses on suicide terrorists rather than simply incidents is encouraged (Sheehan, 2014).

The September 11th suicide attacks sparked significant debate in the Islamic world about the merits of suicide attacks. Sheikh Muhammad Sa'id al-Tantawi, head of Cairo's Al-Azhar, the most prestigious university for Sunni jurisprudence, declared that the Shari'a rejects all attempts at taking human life, and Sheikh Muhammad bin 'Abdallah al-Sabil, a member of the Saudi Council of Islamic Clerics and imam at the Grand Mosque in Mecca, decried the suicide attacks on the basis that Islamic law forbids killing civilians, forbids suicide, and protects Jews and Christians. But both Tantawi and Sabil sidestepped the question of martyrdom operations. Because preserving the life of *dhimmis* (Jews and Christians) is conditional on their acceptance of Muslim rule, suicide attacks upon Israelis or Jews and Christians outside of majority Muslim countries may be permissible. Indeed, other Al-Azhar scholars, for example 'Abd al-'Azim al-Mit'ani, say that it is permissible to kill Israeli civilians in the cause of jihad (Malka, 2003), so one can see that the opinions vary according to the boundaries and definitions used.

Religious Terrorism

Is terrorism carried out based on motivations and goals that have a predominantly religious character? In the modern age, after the decline of ideas such as the divine right of kings and with the rise of nationalism, terrorism has more often been based on anarchism, nihilism, and revolutionary politics. Since 1980, however, there has been an increase in terrorist activity motivated by religion (Hoffman, 1997, 1998).

As the world is witnessing all these problems, psychiatrists and psychologists are asked to comment and to participate in activities designed to counteract terrorism. In doing so, they are at times at risk of being carried into unethical behavior.

ETHICAL CONSIDERATIONS IN THE INTERSECTIONS BETWEEN RELIGION/SPIRITUALITY AND TRADITIONAL BELIEFS AND CULTURES

Nolan, Whetten, and Koenig (2011) have discussed ethics reform by introducing the contribution of religious, spiritual, and traditional beliefs and practices to both subject vulnerability and patient improvement. This contribution is often more relevant in less wealthy countries as the result of many factors including education, cultural standards, and economic factors.

A growing body of evidence suggests that religious, spiritual, and traditional beliefs and practices may provide positive benefits—although in some cases mixed or negative consequences—for mental and physical health. These beliefs and practices add a new level of complexity to ethical deliberations, in terms of what ignoring them may mean for both distributive justice and respect for persons. International ethical guidelines need to be created that are expansive enough to cover an array of social groups and circumstances. It is proposed that these guidelines incorporate the religious, spiritual, and/or traditional principles that characterize a local population. Providing effective mental healthcare requires respecting and understanding how differences, including ones that express a population's religious, spiritual, or traditional belief systems, play into the complex deliberations and negotiations that must be undertaken if researchers are to adhere to ethical imperatives in research and treatment (Nolan et al., 2011).

Case Study 2: Ethics and Healing in Ancient China and India

Ancient Chinese medical ethics is established on the foundation of Confucian ethics. For 2500 years, the Confucian scriptures were essential teaching materials for students, and Confucian ethics was the dominant moral philosophy and ideology of Chinese culture. Many Confucian scholars practiced healing arts and formulated their professional ethics on the bases of Confucian ethics. Medical practice was regarded as one of their many duties. The moral standard for a physician was basically the same as that of an ideal Confucian person: *chun-tzu*, "the superior man." It was widely accepted that a physician's saving his patients' lives and promoting their welfare was as respectable as a Confucian scholar's realizing his moral and political aspirations through ruling the states and bringing peace and prosperity to people (Tsai, 1999). Humaneness (*ren*; in Chinese, 仁) has appeared repeatedly in ancient Chinese medical ethics. Confucius's concept of humaneness has dual meanings: the particular virtue that means love or benevolence, and the general virtue that is the foundation of morality, the basis of all goodness, and the origin of all virtues; hence, the term is also rendered "perfect virtue" or "true humanity." The practice of medicine is the realization of humaneness.

There are many references in Indian philosophical texts to what constitutes an ideal person. Most often, text is quoted from Srimad Bhagavad Gita describing the balanced person as one who has a controlled mind, emotions, and senses. For understanding the concept of mental health, perhaps more important than any one quote is the broad Hindu view of life, as summed up in the well-known four ends or broad aims of life (Purushartha). These are Dharma, Kama, Artha, and Moksha. Dharma is righteousness, virtue, or religious duty. Kama refers to fulfillment of our biological needs or sensual pleasures. Artha refers to fulfillment of our social needs including material gains, acquisition of wealth, and social recognition. Moksha means liberation from worldly bondage and union with ultimate reality. The relationships among these four aims highlight the harmony of different dimensions in life: Kama as the biological dimension, Artha as the social dimension, and Moksha as the spiritual dimension. Dharma is the central axis around which life rotates. If one pursues Kama and Artha without Dharma, the long-term result is suffering for the individual and for others around him (Wig, 1999).

DEVELOPMENT OF GLOBAL ETHICS

With increased human interactions globally and ever more diversity among peoples and cultures in the global age, it has become imperative that ethics as the mode by which peoples understand, evaluate, and direct their action be enriched (McLean, 2007). Since the early 1990s, there have been a number of attempts to formulate a global ethic. These attempts were initiated by ecumenical religious leaders but have subsequently made their way into more general secular discourse, especially within the orbit of the United Nations (Struhl, 2007).

In September 1993, representatives of 120 of the world's religions assembled in Chicago to convene a Parliament of the World's Religions. This marked the 100th anniversary of the 1893 World Parliament of Religions which had initiated a worldwide religious dialogue. The task in the 1993 Parliament was to discuss a draft of a global ethic written by Hans Küng, and the conference adopted the *Declaration Toward a Global Ethic*.[1] The main document discusses four Principles of a Global Ethic. The first principle is that a global ethic is essential for a better global order. Such an ethic, the document states, "can be affirmed by all persons of ethical convictions, whether religiously grounded or not." In short, a global ethic would formulate consensus on a core set of values which all religions, and indeed all persons of reasonable ethical sensibilities, could affirm (Struhl, 2007). The Declaration then begins to

---

1. The full text of the Declaration is available from https://dialogueinstitute.squarespace.com/s/Declaration-of-a-Global-Ethic.pdf.

describe this consensus in its second principle, which is that "every human being must be treated humanely." This principle, the Declaration asserts, can be derived from a fundamental ethical norm found in all the world's religions and ethical systems, an ethical norm known as the Golden Rule, which the Declaration formulates as follows: "What you do not wish to be done to yourself, do not do to others . . . . What you wish done to yourself, do to others" (Struhl, 2007). This principle can be of value in psychiatric practice within various religions and cultures around the world.

The third principle of the Declaration highlights four more specific ethical guidelines which, it claims, follow from the basic principle that every human being must be treated humanely (consistent with the Golden Rule) and which can be found in most of the religions of the world (Struhl, 2007). These are (1) commitment to a culture of nonviolence and respect for life, which includes a concern not just for humans but also for nonhuman animals and plants; (2) commitment to a culture of solidarity and a just economic order, which would oppose totalitarian state socialism and unbridled capitalism and would recognize that peace is not possible without justice; (3) commitment to a culture of tolerance and a life of truthfulness, which presents a challenge to the lies of politicians and business people, to the misinformation and ideological propaganda of mass media, to scientists who allow themselves to be tools of political or economic interests, and to representatives of religion who preach intolerance of other religions; and (4) commitment to a culture of equal rights and partnership between men and women which would oppose sexual discrimination and exploitation. Together, the Declaration declares, these four guidelines, if taken seriously, should be able to transform the world. This leads to the fourth principle of the Declaration, that ethical guidelines by themselves are insufficient and can become a social reality only through a transformation of consciousness (Struhl, 2007). Such a transformation, the Declaration states, is already underway. Without this transformation and the global ethic that would guide it, we cannot solve the global crises which threaten our very existence as a species (Struhl, 2007).

In the same year that the Parliament of the World's Religions discussed Küng's draft, Leonard Swidler, a colleague of Küng at Temple University in Philadelphia, wrote his own draft of a global ethic, which was subsequently presented to a number of international conferences and then posted on the Internet in the hope of reaching a wider audience and of generating responses (Struhl, 2007). His draft on the Internet, entitled *A Universal Declaration of a Global Ethic*, has undergone a number of revisions in the ensuing years. It was preceded by a long discussion entitled *Toward a Universal Declaration of a Global Ethic*. In that discussion, Swidler claimed that humanity is moving from the Age of Monologue to the Age of Global Dialogue, a move that involves a major paradigm shift in consciousness. In this age, Swidler argued, there is a special need for a global ethic insofar as any part of humanity could generate economic, nuclear, or environment disaster for the rest. Thus, there is a need to come to a minimal ethical consensus based on dialogue.

Swidler's *Universal Declaration* takes the Golden Rule as the ultimate basis of this global consensus insofar as some variant of it can be found in every religion and ethical tradition. He then proceeds to list 8 basic principles of a global ethic and 10 middle ethical principles—which are much more specific than the principles of the Parliament's Declaration and seem to be a more Western articulation of a general ethic. For example, the principles affirm that every person should be "free to exercise and develop every capacity, so long as it does not infringe on the rights of other persons"; the right of "freedom of thought, speech, conscience, and religion or belief"; and that all adults should "have the right to a voice in choosing their leaders and holding them accountable" (Struhl, 2007).

Since the drafting of these declarations, several attempts have been made to move the project for a global ethic beyond religious circles (Struhl, 2007). In 1995, the World Commission on Culture and Development issued a UNESCO report which called for a Global Ethic that would provide the basis for a change in attitudes, social priorities, and patterns of consumption necessary to secure "a decent and meaningful life" for all human beings throughout the world. In 1996, the Interaction Council, composed of 30 former heads of state, urged that a global ethics be developed to meet the problems of the 21st century. In 1997, UNESCO initiated a Universal Ethics Project, which brought together philosophers and theologians representing a variety of ethical traditions in order to develop a universal ethic that would be able to confront such problems as poverty, underdevelopment, environmental deterioration, and various forms of intolerance. Such a universal ethic, the document declares, would have a different ontological status from the UN Declaration of Human Rights in that it would provide the philosophical principles from which those rights could be derived.

CLINICAL VIGNETTES

The following vignettes illustrate some of the ethical challenges in the intersection of religion/ spirituality and psychiatry in an international context.

Case 1

A 52-year-old married Muslim patient living in Canada suffered from bipolar affective disorder and was well maintained on lithium. He asked his psychiatrist about discontinuing medication for the month of Ramadan because, he said, he feels very thirsty when fasting. His psychiatrist advised him not to fast and to continue taking lithium, but the patient was reluctant to accept this advice because, according to the Islamic Shari'a, permission not to fast should come from a trustworthy Muslim physician. The psychiatrist was not a Muslim and was not sure of the correct ruling of Islam in this matter.

Questions. (1) Should the psychiatrist only emphasize the importance of continuing lithium? (2) Should the psychiatrist say that he is an atheist? (3) Should the psychiatrist say that he does not know about fasting but knows that the patient needs the medication? (4) Should he ask a colleague or a Muslim religious scholar?

Discussion: Because the religious belief of the psychiatrist is not the central issue in the discussion and focusing on this could represent a crossing of professional boundaries, it will probably be enough to say to the patient, "I know that you need the medication, but I don't know Islam's view on this. Might we consult a Muslim scholar or cleric together about the question of taking medication during Ramadan?"

Case 2

A 20-year-old Muslim university student from Turkey suffering from generalized anxiety disorder asked his treating Jewish psychiatrist in the United States about his sexual needs, as he had no girlfriend and felt he could not watch pornography or masturbate because he was following Islamic rules. The only acceptable option seemed to be marriage, which he could not afford.

Questions: (1) Because there are some similarities between Islam and Judaism, should the psychiatrist proceed to discuss how the situation would be handled in Judaism? (2) Should he simply apologize that he cannot answer this question? (3) Should he advise the patient to have a girlfriend?

Discussion: Raising the question in relation to Judaism is potentially confusing, and simply advising this young man to have a girlfriend is unethical. Masturbation is not forbidden in Islam but rather is not encouraged, which is a significant difference. Apology is an acceptable approach because the question is religious rather than psychiatric. However, the psychiatrist might also offer to work with the patient to develop a solution by learning more about the pertinent issues, potentially consulting and collaborating with a faith leader of the particular Islamic tradition to which this patient belongs.

Case 3

A 25-year-old single Muslim woman in Pakistan suffering from panic disorder became very depressed and guilty because she thought that she had lost her virginity while she was with her boyfriend. Because she was sure it was a sin and dishonoring, she became suicidal. She requested that the psychiatrist examine her to find out if the hymen is still intact or not.

Questions: (1) Can the psychiatrist ethically perform such an examination? (2) How could the psychiatrist reassure her? (3) Is it the duty of the psychiatrist to refer her to a gynecologist? (4) If she does and the hymen is deflorated, can she tell her that?

Discussion: Virginity and premarital sex are major issues from both cultural and religious perspectives for this young lady. In light of this complexity, a psychiatrist should not perform any examination herself but should refer the whole matter to a gynecologist. The result may affect the patient's psychological state, and she could need closer monitoring for suicidal risk.

Case 4

A 42-year-old married construction worker with three children presented to a psychiatrist in Australia with a 2-month history of severe depression. He was reluctant to accept treatment or to discuss the reasons for his state. His wife explained to the psychiatrist that they are Hindu; she stated that her husband believed an evil eye had affected his karma and that the treatment should be directed toward the cause. He had been receiving traditional treatment but was getting worse. When he attempted suicide by trying to take an overdose of pills he had thought everything would be fine after reincarnation. His Christian psychiatrist had little knowledge of Hinduism as practiced in Australia.

Questions: (1) How should the psychiatrist approach this case? (2) Can he ask the traditional healer to come along? (3) Are there any guidelines for approaching such a patient?

Discussion: In Australia, health departments have guidelines for dealing with the health issues of Hindu patients. Hindus believe that all illnesses, whether physical or mental, have biological, psychological, and spiritual elements. Treatments that do not address all three causes may not be considered effective by a Hindu patient. Many Hindus have a strong belief in the concept of the evil eye and may believe it to be a cause of mental illness. Neither involving the traditional healer nor accepting his views is necessary, but explaining that the medication will correct the chemical imbalance caused by the evil eye can help persuade the patient to comply with treatment.

CONCLUSION

In the current global era, a thorough discussion of ethical issues at the intersection between spirituality/religion and psychiatry would not be complete without considering cultural and international variables. This chapter has illustrated some of the opportunities and challenges of such considerations. The development of a global ethic in a multicultural world may be instrumental in advancing this discussion. Although some (e.g., Struhl, 2007) have expressed skepticism about this possibility due to challenges in coming to a minimal consensus on ethical norms globally, McLean (2007) described an approach for the development of such global ethics beginning with a better understanding of the ethics that guide the peoples with whom we now live. This could help to broaden our modes of evaluation in order to take into account not only our own path but those of others. The task of recognizing the uniqueness of peoples, while striving for a unity which will enable them in their diversity to communicate and act cooperatively one with another, will require new avenues of philosophical exploration that are based on many cultural and philosophical traditions, as well as coordinated action on behalf of all. The overall goal is to achieve "diversity in unity" through recognition of divine unity as the point of unity of peoples and the foundation of the sense of good over evil. It is imperative that psychiatry and spirituality/religion be included in such initiatives.

REFERENCES

American Psychiatric Association. (1990). Guidelines regarding possible conflict between psychiatrists' religious commitments and psychiatric practice. Committee on Religion and Psychiatry. *American Journal of Psychiatry, 147*, 542.

Boehnlein, J. K. (2006). Religion and spirituality in psychiatric care: Looking back, looking ahead. *Transcultural Psychiatry, 43*, 634–651.

Cook, C. C. H. (2013). *Recommendations for psychiatrists on spirituality and religion.* Position Statement PS03/2013, Royal College of Psychiatrists. London, England: Royal College of Psychiatrists.

DeAngelis, T. (2009). Understanding terrorism. *Monitor on Psychology, 40*(10), 60.

Hackett, C. P., & Grim, B. J. (2012). *The global religious landscape: A report on the size and distribution of the world's major religious groups as of 2010.* Washington, DC: Pew Research Center, Pew Forum on Religion & Public Life.

Helmchen, H., & Okasha, A. (2000). From the Hawaii Declaration to the Declaration of Madrid. *Acta Psychiatrica Scandinavica Supplementum, 399*, 20–23.

Hoffman, B. (1997). The confluence of international and domestic trends in terrorism. *Terrorism and Political Violence, 9*(2), 1–15.

Hoffman, B. (1998). *Inside terrorism.* New York, NY: Columbia University Press.

Human Rights Watch & Geneva Initiative on Psychiatry. (2002). *Dangerous minds: Political psychiatry in China today and its origins in the Mao era.* New York, NY: Human Rights Watch.

Inglehart, R., Basañez, M., Díez-Medrano, J., Halman, L., & Luijkx, R. (2004). *Human beliefs and values: A cross-cultural sourcebook based upon the 1999-2002 values surveys.* Mexico City, Mexico: Siglo Veintiuno Editores.

Laqueur, W. (1999). *The new terrorism: Fanaticism and the arms of mass destruction.* New York, NY: Oxford University Press.

Lippman, L. H., & McIntosh, H. (2010). *The demographics of spirituality and religiosity among youth.* Child Trends Research Brief. Retrieved from https://www.childtrends.org/wp-content/uploads/01/Spirituality-and-Religiosity-Among-Youth.pdf.

Malka, H. (2003). Must innocents die? The Islamic debate over suicide attacks. *Middle East Quarterly, 10*(2): 19–28.

McLean, G. F. (2007). Introduction. In M. T. Stepanyants (Ed.), *Comparative ethics in a global age.* Washington, DC: The Council for Research in Values and Philosophy.

Moreira-Almeida, A., Sharma, A., Janse van Rensburg, B., Verhagen, P. J., & Cook, C. C. H. (2016). WPA position statement on spirituality and religion in psychiatry. *World Psychiatry, 15*(1), 87–88.

Nolan, J. A., Whetten, K., & Koenig, H. G. (2011). Religious, spiritual, and traditional beliefs and practices and the ethics of mental health research in less wealthy countries. *International Journal of Psychiatry in Medicine, 42*(3), 267–277.

Peteet, J., Abou-Allaban, Y., Dell, M. L., Greenberg, W., Lomax, J., Torres, M., Cowell, V. (2006). *Religious/spiritual commitments and psychiatric practice.* APA Official Actions, American Psychiatric Association. Retrieved from https://www.psychiatry.org/File%20Library/Psychiatrists/Directories/Library-and-Archive/resource_documents/rd2006_Religion.pdf.

Record, J. (2003). *Bounding the global war on terrorism.* Carlisle, PA: Strategic Studies Institute, US Army War College.

Schmid, A. P. (2011). The definition of terrorism. In A. P. Schmid(Ed.). *The Routledge Handbook of Terrorism Research.* New York, NY: Routledge.

Schmid, A. P., & Jongman, A. J. (1988). *Political terrorism: A new guide to actors, authors, concepts, data bases, theories, and literature.* New Brunswick, NJ: Transaction Books.

Sheehan, I. S. (2014). Are suicide terrorists suicidal? A critical assessment of the evidence. *Innovations in Clinical Neuroscience, 11*(9–10), 81–92.

Struhl, K. J. (2007). Is a global ethic possible? In M. T. Stepanyants (Ed.), *Comparative ethics in a global age.* Washington, DC: The Council for Research in Values and Philosophy.

Tsai, D. F. (1999). Ancient Chinese medical ethics and the four principles of biomedical ethics. *Journal of Medical Ethics, 25*(4), 315–321.

Wig, N. N. (1999). Mental health and spiritual values: A view from the east. *International Review of Psychiatry, 11,* 92–96.

Williamson, M. (2009). *Terrorism, war and international law: The legality of the use of force against Afghanistan in 2001.* Hampshire, England: Ashgate Publishing.

World Psychiatric Association. (1996). *Madrid declaration on ethical standards for psychiatric practice.* Geneva: Author.

NINETEEN

Ethical Considerations for Mental Health Providers Responding to Disasters and Emergencies

Samuel B. Thielman, M.D., Ph.D., and Glenn Goss, D.S.W.

DURING THE LAST TWO DECADES, MENTAL HEALTH WORKERS HAVE found themselves involved increasingly in the role of disaster responders. The targeting of civilian populations and the disruption of urban areas during times of war and natural disaster have created a need for large-scale thinking on the part of mental health professionals about how best to respond to populations at risk for psychological harm. Psychiatrists find themselves involved in both civilian and military response efforts—sometimes leading the effort, sometimes playing a supporting role, but always bringing with them their unique training that not only focuses on the medical basis for behavioral disorders but also emphasizes interpersonal skills, group dynamics, and team leadership.

These new challenges have raised a host of ethical issues. In disaster settings, social structures are disrupted, roles become blurred, and the rule of law deteriorates. In such settings, many dilemmas arise that, for individual clinicians, can seem strange or even unprecedented. The purpose of this chapter is to bring to light some ethical issues that commonly arise during disasters and in post-conflict environments and to point to discussions that can help guide our clinical thinking.

DUAL AGENCY AND OTHER CONFLICT-OF-INTEREST CONCERNS

An immediate ethical issue for psychiatrists is that of dual agency or dual loyalty—that is, we can find ourselves working on behalf of two entities, our employer and our patient (Robertson &

Walter, 2008; Sessums, Collen, O'Malley, Jackson, & Roy, 2009; Strasburger, Gutheil, & Brodsky, 1997). For obvious reasons, disaster mental health providers, if they are not volunteers, usually find themselves in the employ of a governmental organization or a non-governmental organization (NGO). Because the survivors are not paying us, there may be pressure to act in ways that do not have the interests of our patient as the first priority.

The principle of "do no harm" comes from classical antiquity (Van der Eijk, 2005) and is deeply rooted in modern medical ethics. Section 8 of the American Psychiatric Association's *Principles of Medical Ethics with Annotations Especially Applicable to Psychiatry* states that "a physician shall, while caring for a patient, regard responsibility to the patient as paramount." Explaining further, it says that, "when the psychiatrist's outside relationships conflict with the clinical needs of the patient, the psychiatrist must always consider the impact of such relationships and strive to resolve conflicts in a manner that the psychiatrist believes is likely to be beneficial to the patient" (American Psychiatric Association [APA], 2013).

Yet organizations and economic pressures sometimes push responders to act in ways that are not aligned with the interest of survivors. One example would be when a government psychiatrist or psychologist, responding to an emergency involving terrorism, is expected to pass along pertinent security information gathered from patients during the provision of care. Another would be a situation in which a worker for a humanitarian organization is pressured to obtain stories from victims that can be used in the service of fund raising, even if eliciting such stories may create unnecessary psychological distress for the victim.

Mental health workers may be under more pressure than most responders with respect to dual role obligations, given that we often have a greater degree of information of use to funding entities. We have access to narratives and socioeconomic data that governments and corporations find interesting and helpful for purposes for manipulating public perceptions. The clear guidance from the APA and other professional organizations on dual role issues can help providers push back against pressures from employers to act in ways not consistent with the patient's best interest.

PSYCHIATRIC COMPETENCIES

For psychiatrists, as for others, a disaster often raises the question of how far to go in using procedures, techniques, or interventions that are not part of one's training or background. There is often great pressure from government and aid agencies to "do something" following an emergency or disaster, especially in terms of psychological support. Because disasters are infrequent and often unanticipated events, planners and responders may or may not have an informed understanding of current thinking on psychological support for disasters. In addition, peer support groups, advocacy organizations, disaster tourists, and well-intended leaders may put pressure on psychiatric responders to offer interventions they perceive to be helpful or useful, regardless of current experts' consensus. This can lead to the use of unproven or disproven therapeutic techniques and to pulling people into "treatment" who may not actually need any sort of mental health (or other) treatment. Such an approach can be both expensive and countertherapeutic.

Should a psychiatrist or other provider make a good faith effort to implement procedures with which he or she has only passing familiarity? John Call and colleagues asserted that ethical guidelines and the law only allow mental health professionals to provide services for which they have been trained and have demonstrated competence, except in the situation where no properly trained person is available and there is a risk of needed services being denied (Call, Pfefferbaum, Jenuwine, & Flynn, 2012). Not all agree. Medical ethicist Edmund G. Howe has taken issue with such a view, noting that, "a care provider's worst defense in court is that he or she did what was legally best for him or herself, when he or she knew that clinically this was suboptimal for the patient. Their very best defense, on the other hand, is most likely that even though they knew that some act might be 'legally wrong,' they did it anyway, because they believed it was best for the patient" (Howe, 2012). The bottom line is that it is critical for an ethical response to be informed by current expert consensus while remaining flexible enough to adapt to unexpected circumstances.

LICENSING AND DOCUMENTATION

In post-disaster and post-conflict environments, especially in the developing world, there are varying degrees of licensing or regulatory frameworks for clinicians. Generally, the emphasis is on self-regulation, and practice is governed by a range of optional international guidelines. And, of course, clinicians working for international NGOs or foreign governments are almost always vetted by their funders and not by the beneficiaries. In fact, the beneficiaries are generally highly vulnerable individuals who have no input into the selection of providers during complex humanitarian emergencies (Pérouse de Montclos, 2012).

Many developing countries do not have the regulatory frameworks that can accommodate an influx of disaster mental health providers. Consequently, international NGO clinical staff often follow—voluntarily—international guidelines that generally have little to say about documentation, usually proposing that mental health staff follow the professional guidelines of the country in which they are licensed. Whereas individual US states sometimes make exceptions to licensing rules when professionals are coming to their state to help in an emergency, such is not necessarily the case in other settings.

Negi and Furman argued that when social workers are involved in transnational social work and when they leave their geographic jurisdiction, they go beyond the authority of their license. Following legal process in the humanitarian sector and law in multiple developing countries requires a complex legal and policy knowledge base that few practitioners possess (Negi & Furman, 2010). In the end, international mental health responders who are fully trained in their host countries are on safest ground when they do what they can to inform themselves of local licensing standards and consult with their local counterparts as they proceed with the response.

INFORMED CONSENT AND CONFIDENTIALITY

Informed consent is an obligation that therapists have with clients to ensure that they are aware of how therapeutic mental health services will proceed (Kanz, 2001). Informed consent is also generally understood to be needed in complex humanitarian emergencies. Mollica and colleagues noted that, in emergencies, informed consent should include individual- and community-shared decision making (Mollica et al., 2004). However, informed consent can be even more difficult with client groups such as refugees, whose self-determination, trust, privacy, security, and identity have been compromised and threatened.

There is no consensus on what constitutes an acceptable standard for obtaining informed consent during a disaster. In fact, during disasters and emergencies, the procedural question of how to obtain informed consent tends to recede into the background in light of the overwhelming needs. Professional organizations rarely offer guidance as to what constitutes informed consent in a disaster or emergency situation (Call et al., 2012). Internationally, the situation is especially cloudy, in that the standards for informed consent vary widely, and in other cultures, notions of personal autonomy and the social authority of the professions diverge significantly from those found in North America and Europe. Philosophically, Enlightenment notions of autonomy are usually absent from traditional societies, and Western notions of informed consent can seem very foreign indeed.

MacKenzie, McDowell, and Pittaway (2007) suggested using "iterative consent" to better take into account the wishes and needs of people who are involved in conflict or disaster, pointing out that it is not enough, and possibly not culturally competent, to simply give a written consent form to sign. Culturally sensitive dialogue needs to take place to ensure that responders consider local values, needs, and concerns.

Frequently, during complex humanitarian emergencies, no real possibility of informed consent exists (Reed, 2002). Once the post-emergency phase is over and people have begun to return to normal life, some sort of informed consent for ongoing care is needed in Western societies. In all situations, responders must give serious consideration to local standards and incorporate these notions into their ongoing response plan. They must take into account current best practices as well as the possibility of unintended consequences of well-meaning interventions.

ETHICS OF EXPLANATORY MODELS

Also important is the notion of whether, how, and what to advocate in terms of explanatory models for psychological conditions. Diagnoses such as posttraumatic stress disorder (PTSD) and depression are extremely powerful. They are often very helpful in disaster settings to assist victims in understanding psychological phenomena occurring after a disaster. A number of observers have pointed out, however, that notions of PTSD, and even bereavement, when overused, can undercut alternative understandings of the symptoms they explain, which some cultures view as messages from ancestors or from the deity (Joshi, Dalton, & O'Donnell, 2008). Likewise, considering behavior such as hypervigilance and reduced emotional reactivity to be pathological makes little sense for people living in constantly dangerous and emotionally overwhelming environments—environments that are common, and commonly prolonged, in a post-disaster setting.

Disaster mental health response work is the focus of one of the most significant controversies relating to psychotherapy harm, namely the debriefing controversy (Lilienfeld, 2007). From the mid-1980s to the early 2000s, critical incident stress debriefing was, in the United States at least, a standard procedure after a disaster or emergency. In 2001, however, Rose and colleagues published an extensive review of the research on critical incident stress debriefing and concluded that single-session individual debriefing was without evidence of effectiveness (Rose, Bisson, Churchill, & Wessely, 2001). They recommended an end to compulsory debriefing of trauma victims. These findings have been reviewed and have continued to be affirmed in subsequent years (Roberts, Kitchiner, Kenardy, & Bisson, 2009). Although some form of debriefing is still used by many humanitarian organizations, expert consensus is that routine debriefing of survivors of disasters and emergencies is unwarranted.

Not only does post-disaster debriefing offer little or nothing in the way of preventing PTSD, it actually exacerbates post-trauma symptoms in vulnerable individuals. In a review of clinical practice guidelines for PTSD involving international expert consensus of seven major professional organizations, we found that *none* of the guidelines recommended routine debriefing for survivors of disasters. Several recommended screening of at-risk individuals; others did not.

A very helpful resource to assist in an ethical response in this regard is psychological first aid (PFA), a widely used first-line mental health effort. PFA can be practiced by nonclinician responders; it focuses on attending to survivors by establishing contact, establishing a level of safety and comfort, stabilizing victims as needed, offering practical assistance, and connecting to sources of usual social support. It is considered an evidence-informed intervention (i.e., there is no *proof* of effectiveness), and expert consensus indicates that it is a useful approach with low risk for harm (Fox et al., 2012; Schafer, Snider, & van Ommeren, 2010; Vernberg et al., 2008).

Mental health providers should carefully consider what, if any, direct role they should play in the initial response to a disaster. The very presence of a mental health provider, under some circumstances, can reinforce a mindset oriented toward psychopathology. On the other hand, providers can often adjust meanings and therapeutic approaches to support local social and cultural factors that promote resilience and healing.

SPECIFIC PSYCHOSOCIAL INTERVENTIONS

In recent years, researchers and practitioners have been concerned about developing "do no harm" guidelines for mass trauma events and for disaster-exposed populations (Mollica, 2006). For example, Weine et al. (2002) worked toward synthesizing best practice standards for psychoeducational training in disaster and conflict areas, specifically including cross-cultural competency, the need for assessment, the imperative for good cooperation, and understanding of complex post-conflict contexts. This research was designed to distill best practice procedures and issues from a number of professionals in psychosocial work with trauma-exposed clients. Additional empirical and consensus-based research is needed to sift through the range of potential interventions used to help survivors and to address issues such as how context and local values should shape planning and training (Weine et al., 2002).

In response to their experiences in the aftermath of the Khmer Rouge genocide and work with torture survivors in Kosovo and America, Mollica et al. (2004) developed a guiding framework in the form of a global mental health action plan. The action plan provides a framework for a psychosocial and mental health response to conflict and disaster. It encompasses the roles of international agencies, human rights, research and evaluation ethics, policy, financing, science-based mental health services, education, and linkage in relation to economic development. This framework, along with emerging documents on best practice and so-called do no harm standards, moves us closer to guidelines on intervention with survivors of mass trauma.

Potential harmful practices connected to cross-cultural misunderstandings and to the more complex misuse of psychosocial approaches, especially when accomplished within a context of conflict or disaster, also must be considered in creating guidelines. Survivors of religious and political persecution, especially refugees, are often vulnerable to potentially harmful practices, benign neglect, or revictimization. For example, Mackenzie et al. (2007) conducted empirical research with 238 refugees and service providers in refugee camps in Kenya, Sri Lanka, and Thailand. Their work revealed breeches in confidentiality and informed consent and abuses of power that led to further oppression and potential exploitation. Once again, critical self-awareness and a proactive ethical stance are needed for an effective intercultural response (Wessels, 2008).

International guidelines developed by the Inter-Agency Standing Committee (IASC) on Mental Health and Psychosocial Support in Emergency Settings also include a section on "do no harm" (IASC, 2007). The experience of NGOs, including our own (Open Doors International), has been that when conflict or disaster strikes a country or region, many organizations converge, resulting in an unhealthy lack of coordination. An entire range of humanitarian interventions, from gold-standard best practices to potentially harmful and even exploitative methods, rapidly mobilize. Guidelines, such has those developed by the IASC, are an important development in the effort to promote an ethical, culturally informed response.

ETHICS OF PSYCHOEDUCATIONAL INTERVENTIONS

Psychoeducation is used widely as a mental health intervention for survivors in conflict and disaster zones. Psychoeducation, as an intervention, includes a mix of education about traumatic stress reactions and problem solving with a strong emphasis on wellness and emotional support (Moller & Rice, 2006; Wessels, 2008). Despite the promise of psychoeducation, scholarly debate remains over whether it is harmful, inert, or helpful (Wessels, 2008). According to Wessels and colleagues, psychoeducation can be more effective if it is tailored to individual or collective group needs (such as those of disaster or conflict survivors), if it seeks to enhance adaptation and resilience, and if it is sensitive to the timing and impact of particular past traumatic events. There are ongoing debates regarding the efficacy of all interventions for trauma survivors (Murray, Davidson, & Schweitzer, 2010). Certainly, psychoeducation can be used to decrease symptoms after trauma and can increase resiliency while helping traumatized persons know what to expect in the weeks and months to come (Krupnick & Green, 2008). Psychoeducational interventions must be used at the right time—that is, not while traumatized persons are in shock (Weine et al., 2002). As with other interventions, psychoeducational interventions should be culturally sensitive, respect individual strengths and human rights, and seek to integrate different perspectives on trauma.

Intervention research regarding refugee and mass trauma is helpful for practitioners, but research combining this information with input on religious or spiritual experience is also needed for effective treatment of survivors of mass conflict. Shoeb, Weinstein, and Halpern (2007) looked at assimilation of refugees and their re-establishment of identity within a new culture, which included identification with their own religious beliefs and practices. In this study, 60 Iraqi Christian and Muslim men and women were interviewed regarding their traumatic experience in Iraq and subsequent migration to the United States. Emerging themes included a struggle to re-establish Iraqi identity, a reshaping of female social roles in a foreign society, a re-establishment of kinship networks, and a way to work through feelings of insecurity and discrimination. On the positive side, the Iraqi participants' faith and sense of transcendence and peace helped them deal with feelings of isolation, insecurity, and uncertainty about the future. Such research provides an example of the need to understand survivors of conflict not only in terms of post-traumatic stress symptoms but also in terms of their reconnection and establishment of meaning through their own religious or spiritual structures.

Similarly, research on survivors of genocide, forced migration, and mass trauma—especially the extensive research on Holocaust survivors—has provided significant insights into the long-term effects of mass trauma and highlighted helpful and hurtful coping styles and interventions. Sensitively conducted narrative interventions, for example, helped Armenian genocide survivors; those who talked about their difficult experiences fared better than those who chose to remain silent. Armenian Christian rituals such as family storytelling, praying, serving others, and keeping family together also promoted healing (Kalayjian & Eugene, 2010). The use of sacred practices to transform lives marred by deeply traumatic experiences into lives that experience meaning, goal attainment, and healing is what is meant when we speak of "positive religious coping" (Raiya, Pargament, Mahoney, & Trevino, 2008).

ETHICAL DIMENSIONS OF NARRATIVE, BELIEF, AND RECONCILIATION APPROACHES

One type of intervention that pushes beyond individual mental health work comprises narrative and reconciliation approaches involving both sides in conflict or complex emergencies where there are tensions between political or religious groups (Zelizer, 2008). According to Kirmeyer, "psychiatry has found a role in the field of peace building and conflict resolution through the provision of mental health services in post-conflict situations" (Kirmayer, 2010, p. 6). Ethically, in such situations, it is difficult to provide individual services and yet ignore the larger issues of communal violence that may have precipitated or occurred concurrently with an event. In terms of religious groups, violence is a subject in the scripture of many of the world's religions, but contained in those same scriptures are strong exhortations to pursue peace and demonstrate compassion (Burns, 2008). Therefore, interventions that include a component of reconciliation and dialogue between groups in conflict appear to be a positive ethical addition (Zelizer, 2008). Maoz (2011) conducted an ethnographic study using empirical data from in-depth interviews, direct observations, and document analysis of planned contact interventions between Palestinian and Israeli groups working to develop personal and collective narratives. He concluded that these groups could increase levels of trust, empathy, and an "understanding of the complexity of the conflict situation" (p. 122). Although the limitation of this narrative model is that storytelling might not lead to any material change in the human rights situation of participants, it is an opportunity for those on opposite sides of a conflict to tell their stories of survival and to work toward potential positive relationships in protracted and tense environments.

Each survivor of conflict or disaster has a rich narrative that includes history, politics, and other larger, systemic issues (George, 2010). Surrounding the narratives of survivors are the twin pillars of historical and structural trauma that encapsulate the meta-narrative or underlying story (Van der Merwe & Gobodo-Madikizela, 2008). Therefore, it is impossible to understand the fullness of the trauma story without understanding what has happened in each area and each generation before and after a mass trauma event. Ethically sound narrative research allows a rich description of the factors affecting survivors and the clinician's reaction to both the terror and the triumph over arduous situations (Grietens, Verschueren, & De Haene, 2010).

ETHICAL DIMENSIONS
OF FOCUSING ON RESILIENCE
AND POSTTRAUMATIC GROWTH

Since the 1980s, there has been a growing interest in the concept of trauma and resilience. In fact, a mental health disaster response informed by concepts of resilience and hardiness has great appeal from an ethical standpoint because such an approach draws from natural sources of support and has significant cross-cultural applicability (Bartone, Kelly, & Matthews, 2013; Rutter, 2013; Southwick & Charney, 2012).

Given the wide range of the nature and severity of disasters and emergencies, predictions of the likelihood of the emergence of persistent posttraumatic symptoms are problematic. Nonetheless, a meta-analysis looking at studies of the trajectory of PTSD found that, of individuals subjected to trauma, about 37% developed PTSD during the following year, and therefore, 63% *never* developed PTSD (Santiago et al., 2013). This finding confirms the common clinical observation that most people do not develop PTSD after a traumatic event and emphasizes the importance of supporting factors that promote natural resilience.

In fact, qualitative studies of resilient disaster survivors highlight the importance of usual sources of support. For example, after Hurricane Katrina, researchers who interviewed resilient survivors found that resilience was promoted by religion, having a church community, and having a job. It was also promoted by the act of helping others, by family and friends, and by the ability to find meaning in adversity (Glandon, Muller, & Almedom, 2008; Lowe, Rhodes, & Waters, 2015). Among traumatized veterans, greater social connectedness, intrinsic religiosity, purpose in life, altruism, gratitude, and an active reading style all were associated with posttraumatic growth, confirming the importance of avoiding a disaster response that focuses on psychiatric pathologies (Tsai, El-Gabalawy, Sledge, Southwick, & Pietrzak, 2014; Tsai, Sippel, Mota, Southwick, & Pietrzak, 2015). Posttraumatic growth refers to positive changes in self-perception, relationships, and view of life that emerge from a traumatic event (and may well co-exist with continuing post-trauma symptoms).

On an international scale, evidence from studies of refugees experiencing persecution shows how resilience can work with survivors of catastrophic events. For example, a study by Kim and Lee (2009) found that North Korean refugees, although severely persecuted, nonetheless experienced posttraumatic growth through telling their stories and through integrating socially with South Koreans. In an empirical study of 23 Holocaust survivors, Lurie-Beck, Liossis, and Gow (2008) also found significant vulnerabilities that included PTSD symptoms but existed concurrently with posttraumatic growth factors (Lurie-Beck, Liossis, & Gow, 2008). With therapeutic interventions that allowed them to process their past traumatic experiences, survivors were able to move toward increased resiliency and posttraumatic growth.

In many cultures, posttraumatic growth seems to be promoted by positive religious coping. For example, Ting and Watson (2007), in a qualitative study of Chinese pastors persecuted for their faith through harsh confinement, found that, despite experiencing serious physical and psychological trauma, the pastors also experienced posttraumatic growth. The authors identified four transformative factors—factors that changed the painful experiences into experiences of growth: a switch of focus from self to the larger good; coming to understand one's own frailty and limits; increased trust in God; and redefinition of personal suffering as something of benefit to oneself. All of the pastors reported that preparing for suffering had helped them to cope. All described active use of Scripture and personal worship as important, and about half of them reported that identifying with the sufferings of Christ also helped (Ting & Watson, 2007). Although these strategies are alien to many in the West, sensitivity to those means by which people transform pain into posttraumatic growth is critical to an ethical mental health response to such survivors. Additionally, a focus on resilience and posttraumatic growth represents a sound approach that is likely to "do no harm" and to promote restoration in a natural way. Disaster responders can use knowledge gained from research on resilience factors, along with insights gleaned from psychological first aid, to craft effective and non-pathologizing mental health support for survivors.

ETHICAL CONSIDERATIONS IN PSYCHIATRIC RESEARCH DURING DISASTERS AND EMERGENCIES

Even with the best research models, utmost care should be taken with vulnerable groups. In addition, the basic human rights of those involved in disaster or conflict need to be taken into consideration. Human rights theory, as it applies to traumatized persons, is the idea that certain abridgements of basic human needs have a substantial impact on marginalized and vulnerable individuals and groups and that a sound approach to ameliorating the situation calls for a combination of legal advocacy and understanding the effects of trauma on such persons. Human rights theory grew out of an increasing moral awareness, in the middle of the last century, of the need for international political and legal protections for survivors of mass trauma and for those whose rights of freedom, conscience, and religion were abridged (Steel, Bateman Steel, & Silove, 2009). With the development of human rights protections came a greater awareness of the need for therapeutic care for victims of mass trauma, further protections of traumatized populations, and the need for cross-cultural competency in trauma care. In the midst of these developments, mental health professions such as social work have included universal human rights as a deeply embedded part of the profession (Healy, 2008). And, the psychiatric profession continues to define and re-define its role while working in complex humanitarian emergencies and conflicts around the world (Kirmayer, 2010).

Miriam George (2010) described colonialist and paternalistic views ingrained in a culture of helping professionals from the West or the global North who attempted to assist those in other diverse cultural groups and nations. Mass trauma, related to refugees and especially to those fleeing religious persecution, is often a result of historical, social, and political influences that recur and overlap. Hence, efforts to devise interventions should be made with consideration of the complex array of racial, cultural, and human rights factors that continue to affect survivors of trauma and forced migration. Steel and colleagues advanced this idea further by outlining the previously mentioned human rights theory that now influences those exposed to mass trauma. The human rights theory includes (1) first-generation rights—civil and political rights (specifically against the use of torture, execution, arbitrary arrest, and forms of discrimination and freedom of religious and other beliefs); (2) second-generation rights—that which is needed for the basic necessities of life, including economic, social, and cultural rights; and (3) third-generation rights—including the idea of protecting human rights of marginalized groups and allowing them to gain control over their society and culture (Steel et al., 2009). The gradual development of human rights protections has serious implications for both protection of victims of religious persecution and the types of psychosocial interventions that are chosen for this group.

Kelly McKinney echoed both George's call to recognize the social and political inequalities affecting refugees, and Steel and colleagues' concern for cultural sensitivity in her ethnographic study of a center offering care to survivors of torture. Her study showed that there can be a power imbalance between elite psychological and medical professionals and biracial counselors (McKinney, 2007). In addition to this power imbalance, she found a lack of advocacy for the torture survivors, which was a serious omission. The need to combine best practices with advocacy on behalf of survivors whose freedoms are ruthlessly attacked in many countries seems obvious. Ethical research should be critically aware of inherent power differentials and the need for cultural competency in order to avoid contributing to an atmosphere of "cultural imperialism and colonial forms of hegemony" (Steel et al., 2009, p. 483).

CONCLUSION

The involvement of Western mental health providers in the response to disasters and emergencies during the last several decades has led to a healthy examination of how our approaches are benefitting survivors. Areas of particular ethical importance include consideration of how to obtain informed consent and respect for local laws. Ethical practice also requires that proper consideration be given to the meaning of common explanatory models for disaster victims who may not be steeped in Western culture. This may well involve seeking additional information about local understandings of religion and spirituality and allowing survivors to identify meaning through means familiar to them—even if these means are unfamiliar or unimportant to responders. Recent guidelines and more sophisticated disaster research are providing a strong framework for ethically informed mental health responses to disasters and emergencies.

REFERENCES

American Psychiatric Association. (2013). *Principles of medical ethics with annotations especially applicable to psychiatry*. Retrieved from https://www.psychiatry.org/psychiatrists/practice/ethics.

Bartone, P. T., Kelly, D. R., & Matthews, M. D. (2013). Psychological hardiness predicts adaptability in military leaders: A prospective study. *International Journal of Selection and Assessment, 21*(2), 200–210. doi:10.1111/ijsa.12029

Burns, C. (2008). *More moral than God: Taking responsibility for religious violence*. London, England: Rowman & Littlefield.

Call, J. A., Pfefferbaum, B., Jenuwine, M. J., & Flynn, B. W. (2012). Practical legal and ethical considerations for the provision of acute disaster mental health services. *Psychiatry, 75*(4), 305–322. doi:10.1521/psyc.2012.75.4.305

Fox, J. H., Burkle, F. M. J., Bass, J., Pia, F. A., Epstein, J. L., & Markenson, D. (2012). The effectiveness of psychological first aid as a disaster intervention tool: Research analysis of peer-reviewed literature from 1990–2010. *Disaster Medicine and Public Health Preparedness, 6*(3), 247–252. doi:doi:10.1001/dmp.2012.39

George, M. (2010). A theoretical understanding of refugee trauma. *Clinical Social Work Journal, 38*(4), 379–387. doi:10.1007/s10615-009-0252-y

Glandon, D. M., Muller, J., & Almedom, A. M. (2008). Resilience in post-Katrina New Orleans, Louisiana: A preliminary study. *African Health Sciences, 8*(Suppl 1), S21–S27.

Grietens, H., Verschueren, K., & De Haene, L. (2010). Holding harm: Narrative methods in mental health research on refugee trauma. *Qualitative Health Research, 20*(12), 1664–1676. doi:10.1177/1049732310376521

Healy, L. M. (2008). Exploring the history of social work as a human rights profession. *International Social Work, 51*(6), 735–748. doi:10.1177/0020872808095247

Howe, E. G. (2012). What legal risks should mental health care providers take during disasters? *Psychiatry, 75*(4), 323–330. doi:10.1521/psyc.2012.75.4.323

Inter-Agency Standing Committee. (2007). *IASC guidelines on mental health and psychosocial support in emergency settings.* Retrieved from https://interagencystandingcommittee.org/system/files/legacy_files/Guidelines%20IASC%20Mental%20Health%20Psychosocial%20%28with%20index%29.pdf.

Joshi, P. T., Dalton, M. E., & O'Donnell, D. A. (2008). Ethical issues in local, national, and international disaster psychiatry. *Child and Adolescent Psychiatric Clinics of North America, 17*(1), 165–185, x-xi. doi:10.1016/j.chc.2007.07.010

Kalayjian, A., & Eugene, D. (2010). *Mass trauma and emotional healing around the world: Rituals and practices for resilience and meaning-making.* Santa Barbara, CA: Praeger.

Kanz, J. E. (2001). Clinical-Supervision.com: Issues in the provision of online supervision. *Professional Psychology: Research and Practice, 32*(4), 415–420. doi:10.1037/0735-7028.32.4.415

Kim, H. K., & Lee, O. J. (2009). A phenomenological study on the experience of North Korean refugees. *Nursing Science Quarterly, 22*(1), 85–88. doi:10.1177/0894318408329242

Kirmayer, L. J. (2010). Peace, conflict, and reconciliation: Contributions of cultural psychiatry. *Transcultural Psychiatry, 47*(1), 5–19. doi:10.1177/1363461510362037

Krupnick, J. L., & Green, B. L. (2008). Psychoeducation to prevent PTSD: A paucity of evidence. *Psychiatry, 71*(4), 329–331. doi:10.1521/psyc.2008.71.4.329

Lilienfeld, S. O. (2007). Psychological treatments that cause harm. *Perspectives on Psychological Science, 2*(1), 53–70.

Lowe, S. R., Rhodes, J. E., & Waters, M. C. (2015). Understanding resilience and other trajectories of psychological distress: A mixed-methods study of low-income mothers who survived Hurricane Katrina. *Current Psychology, 34*(3), 537–550. doi:10.1007/s12144-015-9362-6

Lurie-Beck, J. K., Liossis, P., & Gow, K. (2008). Relationships between psychopathological and demographic variables and posttraumatic growth among Holocaust survivors. *Traumatology, 14*(3), 28–39. doi:10.1177/1534765608320338

Mackenzie, C., McDowell, C., & Pittaway, E. (2007). Beyond 'do no harm': The challenge of constructing ethical relationships in refugee research. *Journal of Refugee Studies, 20*(2), 299–319. doi:10.1093/jrs/fem008

Maoz, I. (2011). Does contact work in protracted asymmetrical conflict? Appraising 20 years of reconciliation-aimed encounters between Israeli Jews and Palestinians. *Journal of Peace Research, 48*, 115–125.

McKinney, K. (2007). Culture, power, and practice in a psychosocial program for survivors of torture and refugee trauma. *Transcultural Psychiatry, 44*(3), 482–503. doi:10.1177/1363461507081643

Moller, M. D., & Rice, M. J. (2006). The BE SMART trauma reframing psychoeducation program. *Archives of Psychiatric Nursing, 20*(1), 21–31. doi:10.1016/j.apnu.2005.08.007

Mollica, R. F. (2006). *Healing invisible wounds: Paths to hope and recovery in a violent world*. Nashville, TN: Vanderbilt University Press.

Mollica, R. F., Cardozo, B. L., Osofsky, H. J., Raphael, B., Ager, A., & Salama, P. (2004). Mental health in complex emergencies. *The Lancet, 364*(9450), 2058–2067. doi:10.1016/S0140-6736(04)17519-3

Murray, K. E., Davidson, G. R., & Schweitzer, R. D. (2010). Review of refugee mental health interventions following resettlement: Best practices and recommendations. *American Journal of Orthopsychiatry, 80*(4), 576–585. doi:10.1111/j.1939-0025.2010.01062.x

Negi, N., & Furman, R. (2010). *Transnational social work practice*. New York, NY: Columbia University Press.

Pérouse de Montclos, M.-A. (2012). Humanitarian action in developing countries: Who evaluates who? *Evaluation and Program Planning, 35*(1), 154–160. doi:10.1016/j.evalprogplan.2010.11.005

Raiya, H. A., Pargament, K. I., Mahoney, A., & Trevino, K. (2008). When Muslims are perceived as a religious threat: Examining the connection between desecration, religious coping, and anti-Muslim attitudes. *Basic and Applied Social Psychology, 30*(4), 311–325. doi:10.1080/01973530802502234

Reed, H. (2002). *Research ethics in complex humanitarian emergencies: Summary of a workshop*. National Research Council Staff Committee on Population. Washington, DC: National Academies Press.

Roberts, N. P., Kitchiner, N. J., Kenardy, J., & Bisson, J. (2009). Multiple session early psychological interventions for the prevention of post-traumatic stress disorder. *Cochrane Database of Systematic Reviews, (3)*, CD006869. doi:10.1002/14651858.CD006869.pub2

Robertson, M. D., & Walter, G. (2008). Many faces of the dual-role dilemma in psychiatric ethics. *Australian and New Zealand Journal of Psychiatry, 42*(3), 228–235. doi:10.1080/00048670701827291

Rose, S., Bisson, J., Churchill, R., & Wessely, S. (2001). Psychological debriefing for preventing post traumatic stress disorder (PTSD). *Cochrane Database of Systematic Reviews, (3)*: CD000560. doi:10.1002/14651858.CD000560

Rutter, M. (2013). Annual research review: Resilience—Clinical implications. *Journal of Child Psychology and Psychiatry, 54*(4), 474–487.

Santiago, P. N., Ursano, R. J., Gray, C. L., Pynoos, R. S., Spiegel, D., Lewis-Fernandez, R., . . . Fullerton, C. S. (2013). A systematic review of PTSD prevalence and trajectories in DSM-5 defined trauma exposed populations: Intentional and non-intentional traumatic events. *PLoS One, 8*(4), e59236. doi:10.1371/journal.pone.0059236

Schafer, A., Snider, L., & van Ommeren, M. (2010). Psychological first aid pilot: Haiti emergency response. *Intervention, 8*(3), 245–254. doi:10.1097/WTF.0b013e32834134cb

Sessums, L. L., Collen, J. F., O'Malley, P. G., Jackson, J. L., & Roy, M. J. (2009). Ethical practice under fire: Deployed physicians in the global war on terrorism. *Military Medicine, 174*(5), 441–447.

Shoeb, M., Weinstein, H. M., & Halpern, J. (2007). Living in religious time and space: Iraqi refugees in Dearborn, Michigan. *Journal of Refugee Studies, 20*(3), 441–460. doi:10.1093/jrs/fem003

Southwick, S. M., & Charney, D. S. (2012). *Resilience: The science of mastering life's greatest challenges*. New York, NY: Cambridge University Press.

Steel, Z., Bateman Steel, C. R., & Silove, D. (2009). Human rights and the trauma model: Genuine partners or uneasy allies? *Journal of Traumatic Stress, 22*(5), 358–365. doi:10.1002/jts.20449

Strasburger, L. H., Gutheil, T. G., & Brodsky, A. (1997). On wearing two hats: Role conflict in serving as both psychotherapist and expert witness. *American Journal of Psychiatry, 154*(4), 448–456.

Ting, R. S.-K., & Watson, T. (2007). Is suffering good? An explorative study on the religious persecution among Chinese pastors. *Journal of Psychology and Theology, 35*, 202–210.

Tsai, J., El-Gabalawy, R., Sledge, W. H., Southwick, S. M., & Pietrzak, R. H. (2014). Post-traumatic growth among veterans in the USA: Results from the National Health and Resilience in Veterans Study. *Psychological Medicine, 45*, 1–15. doi:10.1017/S0033291714001202

Tsai, J., Sippel, L. M., Mota, N., Southwick, S. M., & Pietrzak, R. H. (2015). Longitudinal course of post-traumatic growth among US military veterans: Results from the National Health and Resilience in Veterans Study. *Depression and Anxiety, 33,* 9–18. doi:10.1002/da.22371

Van der Eijk, P. J. (2005). *Medicine and philosophy in classical antiquity: Doctors and philosophers on nature, soul, health and disease.* New York, NY: Cambridge University Press.

Van der Merwe, C., & Gobodo-Madikizela, P. (2008). *Narrating our healing: Perspectives on working through trauma.* Newcastle, England: Cambridge Scholars.

Vernberg, E. M., Steinberg, A. M., Jacobs, A. K., Brymer, M. J., Watson, P. J., Osofsky, J. D., . . . Ruzek, J. I. (2008). Innovations in disaster mental health: Psychological first aid. *Professional Psychology: Research and Practice, 39*(4), 381–388. doi:10.1037/a0012663

Weine, S., Danieli, Y., Silove, D., Van Ommeren, M., Fairbank, J. A., Saul, J., . . . Task Force on International Trauma Training of the Intertional Society for Traumatic Stress, S. (2002). Guidelines for international training in mental health and psychosocial interventions for trauma exposed populations in clinical and community settings. *Psychiatry, 65*(2), 156–164. doi:10.1521/psyc.65.2.156.19936

Wessels, M. (2008). Do no harm: Challenges in organizing psychosocial support to displaced people in emergency settings. *Refuge, 25*(1), 6–14.

Zelizer, C. (2008). Trauma-sensitive peace building: Lessons for theory and practice. *Africa Peace and Conflict Journal, 1*(1), 81–94.

TWENTY

Forensic Psychiatry

Michael A. Norko, M.D., M.A.R.

IN ITS CODE OF MEDICAL ETHICS, THE AMERICAN MEDICAL ASSOCIATION (AMA) notes that "physicians have an obligation to assist in the administration of justice" (AMA, 2016, Chapter 9.7.1). Forensic psychiatry is a subspecialty that is realizing that obligation to its fullest. However, the aims of the administration of justice can often conflict with the traditional aims of medicine at the individual level. For example, an examining forensic psychiatrist is not free to value the best interests of an evaluee above the quest for truth. In treatment practice, the principles of beneficence and nonmaleficence have primacy (Beauchamp & Childress, 2012), but in forensic work they become secondary (Weinstock, 2015). This was the basis for Paul Appelbaum's elucidation of a separate ethics for forensic practice based on truth-telling and respect for persons (Appelbaum, 1997). The Ethics Guidelines of the American Academy of Psychiatry and the Law (AAPL) call for adherence to honesty, striving for objectivity, and respect for persons (AAPL, 2005).

Multiple efforts have been published that expand or otherwise qualify these founding principles (see AAPL, 2015, pp. S4–S5). Some of these have been focused on culture and narrative, with specific references made to religion or religious beliefs and values (Candilis, Martinez, & Dording, 2001; Griffith, 2005; Norko, 2005), and these are explored later in the chapter. But I am aware of no existing literature that specifically attempts to explore ethics considerations at the intersection of forensic psychiatry and religion/spirituality.

This chapter presents a survey of those intersections that I have encountered in the practice of forensic psychiatry. As such, it represents a beginning exploration of several topic areas: religious beliefs and religious delusions in famous legal cases; the concept of forensic empathy and its spiritual connotations; the practice of religion within the restrictions of maximum security settings; and the concepts of remorse and insight as utilized in forensic practice and their relationship to forgiveness and reconciliation.

LEGAL CASES

Several well-known criminal cases have involved religious delusions held by the accused. Each of them invoked questions of morality in one way or another, as the courts and the public were forced to wrestle with issues of criminal and moral responsibility.

Hadfield

A famous case from 1800 England is that of James Hadfield. Mr. Hadfield was a 29-year-old combat veteran who had sustained severe head injuries in battle in France in 1794, after which he was subject to "fits of insanity" (Quen 1974, p. 118). Mr. Hadfield became involved with a millennial cult and came to believe that his death would bring about the Second Coming of Christ (Eigen, 2004). He knew that God would destroy the world, but the sacrifice of his own life would save humanity (Quen, 1969). He decided to shoot at the King at a theater performance in order to be executed for treason, rather than commit the moral wrong of suicide (Quen, 1974). At trial, his attorney, Thomas Erskine, argued against the traditional requirement of "total deprivation of memory and understanding" for acquittal by reason of insanity, contending that "no such madness ever existed in the world" (Quen, 1974, p. 118). He argued instead that Mr. Hadfield's delusion alone marked his insanity and that his act flowed from this illness. The presiding justice charged the jury, "If a man is in a deranged state of mind at the time, he is not criminally answerable for his acts" (Quen, 1974, p. 119). The jury acquitted Mr. Hadfield, who spent the rest of his life confined to Bethlem Hospital (Eigen, 2004).

Although the case might have stood as precedent against the previous narrow interpretation that only "absolute madness" or "perfect insanity" could relieve a defendant of responsibility for his criminal acts, it had very little subsequent effect on English jurisprudence (Quen, 1969). The M'Naghten Rules, established in 1843, set precedent that is still in use today. That set of criteria requires that the defendant's illness has made him unable to know the nature and quality of the act or to know that the act was wrong. Mr. Hadfield committed his act precisely because he knew that the nature of the act and its prohibition would result in his execution—the desired effect of his religious delusional aspirations (Quen, 1969).

Panetti

In 1992, Scott Panetti drove to the Texas home of his estranged wife's parents and shot and killed them. He was tried for capital murder in 1995. He represented himself at trial after being found competent to stand trial and waive counsel despite evidence of his history of psychosis and hospitalizations. He had believed that the devil possessed the family home and had engaged in several rituals to attempt to cleanse the home. Although he presented an insanity defense, he did so ineffectively, in what his standby counsel described as a "judicial farce, and a mockery of self-representation" (*Panetti v. Quarterman,* 2007a, p. 2849). He was convicted and sentenced to death. In December 2003, after his execution date was set for February 2004, Mr. Panetti filed his first claim that he was incompetent to be executed. This was based on the 1986 US Supreme Court ruling that the Eighth Amendment bar of cruel and unusual punishment prohibits execution of the insane (Ford, 1986). In September 2004, the federal district court denied the appeal, saying that Mr. Panetti had failed to demonstrate that he was incompetent, which, in its precedents, required only that he knew the fact of his impending execution and the factual basis for it.

The case eventually reached the U.S. Supreme Court, which reviewed the evidence adduced previously. A mental health expert had diagnosed Mr. Panetti with schizoaffective disorder, noting his delusion that his execution was a "part of spiritual warfare . . . between the demons and the forces of the darkness and God and the angels and the forces of light" (*Panetti v. Quarterman,* 2007a, p. 2859). Although Mr. Panetti understood that the government stated that his execution was punishment for the murder convictions, he believed that this was a sham. He asserted that the state wanted to execute him in order "to stop him from preaching" (*Panetti v. Quarterman,* 2007a, p. 2859) and that the state was "in league with the forces of evil that have conspired against him" (*Panetti v. Quarterman,* 2007a, p. 2863). The American Psychological Association, American Psychiatric Association, and National Alliance on Mental Illness submitted a joint brief arguing that the Fifth Circuit's narrow interpretation of the limits imposed by *Ford* permitted "the execution of individuals who lack any meaningful understanding of the nature and purpose of their punishment" (*Panetti v. Quarterman,* 2007b).

In its 5-4 decision, the Supreme Court reasoned that "A prisoner's awareness of the State's rationale for an execution is not the same as a rational understanding of it" (*Panetti v. Quarterman,* 2007a, p. 2862). The Court remanded the case for further proceedings, observing, "Expert evidence may clarify the extent to which severe delusions may render a subject's perception of reality so distorted that he should be deemed incompetent" (*Panetti v. Quarterman,* 2007a, p. 2863).

On remand, the federal district court found that Mr. Panetti was mentally ill at the time of the crime and up to the present, but that his delusions did not prevent his rational understanding of the connection between the murders and his death sentence (*Panetti v. Quarterman,* 2008). However, the court stayed his execution pending appeal. The Fifth Circuit Court of Appeals eventually received that appeal and in December 2014 stayed the execution to permit it to "fully consider" the "complex legal questions at issue in this matter" (*Panetti v. Stephens,* 2014). After 22 years of legal proceedings, the matter remains open; in July 2017 the Fifth Circuit Court of Appeals reversed the district court's denial of counsel and funding for experts, vacated its finding of Mr. Panetti's competence to be executed, and remanded the case for further investigation and expert assistance and a new determination of his competency to be executed (*Panetti v. Davis.* 2017).

The US Supreme Court has not barred the execution of individuals with severe mental illness per se. The moral arguments continue to focus on how much of an understanding of the nature of and reason for the punishment of death is necessary for an execution to be unimpeded by the Eighth Amendment.

Filicide Cases

In 2001, Andrea Yates was a Texas mother of five children, aged 7 months to 7 years. Two years earlier, she had come to believe that Satan wanted to kill her children. She attempted suicide twice and had four psychiatric hospitalizations over the next 2 years—the last two occurring months after the birth of her fifth child. She had several paranoid delusional beliefs and was depressed and suicidal. She came to believe that Satan was within her, that he was torturing her and her children, and that he would take her children to burn in hell (Resnick, 2007). On June 20, 2011, Ms. Yates drowned all five children in the bathtub, thinking that she was "doing what was right for her children by arranging for them to go to heaven while they were still 'innocent'" (Resnick, 2007, p. 150). She also believed that when she was executed, Satan would be executed as well (Resnick, 2007). She called the police and her husband after killing the children.

A total of 10 psychiatrists and two psychologists testified at Ms. Yates's trial. Four of the psychiatrists and one psychologist had treated her previously; the others were asked to evaluate her after her arrest. Of those who evaluated her after arrest, all but one psychiatrist testified that she did not know her acts were wrong. The psychiatrist retained by the prosecution, like all the others, believed that she was psychotic but knew that what she had done was wrong (*Yates v. State,* 2005). The prosecution witness reasoned that Ms. Yates knew these thoughts were coming from Satan and therefore "must have known they were wrong" (Yates, 2005, p. 218), seemingly applying a criterion of reason to an irrational belief. The chief forensic psychiatrist for the defense offered further explanations of Ms. Yates's religious delusions and their effect on her behavior and thought in reaching his conclusion (Resnick, 2007).

In 2002, the jury found Ms. Yates guilty under the Texas version of the M'Naghten Rules but rejected the death penalty; she was sentenced to life in prison. However, in 2005, her conviction was overturned because the prosecution failed to reveal to the jury that its chief witness acknowledged an error in his testimony that the prosecutor emphasized in his arguments (Yates, 2005). A second trial in 2006 resulted in a finding of not guilty by reason of insanity (NGRI). The jury foreman explained to reporters the jury's opinion that Ms. Yates knew her actions were legally wrong but that because of her delusions she thought they were right (Resnick, 2007). Ms. Yates was committed to a state psychiatric hospital. Doctors there recommended in 2012 that she be allowed brief passes to attend church services, but that request was denied by the judge (Hlavaty, 2014). A 2014 request for her to attend supervised group outings from the hospital was withdrawn due to negative attention from the media and public scrutiny ("Andrea Yates Fast Facts," 2017).

Between the first and second Yates trials, two other Texas mothers had been found NGRI for killing their children. On May 9, 2003, Deanna Laney killed her two sons, ages 8 and 6, by beating their heads with a rock; she also beat her 15-month-old son but stopped before killing him. She believed that God had told her the world was going to end and she needed to "get her house in order"; killing the children was part of that command ("Attorney," 2004). Five mental health experts testified at her trial that she was experiencing delusions at the time of the acts and did not know right from wrong. She believed that she and Andrea Yates were "chosen by God to bear witness to the imminent end of the world" (Springer, 2004). She struggled between obeying God's commands to kill the boys in increasingly violent ways and her desire to love and nurture them. She was found NGRI in April 2004.

Ms. Laney was allowed passes outside the hospital starting in 2005, but when prosecutors objected in court in 2007, a judge ordered that the passes cease (Worchel, 2012). She was ordered released to outpatient treatment in May 2012, after testimony that she was not a danger to herself or others ("Another Closed Hearing," 2013).

Dena Schlosser was the second Texas mother found NGRI of killing her child between the two trials of Andrea Yates. Ms. Schlosser cut the arms off her 10-month-old daughter, then cut deeply into her own shoulder with a knife, believing that she was commanded by God to cut the baby's arms off, then her own, and then her legs and head in order to give them to God (Associated Press, 2006a). Ms. Schlosser had a history of postpartum depression and treatment with antidepressants, which she did not take regularly. She and her husband were devoted followers of the Water of Life Church, located about 60 miles from their home, where they attended services several times a week. The preacher at the church taught that mental illness was caused by demons and that medication could not cure it (Whitley, 2006).

A trial jury was deadlocked in February 2006. In a second trial in April 2006, the judge found Ms. Schlosser NGRI based on psychiatric testimony at the previous trial (Associated Press, 2006b). Ms. Schlosser was released from the state hospital in 2008 but ordered back to the hospital in 2010 after being found wandering the street at 2 AM by local firefighters (Crawford, 2010).

Two reports on maternal filicide (Hatters Friedman, Hrouda, Holden, Noffsinger, & Resnick, 2005; Lewis & Bunce, 2003) found that more than a quarter of the women studied had religious delusions (Falkenberg, 2004). In a study in Michigan of 55 filicidal mothers evaluated for forensic purposes, 53% had psychotic symptoms at the time of the act (Lewis & Bunce, 2003). In a study of 39 women found NGRI in Michigan and Ohio of filicide, 82% were psychotic at the time of the act. More than half of the women thought they were acting in the best interests of their children, but for 85% of them, the motivation was psychotic in nature (Hatters Friedman et al., 2005). The horrific nature of these stories tends to raise questions about the equitableness of the insanity defense (from divergent perspectives), the stigma of mental illness, and the potential dangers of religion and its relationship to mental healthcare.

Refusal of Treatment

A very different type of case raises the bioethics question of autonomy in the context of sincerely held religious beliefs. In 1963, Jesse Jones, a 25-year-old mother of a 7-month-old infant, was brought to the emergency department of a hospital with a ruptured gastric ulcer and severe blood loss. The doctors could not control the bleeding and wished to transfuse her. Ms. Jones and her husband were Jehovah's Witnesses and declined permission for the blood transfusion. Attorneys for the hospital applied to the court for an order to permit the physician to transfuse Ms. Jones. The original judge refused to sign such an order, and the case was brought to an appeals court judge at 4 PM. The judge first spoke to the doctors and then traveled to the hospital, where he spoke with Mr. Jones and attempted to question Ms. Jones. Mr. Jones told the judge he would not approve the transfusion on religious grounds, but said that, if the court ordered it, it would not be his responsibility (*Application*, 1964). In her severely debilitated condition, Ms. Jones was only able to say "against my will" in response to the judge's questions. The judge later wrote that, "as best [he] could make out," Ms. Jones also indicated it would not be her responsibility were the court to order the transfusion (*Application*, 1964, p. 1007). It is not clear from the decision how the judge knew this.

By 5:20 PM, the judge issued an order permitting the physicians to administer the transfusion in order to save Ms. Jones's life and preserve the status quo of the legal arguments involving autonomy and religious liberty. He gave four reasons for this decision. First, the husband had no power to prevent the saving of his wife's life, in the same way a parent has no right to prevent life-saving treatment of a child. He saw Ms. Jones at that moment as incompetent to decide for herself, "as any child would be" (*Application*, 1964, p. 1008). Second, the state does not allow a parent to abandon a child, so he could not allow this mother to abandon permanently her infant child. Third, it was not clear, as a matter of law, that Ms. Jones had the authority to place the doctors and the hospital in an impossible position. He expanded on this point to note that the religious liberty objection was mitigated by the fact that a court-ordered transfusion would not create a problem in regard to her religious practice. He also reasoned that Ms. Jones did not wish to die anyway; her death "was not a religiously-commanded goal, but an unwanted side effect of a religious scruple" (*Application*, 1964, p. 1009). Finally, the judge noted that the most compelling reason for his decision was that "a life hung in the balance" and "Death could have mooted the cause in a matter of minutes, if action were not taken to preserve the status quo . . . . To refuse to act, only to find later that the law required action, was a risk I was unwilling to accept. I determined to act on the side of life" (*Application*, 1964, pp. 1009–1010).

The theme of colliding values between medicine and religion was explored in an article by Nada Stotland describing a similar situation with a patient in need of transfusion who refused because she was a Jehovah's Witness (Stotland, 1999). The hospital physicians and nursing staff were frustrated at their inability to save a life, the hospital administrator was concerned over the hospital's liability, and tensions arose between the hospital staff and family members. A psychiatrist was called in with some hope that there might be "some pretext for declaring [the patient] incompetent" to refuse treatment (Stotland, 1999, p. 306). Weeks after the woman's death, a grand rounds was held to discuss the case, with guests from the Jehovah's Witness Church. Hospital staff were surprised to learn of the Jehovah's Witnesses' empathic understanding of their situation; they were "well aware of the problems their beliefs caused for the medical profession" and that it was "somewhat unfair" to ask them to watch their patients die (Stotland, 1999, p. 307). Recent changes in the policy of Jehovah's Witnesses toward blood products allows for potentially greater freedom of individual conscience of adherents; clinicians need to understand the options available and conduct individualized assessments of treatment refusal (Muramoto, 2001).

The evaluation of capacity to give or withhold informed consent to treatment is a forensic matter that is often encountered when a patient's religious/spiritual beliefs conflict with treatment proposals (Waldfogel, 1996). Such evaluations require a level of comfort with religion/spirituality; the distinction between irrational thoughts and different worldview orientations also requires knowledge, which may necessitate consultation with the patient's faith community (Waldfogel 1996). Resources are available to help the clinician distinguish religious belief from delusional belief when questions arise (Brun, 2005; Pierre, 2001; Rieben et al., 2013; Siddle, Haddock, Tarrier, & Fargher, 2001; Waldfogel, 1996; see also Chapters 4, 5, and 17).

FORENSIC EMPATHY

The principles of truth-telling and striving for objectivity in forensic work might be interpreted as a rigid requirement of cold neutrality. But the conjoined principle of respect for persons, as described earlier, entails a broader reading of the task. Ezra Griffith and colleagues conceptualized the performative narrative of a person's story and giving voice to the evaluee as elements of respect for the person (Griffith, Stankovic, & Baranoski, 2010). Kenneth Appelbaum (2010) extended that notion to describe forensic empathy as an effort to strive for "an awareness of the perspectives and experiences of interviewees." Without such empathy, he wrote, "how can we hope to understand and explain the effect of a mental illness, such as a psychotic disorder, on an individual's behavior or how a competent person's unique background and experiences may lead him to make otherwise unexpected choices?" (Appelbaum, 2010, p. 44). The cases described previously are apt illustrations of this point. Appelbaum emphasized the importance of assessing the religious and cultural background of evaluees by interviewing their clergy, family, and friends about their beliefs and experiences.

Daniel Shuman distinguished this type of forensic empathy, which he called "receptive empathy," from "reflective empathy" in forensic work (Shuman, 1993, p. 298). The former is necessary to understand the cognitive and affective experiences of the evaluee in a way that is useful or relevant to a court (as demonstrated, for example, by the deeper analysis of Ms. Yates's religious beliefs described earlier). The latter, however, crosses "a bright ethical line" in that it is a technique used to foster therapeutic alliance and thus unfairly invites the evaluee to forget the forensic examiner's warnings about the lack of a treatment relationship and confidentiality (Shuman, 1993, p. 298).

Philip Candilis and colleagues discussed this type of receptive empathy, in the broader context of the "compassionate professional," in a description of a challenging forensic evaluation of a formerly active and vibrant woman who suffered a brainstem stroke (Candilis et al., 2001). The stroke left her paralyzed and able to communicate only by raising her eyebrows. After 2½ years of attempted rehabilitation, the woman chose to refuse her tube feedings to end her life. The forensic psychiatrist was asked by the probate court to evaluate the woman's decision-making capacity. The family dynamics were complicated and contrary, with an Eastern Orthodox parent objecting to her daughter's plan as suicide and a brother expressing Adventist views that her decision was sinful. The authors argued that a "robust view" of the professional role in this case entailed "elements of counseling, education, conflict resolution and referral for spiritual guidance" (Candilis et al., 2001, pp. 170, 173). The latter was facilitated by the psychiatrist's own Eastern Orthodox roots (see Chapter 9). The court ultimately allowed the woman's decision to end feedings, and the family developed a level of "reluctant support" (Candilis et al., 2001, p. 173) of the decision; she died 10 days later. The stance that Candilis and colleagues advocated was a narrative, humanistic approach to being in the presence of suffering—a stance they distinguished from a "disengaged and objective" professional role, which they would have found troubling in such a situation (Candilis et al., 2001, p. 172).

In a similar way, Griffith described his approach to forensic work, in which the clinician is sensitive to the pain and suffering of evaluees, "recognizing them as one of us" and "connect[ing] to them empathically" (Griffith, 2005, p. 380). This, he argued, is part of the narrative approach to the work, where truth-telling and objectivity are "leavened with humanity and generosity" (p. 381). He called for attention to community and compassion for and service to the needs of "the least of my brothers," referring to the message in the Gospel of Matthew (Matthew 25:40) while noting that other religions similarly preach compassion for one's neighbors.

In my commentary on Griffith's paper, I argued that compassion was a powerful and universal principle of all sacred beliefs and ethics and was thus suitable as a "moral foundation for forensic work" (Norko, 2005, 388). A compassionate engagement with all evaluees permits "an approach to justice that allows us to attend to and engage the humanity of all the subjects of our evaluations" (Norko, 2005, p. 388). Conceptualizing the work in such a way does less to separate the role and ethics of forensic psychiatry from its roots in medicine than do the efforts described at the beginning of this chapter to articulate special ethics for forensic psychiatry. The Physician's Oath adopted by the World Medical Association in their 1948 *Declaration of Geneva* includes these provisions: "I solemnly pledge to consecrate my life to the service of humanity . . . . I will maintain the utmost respect for human life . . . . I will not use my medical knowledge to violate human rights and civil liberties, even under threat . . . . " (World Medical Association, 2006). Adopting compassion as a core element of forensic work strengthens its connections to the values underlying all medical care. It may also be understood, in its spiritual dimensions, as an openness to being in the presence of suffering and bearing witness to it.

Simone Weil, the 20th century French philosopher, activist, and mystic, observed that "Every created thing is an object for compassion because it is ephemeral. Every created thing is an object for compassion because it is limited" (Weil, 1998, p. 143). Forensic psychiatry is so often focused on human limitations and so often reminds us of the ephemeral nature of our being.

Griffith reminds us that the subjects of forensic evaluations are "one of us." The self-recognition of the psychiatrist's limits is a participation in that oneness. As Weil put it, "Compassion directed toward oneself is humility" (Weil, 1998, p. 143).

SECURE INPATIENT CARE

The values of forensic empathy and compassion ideally find their way into forensic treatment as well as forensic evaluation. The management of secure inpatient settings requires a delicate balancing of therapeutic and security needs so that patients and staff may all feel safe and thus be able to participate in a therapeutic environment (Scales, Phillips, & Crysler, 1989). Attending to the religious and spiritual needs of patients in secure forensic treatment settings necessitates careful consideration of multiple boundaries in addition to usual concerns (see Chapter 6).

Part of the management of secure settings is attention to keeping contraband materials out of the milieu (Norko & Dike, 2009). Although patients are encouraged to participate in religious and other activities, some prayer items may be prohibited from secure environments due to their potential use in harmful acts, including phylacteries and rosaries or prayer beads. One patient who made repeated and insistent requests to possess and use phylacteries on a maximum security unit (in addition to demanding kosher meals) belied the seriousness of his religious intentions when he ordered and enjoyed a pepperoni pizza on the unit's monthly pizza night. But even had he not done so, it would not have been possible to allow the possession of lengths of leather straps in an environment of dangerous offenders.

Secure forensic treatment facilities that are accredited by The Joint Commission are expected to accommodate the patient's "right to religious and other spiritual services," as well as the patient's religious food preferences, and to assess the patient's religious/spiritual needs and beliefs (The Joint Commission, 2014). In correctional facilities, psychiatrists and other clinicians are encouraged to routinely assess inmates' spirituality and religious practice as a way of providing support and a potential source of strength and meaning (American Psychiatric Association, 2015, p. 70).

Efforts are generally made to arrange for regular religious services in secure environments but may be limited by the availability of willing clergy. When clergy are available, traditional Sunday services may take place on a weekday, for example. Chaplains may provide services in interfaith or ecumenical settings. Wine is not used in communion services. Visits from outside clergy are permitted. In Connecticut, for example, state law requires that a psychiatric patient's "clergyman" be permitted to visit "at any reasonable time" (Connecticut Code, 2012).

Many years ago, when I was the director of a maximum security forensic hospital, one patient had a particularly engaged and energetic minister, who advocated strongly that the patient be permitted to receive the assistance of prayer alone in healing his illness. In response to the minister's advocacy with government officials, I was asked to write an amendment to our statutes on medication addressing this issue, which was passed that year by the legislature. The law reads, "Unless there is a serious risk of harm to the patient or others, based upon the patient's past history or current condition, nothing in this section authorizes any form of involuntary medical, psychological or psychiatric treatment of any patient who in the sincere practice of his or her religious beliefs is being treated by prayer alone in accordance with the principles and practices of a church or religious denomination by a duly accredited practitioner or ordained minister, priest or rabbi thereof" (Connecticut Code, 2011). In a forensic setting, most patients have posed some risk to others, so the attempt to invoke the statute would likely entail consideration of the imminence of potential risk. Clinicians could well face the dilemma of being constrained in using involuntary treatment to prevent not only self-harm but also harm to others. As evidenced in the discussion of forensic cases in this chapter, religious delusions can be seriously dangerous. To my knowledge, the statute has never been invoked except in the case of the original patient and his minister.

Religion and spirituality can be a source of comfort and support for forensic patients, particularly as they look forward to reintegration into the community. Patients sometimes find supportive faith communities to assist them, and guidance is now available to faith communities to help them understand the needs of persons with mental illness (American Psychiatric Association Foundation, 2015). The question of how much information the patient should share with the community about his violent past can be a delicate matter. It is not likely that the community will never learn of the patient's past, given the level of public and media scrutiny attached to the release of many forensic patients. And yet it is hard to ask anyone to begin new relationships with fellow believers by leading with that information. At some point, the information must be revealed to some portion of the faith community, hopefully at a time and in a way that minimizes the potential shock and maximizes compassionate acceptance by the community members. Responsive faith communities may also face scorn and even threats from other segments of the population for their acceptance of someone with a violent past into their midst. There are no easy answers to assisting patients with such negotiations, but the efforts often require clinical and diplomatic skills.

FORGIVENESS, RECONCILIATION, REMORSE, AND INSIGHT

I will close with some brief reflections on the use of the concepts of remorse and insight in forensic psychiatry and the related concepts of forgiveness and reconciliation, which are commonly used in religious/spiritual discussion but not in forensic psychiatry. These considerations can be illustrated in a hypothetical ideal situation of successful management of a violent insanity acquittee in a forensic setting.

The ideal patient of this type is someone who had committed a violent act in the throes of psychosis and was found not to be morally blameworthy (or criminally responsible) on the basis of his irrational state of mind at the time of the violent act. The patient accepted treatment, psychotic symptoms waned, and over time the patient developed insight into the nature of his mental illness and his need for continued treatment. Along with that insight came a sense of remorse for his act that was hurtful to others. The development of such insight and remorse allows others to more readily accept the patient's exculpation and to be less concerned about the preparation for the patient's re-entry into the community. Within that acceptance are elements of forgiveness and reconciliation that we do not typically acknowledge or articulate explicitly.

The trajectory of this ideal type is strikingly similar to the description of remorse and reparation in a chapter on classical Greece contained within a series of texts on forensic psychotherapy:

> [R]emorse and its concomitant desire to make reparation (and elicit forgiveness) are fundamental strategies in the maintenance of co-operation—one accepts one's own responsibility while

acknowledging the legitimacy of others' criticism, and thus declares oneself an acceptable, moral interlocutor, ready to resume co-operation. Some such strategy is to be expected wherever co-operation occurs, since all societies will demand that errant individuals demonstrate an awareness of the unacceptable nature of past behavior and a willingness to co-operate in [the] future. (Cairns, 1999, p. 172)

Real cases reveal wide variance from this ideal type. For one thing, many patients never develop insight; some, in fact, deny both that they committed the act and that they are mentally ill, despite those admissions being the *sine qua non* of offering an insanity defense (Zonana & Norko, 1993). Some patients may overcome their denial and begin to make progress. These processes do not necessarily proceed in a linear or predictable fashion, but they do occur for most patients at some observable pace.

Insight and remorse, when they develop, facilitate the patient's continued progress back to the community. If they do not develop, the argument for advancement to less restrictive levels of care is more vigorously challenged. Sustained appropriate behavior, without proper insight, is held suspect as an indication for movement. Yet, deficits in insight are a well-described aspect of schizophrenia, for example, which is a common basis for a successful insanity defense. Is it fair, then, to insist on the attainment of insight as the main legitimization of recovery? Remorse may also be difficult to achieve, such as when the patient's only memory of the event is a collection of scattered, disorganized, and fearful thoughts. The patient may not be able to integrate a memory of his victim as a fellow human being but may be able to empathize with the victim's family members, who can be perceived anew in the light of a reasonably restored mental state.

Individual and communal reconciliation rituals and services are part of many faith traditions. The bond of brokenness that we all share as human beings is familiar to many people of faith. And so is the bond of forgiveness. What is still hard for communities is the ability to overcome fear and see the humanity of people who have committed severe acts of violence.

I have evaluated or treated many people who have killed. In fact, I have a T-shirt signed by 13 such individuals—a parting gift from my patients when I left a treatment unit at a maximum security unit. Some of them have re-entered the community, some have since died, and some—after more than 20 years—are still patients in the maximum security hospital. Those who have attracted media attention have had a particularly difficult time in their recovery because that attention generally amplifies fears and fans the flames of public resistance.

The filmmaker John Kastner (2014) demonstrated that this need not be the case, that very open attention to the stories of people acquitted by reason of insanity of terrible crimes can bring healing and forgiveness. Kastner produced two documentaries about patients at the Brockville Psychiatric Hospital, a forensic facility in Ontario: *NCR: Not Criminally Responsible* and *Out of Mind, Out of Sight*. They are moving narratives that document the stories of forensic patients and their interconnection with others, including their victims and the wider community. As Kastner wrote:

We have demonstrated that our films can help. They can actually change closed minds. Take the remarkable response to Sean Clifton, principal subject of *NCR,* who tried to stab a woman to death. Post-telecast, he has not had a single negative reaction, only well-wishers approaching him in the street. When he attended a Toronto screening the audience of 750 gave him a standing ovation. Best of all, his victim and her family forgave him after seeing the film and now spread the word at public appearances.

Some victims even go beyond forgiveness: "There is nothing to forgive," I was told by a family member of the victim of Michael Stewart, a patient in *Out of Mind, Out of Sight*. "He was ill. You don't forgive someone for contracting cancer."

I have known families who have forgiven and families who have held tightly to their anger and hostility. I have seen faith communities proclaim a welcoming call from the community and others close their doors to the outcast. I have witnessed people of faith unable to let go of their fear and anger in the aftermath of violent offense and people of no particular faith show kindness and compassion to those who have caused much harm. Compassion, as Kastner demonstrated so well, is the ultimate healing energy of successful forensic treatment—and it takes a village to truly realize that healing.

REFERENCES

American Academy of Psychiatry and the Law. (2005). *Ethics guidelines for the practice of forensic psychiatry*. Retrieved from http://aapl.org/ethics.htm.

American Academy of Psychiatry and the Law. (2015). AAPL practice guideline for the forensic assessment. *Journal of the American Academy of Psychiatry and the Law, 43*(2), S3–S53.

American Medical Association. (2016). Code of Medical Ethics, Chapter 9.7.1 Medical Testimony. Retrieved from https://www.ama-assn.org/delivering-care/ama-code-medical-ethics#Chapter%20 9:%20Opinions%20on%20Professional%20Self-regulation.

American Psychiatric Association. (2015). *Psychiatric services in correctional facilities* (3rd ed.). Arlington, VA: Author.

American Psychiatric Association Foundation. (2015). Mental health: A guide for faith leaders. Retrieved from psychiatry.org/faith.

Andrea Yates fast facts. (2017, June 22). Retrieved from http://www.cnn.com/2013/03/25/us/andrea-yates-fast-facts/.

Another closed hearing for East Texas mother acquitted of murdering her children. (2013, Aug 9). KLTV. Retrieved from http://apmobile.worldnow.com/story/22552528/another-closed-hearing-for-east-texas-mother-acquitted-of-murdering-her-children.

Appelbaum, K. L. (2010). Commentary: The art of forensic report writing. *Journal of the American Academy of Psychiatry and the Law, 38*, 43–45.

Appelbaum, P. S. (1997). A theory of ethics for forensic psychiatry. *Journal of the American Academy of Psychiatry and the Law, 25*, 233–247.

Application of President and Directors of Georgetown College. (1964). 331 F.2d 1000 (D.C. Cir. 1964).

Associated Press. (2006a, Feb 21). Mother says God told her to cut baby. *The Washington Post*. Retrieved from http://www.washingtonpost.com/wp-dyn/content/article/2006/02/20/AR2006022001197.html.

Associated Press. (2006b, April 8). Texas mother who killed baby is acquitted on insanity grounds. *The New York Times*. Retrieved from http://www.nytimes.com/2006/04/08/us/08baby.html?pagewanted=print&_r=0.

Attorney: Woman thought God told her to kill sons. (2004, March 30). Retrieved from http://www.cnn.com/2004/LAW/03/29/children.slain/index.html?iref=newssearch.

Beauchamp, T. L., & Childress, J. F. (2012). *Principles of biomedical ethics* (7th ed.). New York, NY: Oxford University Press.

Brun, W. L. (2005). A proposed diagnostic schema for religious/spiritual concerns. *The Journal of Pastoral Care & Counseling, 59*, 425–440.

Cairns, D. L. (1999). Representations of remorse and reparation in classical Greece. In M. Cox (Ed.), *Remorse and reparations* (pp. 171–178). London, England: Jessica Kingsley.

Candilis, P. J., Martinez, R., and Dording, C. (2001). Principles and narrative in forensic psychiatry: Toward a robust view of professional role. *Journal of the American Academy of Psychiatry and the Law, 29*, 167–73.

Connecticut Code. (2011). Title 17a, Chapter 319i, Sec. 17a-543(i). Retrieved from http://law.justia.com/codes/connecticut/2011/title17a/chap319i/Sec17a-543.html.

Connecticut Code. (2012). Title 17a, Chapter 319i, Sec. 17a-547. Retrieved from http://law.justia.com/codes/connecticut/2012/title-17a/chapter-319i/section-17a-547.

Crawford, S. (2010, April 24): Plano mother who cut baby's arms off ordered back into state mental hospital. *The Dalls Morning News*. Retrieved from https://www.dallasnews.com/news/plano/2010/04/24/Plano-mother-who-cut-baby-s-2446.

Eigen, J. P. (2004). Hadfield, James (1771/2–1841). *Oxford Dictionary of National Biography*. Oxford University Press. Retrieved from http://www.oxforddnb.com/view/article/41013.

Falkenberg, L. (2004, Dec 13). Religiosity common among mothers who kill children. *San Antonio Express-News*. Retrieved from http://today.uchc.edu/headlines/2004/dec04/religiosity.html.

Ford v. Wainwright. (1986). 477 U.S. 399.

Griffith, E. E. (2005). Personal narrative and an African-American perspective on medical ethics. *Journal of the American Academy of Psychiatry and the Law, 33*, 371–381.

Griffith, E. E., Stankovic, A., & Baranoski, M. (2010). Conceptualizing the forensic psychiatry report as performative narrative. *Journal of the American Academy of Psychiatry and the Law, 38*, 32–42.

Hatters Friedman, S, Hrouda, D. R., Holden, C. E., Noffsinger, S. G., & Resnick, P. J. (2005). Child murder committed by severely mentally ill mothers: An examination of mothers found not guilty by reason of insanity. *Journal of Forensic Sciences, 50*, 1466–1471.

Hlavaty, C. (2014, Feb 15). Doctors say Andrea Yates ready for group outings. *Houston Chronicle*. Retrieved from http://www.chron.com/news/houston-texas/houston/article/Doctors-say-Andrea-Yates-ready-for-group-outings-5239049.php.

The Joint Commission. (2014). *A crosswalk of the National Standards for Culturally and Linguistically Appropriate Services (CLAS) in health and health care to The Joint Commission Ambulatory Health Care Accreditation Standards*. Retrieved from https://www.jointcommission.org/assets/1/6/Crosswalk_CLAS_AHC_20141110.pdf.

Kastner, J. (2014, April 25). Forensic psychiatric patients are ill, not evil—and we should stop hiding them. *The Globe and Mail*. Retrieved from http://www.theglobeandmail.com/globe-debate/forensic-psychiatric-patients-are-ill-not-evil---and-we-should-stop-hiding-them/article18205568/.

Lewis, C. F., & Bunce, S. C. (2003). Filicidal mothers and the impact of psychosis on maternal filicide. *Journal of the American Academy of Psychiatry and the Law, 31*, 459–470.

Muramoto, O. (2001). Bioethical aspects of the recent changes in the policy of refusal of blood by Jehovah's Witnesses. *BMJ, 322*, 37–39.

Norko, M. A. (2005). Compassion at the core of forensic ethics. *Journal of the American Academy of Psychiatry and the Law, 33*, 386–389.

Norko, M. A., & Dike, C. C. (2009). The forensic unit. In S. S. Sharfstein, F. B. Dickerson, & J. M. Oldham (Eds.), *Textbook of Hospital Psychiatry* (pp. 185–195). Washington, DC: American Psychiatric Publishing.

Paneteti v. Davis, No. 14-70037, 5th Cir., July 11, 2017.

Panetti v. Quarterman. (2007a). 127 S. Ct. 2842.

Panetti v. Quarterman. (2007b). Brief for *Amici Curiae* American Psychological Association, American Psychiatric Association, and National Alliance on Mental Illness in support of petitioner. No. 06-6407 in the Supreme Court of the United States.

Panetti v. Quarterman. (2008). U.S. Dist. LEXIS 107438 (2008 WL 2338498)

Panetti v. Stephens. (2014). 586 Fed. Appx. 163.

Pierre, J. M. (2001). Faith or delusion? At the crossroads of religion and psychosis. *Journal of Psychiatric Practice, 7*, 163–172.

Quen, J. M. (1969). James Hadfield and medical jurisprudence of insanity. *New York State Journal of Medicine, 69*, 1221–1226.

Quen, J. M. (1974). Anglo-American criminal insanity: An historical perspective. *Bulletin of the American Academy of Psychiatry and the Law, 2*, 115–123.

Resnick, P. J. (2007). The Andrea Yates case: Insanity on trial. *Cleveland State Law Review, 55*, 147–156.

Rieben, I., Mohr, S. Borras, L. Gillieron, C. Brandt, P.-Y., Perroud, N., & Huguelet, P. (2013). A thematic analysis of delusion with religious contents in schizophrenia. *The Journal of Nervous and Mental Disease, 201*, 665–673.

Scales, C. J., Phillips, R. T. M., & Crysler, D. (1989). Security aspects of clinical care. *American Journal of Forensic Psychology, 7*, 49–57.

Shuman, D. W. (1993). The use of empathy in forensic examinations. *Ethics & Behavior, 3*, 289–302.

Siddle, R., Haddock, G., Tarrier, N., & Faragher, E. B. (2001). Religious delusions in patients admitted to hospital with schizophrenia. *Social Psychiatry and Psychiatric Epidemiology, 37*, 130–138.

Springer, J. (2004, April 1). In interview, mother details delusions that spurred her to kill sons." *CNN.com*. http://www.cnn.com/2004/LAW/04/01/laney/. Accessed December 1, 2015.

Stotland, N. L. (1999). When religion collides with medicine. *American Journal of Psychiatry, 156*, 304–307.

Waldfogel, S., & Meadows, S. (1996). Religious issues in the capacity evaluation. *General Hospital Psychiatry, 18*, 173–182.

Weil, S. (1998). *Writings selected with an introduction by Eric O. Springsted*. Maryknoll, NY: Orbis Books.

Weinstock, R. (2015). Dialectical principlism: An approach to finding the most ethical action. *Journal of the American Academy of Psychiatry and the Law, 43*, 10–20.

Whitley, G. (2006, May 18). The Devil and Doyle Davidson. *Dallas Observer*. Retrieved from www.dallasobserver.com/news/the-devil-and-doyle-davidson-6408771.

Worchel, D. (2012, May 25). Deanna Laney released from state hospital. *Tyler Morning Telegraph*, Tyler, TX.

World Medical Association. (2006). WMA Declaration of Geneva. Retrieved from https://www.wma.net/policies-post/wma-declaration-of-geneva/.

Yates v. State. (2005). 171 S. W. 3d 215 (Court of Appeals of Texas, First District).

Zonana, H. V., & Norko, M. A. (1993). Mandated treatment. In W. R. Sledge & A. Tasman (Eds.), *Clinical Challenges in Psychiatry* (pp. 249–291). Washington DC: American Psychiatric Press.

TWENTY-ONE

Ethical Considerations Regarding Religion/Spirituality in Psychiatric Research

Alexander Moreira-Almeida, M.D., Ph.D., Quirino Cordeiro, M.D., Ph.D., and Harold G. Koenig, M.D., M.H.Sc.

INTRODUCTION

Two unwarranted assumptions often impair discussions of the relationship between science and religion/spirituality. First, it is often assumed that religion and spirituality have permanently and inevitably been in conflict with science. A second assumption is that religion/spirituality and science are completely separate domains, making impossible any scientific study of religion/spirituality or any fruitful interaction between them (Barbour, 1998).

Several high-level historical studies with primary sources have shown convincingly that the interactions between science and religion are much more interesting, complex, and often positive than is usually assumed. It is now clear that the notion of an inevitable conflict between science and religion is a myth largely developed during the end of the 19th century (Brooke, 1991; Numbers, 2009). For example, Ronald Numbers, editor of a book summarizing some of the main historical studies on religion and science, commented on the issue of scientists being murdered by religious fanatics: "[N]o scientist, to our knowledge, ever lost his life because of his scientific views" (Numbers, 2009, p. 8).

Regarding the impossibility of scientific studies on religious/spiritual, this claim has been challenged by the more than 3000 original studies identified by two systematic reviews of empirical scientific studies performed on religious/spiritual and health during 20th and 21st centuries (Koenig, McCullough, & Larson, 2001; Koenig, King, & Carson, 2012). If we understand science as a rational and empirical investigation of the universe (nature in the broad sense), all things happening in the universe that have empirical expressions (i.e., those that are observable or notable by sense experience) can be subject to scientific investigation. Regardless of one's attitudes regarding the ultimate nature of religious/spiritual beliefs and experiences, they have empirical dimensions that can be assessed in scientific studies and correlated with other variables, such as health outcomes. Among the expressions of religion/spirituality that can be measured are behavioral/social expressions (e.g., church attendance, prayer, meditation, reading religious texts, voluntary work) and mental/cognitive ones (e.g., attitudes, beliefs, trances).

Because it is possible to conduct studies on religion/spirituality and health, this sort of investigation needs to follow international ethical and methodological guidelines for studies involving human subjects (World Medical Association, 2013). Although this chapter does not cover the general principles for good scientific practice, it discusses relevant ethical issues related to research on religion/spirituality and mental health.

THE ETHICAL DUTY OF STUDYING RELIGION/SPIRITUALITY IN PSYCHIATRY

We believe that psychiatry not only can but actually should investigate religion/spirituality, based on the following arguments:

- In a quest to decrease suffering and promote mental health, it is our duty as mental health professionals (researchers and clinicians) to study all factors that influence mental health and well-being.
- Religion/spirituality is relevant to most of humanity because 84% of the world's population is affiliated with a religious faith (Pew Research Center, 2012).
- Religion/spirituality has consistent impacts on health outcomes; it affects prevention, treatment seeking, treatment strategies, and patient outcomes (Koenig et al., 2001, 2012).
- Religion/spirituality is a topic valued by psychiatric patients, and many would like this topic to be included in preventive and therapeutic interventions (Moreira-Almeida, Koenig, & Lucchetti, 2014).
- Neglecting investigation on religion/spirituality may deprive psychiatric patients of valuable knowledge and effective interventions that could decrease the burden and suffering associated with mental illness as well as increase well-being and quality of life.

Based on these and other considerations, the World Psychiatric Association (WPA) recently released a position statement on spirituality and religion in psychiatry stressing that, for a comprehensive and person-centered approach, religion/spirituality should be considered in research, training, and clinical care (Moreira-Almeida, Sharma, van Rensburg, Verhagen, & Cook, 2016). The following recommendations are especially relevant to research:

A consideration of their [religious/spiritual] relevance to the origins, understanding and treatment of psychiatric disorders and the patient's attitude toward illness should therefore be central to clinical and academic psychiatry . . . . There is a need for more research on both religion and spirituality in psychiatry, especially on their clinical applications. These studies should cover a wide diversity of cultural and geographical backgrounds.

BIAS AND CONFLICT OF INTEREST BASED ON SPIRITUAL/ ANTI-SPIRITUAL RESEARCHER'S VIEWS

When discussing scientific studies on religious/spiritual, the attention of critics is often focused on researchers' religious or anti-religious beliefs. It is done in a way that suggests that these are key factors in judging the validity and credibility of the scientific investigation or finding. In testing the veracity of a scientific statement, it is important to check the statement itself and not the source of the statement. As argued by the philosopher of science Karl Popper (1995, pp. 24–25):

> In general we do not test the validity of an assertion or information by tracing its sources or its origin, but we test it, much more directly, by a critical examination of what has been asserted—of the asserted facts themselves.

Two logical fallacies are usual when accepting or rejecting scientific findings. The first is the *ad hominem* attack: rejecting a statement by attacking the person who states it (e.g., refuting a study because the scientist is religious or atheist). The second is appeal to authority: accepting a statement because of the position or authority of the person who states it, neglecting the evidence needed to support the claim.

An example that relates to our topic here might be accepting a claim on religion/spirituality because it came from an authority in another field, such as a reputable physicist or neuroscientist outside the health field, who did not provide supporting evidence for the claim.

Recognizing that science is conducted by human beings holding various convictions, Popper stated that "the *objectivity* of scientific statements lies in the fact that they can be inter-subjectively tested." The subjectivity is controlled by "the more general idea of inter-subjective criticism, or, in other words, of the idea of mutual rational control by critical discussion" (Popper, 2002, p. 22).

There has been growing attention to the disclosure of financial conflicts of interest (COI) with regard to academic activities. More recently, there has been discussion of non-financial forms of COI. These can be as diverse as personal, political, academic, ideological, or religious. It has been acknowledged that these COI may impact scientific practice, so the major problem has been how to manage them (*PLoS Medicine* Editors, 2008). COI are so ubiquitous (affecting virtually every scientific work) that they are hard to define and operationalize. Consequently, several top medical journals and the International Committee of Medical Journal Editors (ICMJE) decided not create specific guidelines for non-financial COI (Drazen et al., 2010; *PLoS Medicine* Editors, 2008). If taken to the extreme, non-financial COI would require disclosure of personal experiences, beliefs, and values related to drugs, sex, academic training, philosophy, religion, science, and so on. Virtually every aspect of our personal history may influence our judgment and decisions.

A wide range of personal factors (e.g., personality, ideology, cultural background, previous traumatic or positive experiences related to the topic) may influence one's interpretation of daily experiences (including scientific experiments) and the acceptance or rejection of political, religious, or scientific views. Because we are usually unable to track and evaluate the beliefs and other personal factors in a scientist's background, the philosopher of science Alan Chalmers (1990) proposed that they are not of great value when evaluating a scientific study. Such evaluations should be based on the arguments offered and methods used, not on the beliefs of involved scientists. For example, during mid-19th Century, there was a heated debate about whether germs could cause diseases. However, the fact that John Snow previously accepted germ theory cannot fairly be used to invalidate his conclusions of his studies of the relationship between cholera cases and the water supply in London, which favored the germ theory (Vandenbroucke et al., 1991). To judge the validity of scientists' claims, it is important to investigate their methods and try to replicate their findings. An interesting example that illustrates the complexity of the history of the relationship between science and religion and the inadequacy of focusing on scientists' backgrounds is the Voltaire–Needham dispute. The self-proclaimed champion of reason and science, Voltaire, violently attacked the studies on generation of life developed by the naturalist John Needham. Instead of pointing out problems in Needham's methodology or reasoning, Voltaire attacked him mainly for being a Catholic priest and for, according to Voltaire, promoting atheist ideas (Roe, 1985).

A few years ago, the ICMJE removed from the COI form "queries about potential competing interests of authors' spouses and minor children and about nonfinancial competing interests," because of "concerns about the ethics of inquiring about nonfinancial associations" and the negative feedback they received, stating that "there is immense difficulty in defining competing interests beyond those that involve the direct exchange of money from an interested party to an individual author or the author's institution." Currently the form simply asks: "Are there any other relationships or activities that readers could perceive to influence, or that give the appearance of potentially influencing, what you wrote in the submitted work?" (Drazen et al., 2010, p. 188).

The discussion of non-financial COI may also bring to the table a prejudice against religion/ spirituality. There is a common belief that a true scientist needs to be non-religious. According to this view, science has proved that matter and physical forces are everything that exists in the universe, and as a result, religious/spiritual beliefs are anti-scientific superstitions. A related assumption is that atheism and materialism are the default or neutral positions, whereas spiritual and non-materialist perspectives are biased stances. These positions are based on faulty assumptions that have been exposed in various studies (Barbour, 1998). First of all, most of the founders of modern science (e.g., Bacon, Descartes, Galileo, Kepler, Newton, Boyle) not only were religious but had spiritual motivations that undergirded their efforts to conduct scientific studies. They saw scientific study of nature as a way to "provide knowledge of the wisdom and intelligence of the creator" (Osler, 2009, p. 96). Second, as John Haught (2005) has discussed, although it is a widespread belief that science (a method of exploration) is inseparable from a materialistic ideology (a worldview called *materialist scientism*), "it is not written anywhere that the rest of us who appreciate science have to believe that. In fact, most of the great founders of modern science did not" (Haught, 2005, p. 367). The materialist ideology, although respectable, is not necessarily a logical conclusion of scientific activity (Araujo, 2012; Barbour, 1998). Therefore, we need to avoid the conflation of science with materialism in discussions involving religion/spirituality and science. Materialist perspectives of mind, human beings, and spiritual experiences are not neutral; they are but one among several valid positions on these subjects. Along this line, it is also important to distinguish true skepticism (i.e., doubts about the accuracy of knowledge, a sort of agnosticism) from the position of self-proclaimed "skeptics" or "rationalists" (e.g., militant atheists who systematic deny spirituality because they hold to an ideology of materialist scientism).

An illustrative example is the proposition by the cosmologist George Lemaitre of an expanding universe starting from a "primeval atom." Many atheists dismissed this theory as an attempt by religious people (Lemaitre was also a Catholic priest) to promote religious ideas; to mock the theory, they called it the "Big Bang" theory—the name by which it is well known today. This theory was even banned from atheist Soviet Union because it was considered a "reactionary [and] clerical . . . fairy tale" (Kragh, 2008).

In summary, non-financial COI are relevant to science but very hard to define and to manage. If non-financial COI are to be regularly disclosed, they should include all potential types (e.g., personal, political, academic, ideological) and not be limited only to religious forms. A similar point was made by Cook (2010). Probably the best way to proceed is to follow Popper's recommendations of intersubjective criticism: Clearly present the methods, data, and discussion to a wide range of high-quality audiences. The focus should be more on the science than on the scientists.

THE NEED TO RESPECT PATIENTS' RELIGIOSITY/SPIRITUALITY IN DESIGNING AND DISCUSSING A STUDY

All types of research must be ethically patient-centered. Therefore, researchers should ask about and respect patients' beliefs when designing and performing a clinical trial. This includes their religious or spiritual beliefs.

Another important ethical issue involving religious/spiritual is related to the publication of results showing, for example, that a specific type of religious or anti-religious belief may be related to negative coping. Although potentially problematic, this result may be important to fully understanding the relationship between religion and health. Researchers therefore have an obligation to publish the results of such investigations, even if they do not confirm their initial hypotheses.

According to the *World Medical Association Declaration of Helsinki: Ethical Principles for Medical Research Involving Human Subjects* (World Medical Association, 2013):

> [R]esearchers have a duty to make publicly available the results of their research on human subjects and are accountable for the completeness and accuracy of their reports . . . . [N]egative and inconclusive as well as positive results must be published or otherwise made publicly available.

In order to avoid the concealing of negative or unwanted effects uncovered by clinical research, the scientific community has initiated some procedures. In 1997, a joint initiative of the US Food and Drug Administration and the Department of Health and Human Services created the Web site, ClinicalTrials.gov. The objective was to create a platform for recording information on clinical trials performed by public and private institutions. The Food and Drug Administration Modernization Act (FDAMA) made compulsory the registration of clinical trials in order to make them widely available to the medical community, researchers, and general society (SciELO in Perspective, 2015). Thus, it is clear that researchers have an obligation to publish the results of studies they conduct. This must be done carefully and in a sensible way so as not to generate academic and social harm.

ETHICS OF PERFORMING INTERVENTIONS INVOLVING SPIRITUALITY IN THE CONTEXT OF RESEARCH

Concerns exist about how ethically acceptable it is to investigate and, in particular, to use a therapeutic intervention that seeks to affect a patient's religious/spiritual beliefs or practices. Here, we discuss two situations in which such issues are raised: in psychotherapy and in dealing with patients suffering from severe mental disorders.

Religion/Spirituality and Psychotherapy

All forms of psychotherapy involve efforts to influence beliefs, attitudes, and behaviors, including values and worldviews. The patient's beliefs, attitudes, and behaviors are often the problem that is driving the psychopathology for which they need psychotherapy. The patient comes in for treatment seeking help to change those beliefs, attitudes, and behaviors into healthier ones that lead to greater fulfillment in life and better relationships. The question is whether there is anything unique about religious/spiritual beliefs (or lack thereof) that makes them a special category that mental health professionals should not touch. This was certainly not the view of Freud, who made it clear that such beliefs were neurotic and could be the subject of therapy (Freud, 1927/2010). Utilizing and strengthening patients' own positive religious/spiritual beliefs and behaviors in order to enhance their functioning and well-being and improve their relationships would fall into the category of ethical treatment. The WPA's *Madrid Declaration on Ethical Standards for Psychiatric Practice*, at the topic "Ethics of Psychotherapy," states that the approach employed should be sensitive to religious and cultural factors (Okasha, 2003).

Based on this premise, several forms of spiritually integrated psychotherapies have been developed that stimulate patients' positive religious coping strategies. Dozens of clinical trials have been conducted and have shown that this type of therapy tends to be well accepted by patients and has similar or superior efficacy compared with conventional psychotherapies (Koenig et al., 2015; Worthington, Hook, Davis, & McDaniel, 2011). The use of a spiritually integrated approach needs to be carefully explained to the patient beforehand, and the patient must agree to such therapy. This approach, called *full disclosure*, must be taken by both the professional who assists the patient and the researcher who conducts an investigation using this type of psychotherapy. Spiritually integrated psychotherapies, in the context of clinical practice and research, need to be patient-centered. Therapists and researchers must focus on the positive religious/spiritual beliefs of the patient and not introduce a new belief system that is foreign to the patient and conflicts with existing beliefs. In other words, proselytizing or trying to convert a patient to another belief system (particularly, the belief system of the therapist) is unethical (Moreira-Almeida et al., 2014).

In addition to avoidance of proselytism, clinicians must also pay attention to practices that are not part of their professional role. The extent to which religious/spiritual beliefs and practices are integrated into mental health care has been a source of increasing controversy. An example is a clinician praying with a patient. In 2011, *The British Journal of Psychiatry* published a debate about whether praying with patients constituted a breach of professional boundaries in psychiatric practice (Poole & Cook, 2011). Systematic research indicates that religious patients often wish clinicians to pray with them (King & Bushwick, 1994; MacLean et al., 2003; Siatkowski, Cannon, & Farris, 2008). In general, a mental health professional's response to a patient's request for prayer depends on both the patient and the health professional. If both are religious, especially if they are from the same religion, and there is no clear clinical reason for objecting to this request, then we think it is appropriate for the clinician to say a short, simple prayer with the patient (alternatively, the clinician may ask the patient to say the prayer). Before granting this request, however, the clinician should ask the patient what he or she would like prayer for, and useful information can be learned from the response. Even if the patient and the mental health professional are not from the same religion, this may be permissible (Sulmasy, 2009). However, in some circumstances, the mental health professional may not be comfortable praying with patients. In such situations, clinicians may decline and gently explain why (e.g., no religious conviction, discomfort engaging in a particular type of prayer, worry about the effect of such intimate sharing on the physician–patient relationship) (Sulmasy, 2009).

Clinicians should never force prayer on patients, and they need to be careful not to prey on the vulnerabilities of patients (Sulmasy, 2009). Proselytizing has no role in the relationship between patients and health care professionals. The vulnerability of the patient and the power imbalance between clinician and patient limit such decisions. Mental health professionals should respect the vulnerable condition of patients and take care not to impose their personal (religious or non-religious) beliefs (Sulmasy, 2009). Furthermore, when professionals offer to pray with patients, this may give the impression that the clinician is desperate and that nothing else can be done to help the patient. If this is so—and admittedly is probably rare—it may compromise the health care–patient relationship. Bear in mind, however, that most of the key points in this discussion are based on expert opinion. Besides common sense, there is very little research supporting these suggestions. As a result, research is extremely important in this area to guide clinical decision making.

Religion/Spirituality and Patients with Severe Mental Disorders

Studies have reported conflicting results regarding the role of religion/spirituality in severe mental disorders (especially psychotic disorders) in terms of the etiology of psychopathology, treatment-seeking behavior, treatment adherence, and illness outcome. Therefore, research in this area is extremely important. However, because of a variety of ethical issues that touch on this subject, researchers need to be mindful of the complexities. Two major concerns are the potential harmful effects of addressing religious/spiritual issues with psychotic patients and whether such patients have the capacity to consent to an religious/spiritual intervention.

There is growing research indicating that religion/spirituality is important to many patients with schizophrenia and other psychotic disorders. As in patients with general medical conditions or other mental disorders, psychotic patients often use religion/spirituality to cope with their symptoms and living circumstances. These strategies may have either a positive or a negative influence on their psychiatric symptoms. Mohr et al. (2011) assessed the value of positive and negative uses of religion to cope with schizophrenia or schizoaffective disorder. For patients using positive religious coping strategies at baseline, importance of spirituality predicted fewer negative symptoms, better clinical global impression, increased social functioning, and higher quality of life. For patients using negative religious coping at baseline, no relationships were found. The authors concluded that positive forms of religious/spiritual coping, but not negative forms, predicted better outcomes. According to the authors, religion/spirituality may contribute to recovery by providing resources for coping with symptoms. In some situations, however, religion/spirituality may also serve as a source of suffering. In a systematic review of this literature, Gearing et al. (2011) found that religion can act as both a risk factor and a protective factor because it interacts with symptoms involving hallucinations and delusions.

In a review paper on the relationship between schizophrenia and religion/spirituality and its implications for clinical care, Mohr and Huguelet (2004) also reported that religion/spirituality has an impact, usually but not always positive, on patients with schizophrenia associated with substance abuse and suicidal attempts. On the one hand, religion/spirituality plays an important role in the processes of reconstructing a sense of self and recovery for many patients. In some cases, patients are helped by their faith community, uplifted by spiritual activities, and comforted by their religious beliefs. On the other hand, patients may be rejected by their faith community, burdened by spiritual activities, or disappointed and demoralized by their beliefs. In general, though, religion/spirituality is relevant for the treatment of many patients with schizophrenia, helping to reduce symptoms, enhance coping, and foster recovery. Mohr and Huguelet suggested that when one is treating patients with schizophrenia, it is useful to tolerate diversity, respect patients' beliefs, ban proselytizing, and have a good knowledge of one's own spiritual identity.

Because religion/spirituality can affect outcome in psychotic patients, clinicians should address it as part of clinical care. Interventions may involve supporting positive religious coping strategies and modifying negative ones. There has been concern that approaching religion/spirituality in psychotic patients may exacerbate delusions and hallucinations. Although more research is needed, there is no consistent evidence to support this view, especially when religion/spirituality is addressed in a thoughtful, sensitive manner (Koenig, 2007). An example was provided by Kehoe (2007), who described her experiences gained over more than 20 years of conducting group therapy for patients with chronic mental illness that focused on spiritual beliefs and values. Group therapy that is focused on religious/spiritual issues may provide, even for seriously mentally ill persons, an opportunity to explore this topic which is usually ignored during regular mental health practice. Kehoe reported that negative effects occurred only rarely, and delusions were not exacerbated. The feasibility and impact of interventions involving religion/spirituality in psychosis and other severe mental disorders are topics with an urgent need for more rigorous studies.

Another ethical concern is whether the religious beliefs of patients compromise their clinical treatment. Here it is important to observe the principles of autonomy, beneficence, and non-maleficence. When conducting research in this field, investigators should also take these ethical principles into account. One of the most important goals of contemporary interventions in mental healthcare (clinical and research) is to preserve and promote the autonomy of patients. However, it is essential that such practices also be consistent with the ethical principles of beneficence and non-maleficence. Patients with severe mental disorders may be impaired in their ability to make autonomous decisions. Therefore, it is important to establish the line between respect for patients' autonomous decision making and protection of those whose ability to make decisions for themselves is impaired. Individuals with severe mental disorders may in some circumstances have reduced autonomy, which can influence their decision making processes (Eike-Henner, 2008).

Eike-Henner (2008) recommended that patients whose autonomy is impaired should not be treated in the same way as those whose autonomy is intact. Gessert (2008) argued that the extreme importance given in recent times to patients' autonomy may have an adverse effect on these individuals. The right to autonomy must be respected in situations in which patients are lucid and knowledgeable adults. However, extremely vulnerable patients may often be put in situations where they cannot act autonomously. Thus, the simple application of the principle of autonomy to patients with severe mental disorders with reduced power to make autonomous decisions may be a problem. This context may require a clinical and research approach based on ethical principles of beneficence and non-maleficence by a staff that is in touch with the patients. Attitudes that are based on these principles seek to ensure that the interests of patients with reduced autonomy are achieved. These ethical principles are applicable not only to clinical contexts but to research contexts as well. However, ethical principles should not be considered in a hierarchical manner and must be regarded *prima facie*. Therefore, the choice for using one principle over the other should take place on a case-by-case basis.

In addition to the three ethical principles just discussed, the principle of justice deserves respect when conducting research involving religion/spirituality issues in the field of mental health. In the scientific arena, biomedical ethics has provided more emphasis on interpersonal relationships between researcher and research participant, where autonomy, beneficence, and non-maleficence have played a prominent role, thereby undervaluing the principle of justice. That principle has been associated preferentially with social groups and concern with appropriate and equitable way to treat people in biomedical studies. Different questions appear when justice is discussed in the research context. One point relates to the participation of subjects in scientific studies. Participants shall not be selected, whether intentionally or inadvertently, according to culture, language, race, disability, sexual orientation, ethnicity, linguistic proficiency, gender, age, or religion, unless justified by study objectives. Moreover, researchers shall not exclude individuals from the opportunity to participate in research on the basis of such attributes unless there is a valid scientific reason for the exclusion. So, the ethical principle of justice imposes a duty on researchers not to exclude individuals or groups from participation in investigations for reasons that are not related to the study. If groups of individuals (e.g., religious people) are excluded, the results of research may not be generalized easily to real-life situations. The results may not be applicable to the more usual patient found in clinical practice. Another important point related to the ethical principle of justice concerns the collection and analysis of research data. In many clinical and epidemiological studies, the investigation of religious variables has been neglected. As a result, appropriate information about certain groups is not available to the scientific and clinical community, which may disadvantage people in those groups. Unfortunately, this issue has not received the attention it deserves from the scientific community.

SCIENCE POPULARIZATION IN RELIGION/SPIRITUALITY

It is society that sponsors scientific investigations, and scientists cannot stay in an ivory tower. We have an ethical duty to make results available to the community that ultimately funds scientific activity. Scientific studies on religion/spirituality and mental health, like several other sensitive areas (e.g., gender, substance use), are related to deeply held values and beliefs and often generate extreme reactions from academic and lay audiences.

Scientific studies on religion/spirituality are usually highly valued by the media and the general population. As in other scientific areas, news about such studies frequently suffers from sensationalism or distortion. Studies are often presented as providing proof of a religious claim (e.g., the existence of heaven based on reports of spiritual experiences) or as exposing spiritual experiences as nothing more than the firing of neurons from a certain region of the brain.

The participation of healthcare professionals in discussing matters related to their research with representatives of the media should be guided by the accurate reporting of findings and their implications, with care taken not to stimulate sensationalism or self-promotion. Researchers are obligated to ensure that what they report is based on the actual study findings that are relevant to the public interest.

Here are some guidelines we recommend:

- Researchers must be able to back up whatever they say in the media with solid research data. Research rarely "proves" anything; rather, it identifies correlations and tests hypotheses. Religion/spirituality may predict changes in mental health, and religious/spiritual interventions my improve outcomes, but it is usually not appropriate to say that a specific research project proves something.
- Avoid simplistic explanations for the effects of religion/spirituality on health, as if they fully explained or ultimately caused or were caused by a biological or psychological process (e.g., brain activation, cognitive style, psychological projection).
- Be careful when interpreting findings, always mentioning the limitations and alternative explanations. Display extra caution when discussing whether scientific data support or disprove religious beliefs or explain them away.
- Be careful when discussing research that compares different religious traditions to avoid stereotyping or fostering competition or animosity between religious groups.

CONCLUSIONS

Psychiatric research in religion/spirituality is a challenging topic that has received growing attention from both academic and general audiences. The ethical considerations raised by this sort of investigation are similar to those of other topics in psychiatry because our field often deals with values, beliefs, and behavior.

It is essential to remember that values and beliefs are related not only to religion/spirituality but also to any sort of philosophy, ideology, or cosmology. In essence, we recommend treating religion/spirituality as we treat other aspects of humans' culture, whether in relation to patients or to researchers themselves. In summary, religious/spiritual values, beliefs, and behaviors should be carefully addressed, investigated, and respected, as should any values, beliefs, and behaviors.

REFERENCES

Araujo, S. F. (2012). Materialism's eternal return: Recurrent patterns of materialistic explanations of mental phenomena. In A. Moreira-Almeida & F. S. Santos (Eds.), *Exploring frontiers of the mind-brain relationship* (pp. 3–15). New York, NY: Springer. doi:10.1007/978-1-4614-0647-1_1

Barbour, I. G. (1998). *Religion and science: Historical and contemporary issues.* London, England: SCM Press.

Brooke, J. H. (1991). *Science and religion: Some historical perspectives.* Cambridge, England: Cambridge University Press.

Chalmers, A. (1990). *Science and its fabrication.* Minneapolis, MN: University of Minnesota Press.

Cook, C. C. (2010). Re: A common standard for conflict of interest disclosure in addiction journals. *Addiction, 105*(4), 760–761. doi:10.1111/j.1360-0443.2010.02921.

Drazen, J. M., de Leeuw, P. W., Laine, C., Mulrow, C., DeAngelis, C. D., Frizelle, F. A., . . . Zhaori, G. (2010). Toward more uniform conflict disclosures: The updated ICMJE conflict of interest reporting form. *The New England Journal of Medicine, 363,* 188–189. doi:10.1056/NEJMe1006030

Eike-Henner, W. (2008). Incompetent patient, substitute decision making and quality of life: Some ethical considerations. *Medscape Journal of Medicine, 10,* 237.

Freud, S. (1927/2010). *The future of an illusion.* Seattle, WA: Pacific Publishing Studio.

Gearing, R. E., Alonzo, D., Smolak, A., McHugh, K., Harmon, S., & Baldwin, S. (2011). Association of religion with delusions and hallucinations in the context of schizophrenia: Implications for engagement and adherence. *Schizophrenia Research, 126*(1–3), 150–163. doi:10.1016/j.schres.2010.11.005

Gessert, C. E. (2008). The problem with autonomy. *Minnesota Medicine, 91*(4), 40–42.

Haught, J. F. (2005). Science and scientism: The importance of a distinction. *Zygon: Journal of Religion and Science, 40,* 363–368.

Kehoe, N. (2007). Spirituality groups in serious mental illness. *Southern Medical Journal, 100*(6), 647–648.

King, D. E., & Bushwick, B. (1994). Beliefs and attitudes of hospital inpatients about faith healing and prayer. *Journal of Family Practice, 39,* 349–352.

Koenig, H. G. (2007). Religion, spirituality and psychotic disorders. *Revista de Psiquiatria Clinica, 34*(Suppl 1), 95–104. doi:dx.doi.org/10.1590/S0101-60832007000700013

Koenig, H. G., King, D., & Carson, V. B. (2012). *Handbook of religion and health* (2nd ed.). New York, NY: Oxford University Press.

Koenig, H. G., McCullough, M. E., & Larson, D. B. (2001). *Handbook of religion and health.* New York, NY: Oxford University Press.

Koenig, H. G., Pearce, M. J., Nelson, B., Shaw, S. F., Robins, C. J., Daher, N., . . . King, M. B. (2015). Religious vs. conventional cognitive-behavioral therapy for major depression in persons with chronic medical illness. *Journal of Nervous and Mental Disease, 203*(4), 243–251. doi:10.1097/NMD.0000000000000273

Kragh, H. S. (2008). *Entropic creation: Religious contexts of thermodynamics and cosmology.* Hampshire, England: Ashgate.

MacLean, C. D., Susi, B., Phifer, N., Schultz, L., Bynum, D., Franco, M., . . . Cykert, S. (2003). Patient preference for physician discussion and practice of spirituality. *Journal of General Internal Medicine, 18,* 38–43.

Mohr, S., & Huguelet, P. (2004). The relationship between schizophrenia and religion and its implications for care. *Swiss Medical Weekly, 134,* 369–376.

Mohr, S., Perroud, N., Gillieron, C., Brandt, P. Y., Rieben, I., Borras, L., & Huguelet, P. (2011). Spirituality and religiousness as predictive factors of outcome in schizophrenia and schizo-affective disorders. *Psychiatry Research, 186*(2–3), 177–182. doi:10.1016/j.psychres.2010.08.012

Moreira-Almeida, A., Koenig, H. G., & Lucchetti, G. (2014). Clinical implications of spirituality to mental health: Review of evidence and practical guidelines. *Revista Brasileira de Psiquiatria, 36*(2), 176–182. doi:dx.doi.org/10.1590/1516-4446-2013-1255

Moreira-Almeida, A., Sharma, A., van Rensburg, B. J., Verhagen, P. J., & Cook, C. C. H. (2016). WPA position statement on spirituality and religion in psychiatry. *World Psychiatry, 15*(1), 87–88.

Numbers, R. L. (Ed.). (2009). *Galileo goes to jail and other myths about science and religion.* Cambridge, MA: Harvard University Press.

Okasha, A. (2003). The Declaration of Madrid and its implementation: An update. *World Psychiatry*, *2*(2), 65–67.

Osler, M. J. (2009). Myth 10: That the scientific revolution liberated science from religion. In R. L. Numbers (Ed.), *Galileo goes to jail and other myths about science and religion* (pp. 90–98). Cambridge, MA: Harvard University Press.

Pew Research Center. (2012). *The global religious landscape*. Retrieved from http://www.pewforum.org/2012/12/18/global-religious-landscape-exec.

PLoS Medicine Editors. (2008). Making sense of non-financial competing interests. *PLoS Medicine* 5:e199. doi:10.1371/journal.pmed.0050199

Poole, R., & Cook, C. C. (2011). Praying with a patient constitutes a breach of professional boundaries in psychiatric practice. *British Journal of Psychiatry*, *199*(2), 94–98. doi:10.1192/bjp.bp.111.096529

Popper, K. R. (1995). *Conjectures and refutations: The growth of scientific knowledge* (5th ed.). London, England: Routledge.

Popper, K. R. (2002). *The logic of scientific discovery*. London, England: Routledge Classics.

Roe, S. A. (1985). Voltaire versus Needham: Atheism, materialism, and the generation of life. *Journal of the History of Ideas*, *46*(1), 65–87.

SciELO in Perspective. (2017). Blog. Retrieved from http://blog.scielo.org/en/#.WYnvs7pFw5s.

Siatkowski, R. M., Cannon, S. L., & Farris, B. K. (2008). Patients' perception of physician-initiated prayer prior to elective ophthalmologic surgery. *Southern Medical Journal*, *101*, 138–141. doi:10.1097/SMJ.0b013e3181612128

Sulmasy, D. P. (2009). Spirituality, religion and clinical care. *Chest*, *135*(6), 1634–1642. doi:10.1378/chest.08-2241

Vandenbroucke, J. P., Eelkman Rooda, H. M., & Beukers, H. (1991). Who made John Snow a hero? *American Journal of Epidemiology*, *133*(10), 967–973

World Medical Association. (2013). World Medical Association Declaration of Helsinki: Ethical principles for medical research involving human subjects. *JAMA*, *310*(20), 2191–2194. doi:10.1001/jama.2013.281053

Worthington, E. L., Hook, J. N., Davis, D. E., & McDaniel, M. A. (2011). Religion and spirituality. In J. C. Norcross (Ed.), *Psychotherapy relationships that work* (2nd ed., pp. 402–419). New York, NY: Oxford University Press.

TWENTY-TWO

Psychiatric Education

Gerrit Glas, M.D., M.A., Ph.D.

INTRODUCTION

How should residents learn to deal with the ethical impact of religion and spirituality in the lives of their patients? What is the role of the psychiatric educator with respect to the resident whose moral and religious views interfere with his clinical and psychotherapeutic work? Are clinicians allowed to express their own religious and moral views to provide a rationale for their stance with respect to treatment-related issues? Should a female resident be allowed to wear a headscarf when performing her clinical work?

These are some of the questions psychiatric educators have to deal with when they teach, supervise, and set up their training programs. This chapter focuses predominantly on how to teach residents to understand and deal with religion and spirituality in an ethically responsible and sensitive way. There are a number of issues that come to mind in this context. One is about what residents need to learn about their role and professional attitude with respect to religious/spiritual issues in patients. Another is about the task of the psychiatric educator when religious/spiritual issues intersect with the resident's role as a professional. What kind of competence needs to be developed in the resident? And, given the sensitivity of the subject, how should psychiatric educators themselves develop the skills that are needed to teach residents to adequately deal with religious/spiritual issues? A related and more fundamental question is how the profession should make sense of the competence of professionalism in this respect. In documents on medical specialist training, it is generally agreed that training involves more than enhancing medical knowledge, practical skills, and scholarship and that it should involve training in a whole range of other competences, including communication, collaboration, and professionalism. Professionalism is then defined as a competence that enables the trainee to reflect on her own functioning, to identify her educational needs, and to behave in an ethically responsible way (Gabbard et al., 2012). However, the question of what the competence of professionalism implies with respect to the resident's ability to deal with religious/spiritual issues, her own religious/spiritual issues included, still needs further investigation (Sloan et al., 2000).

So far, there are three questions on the table: one about what it means for a resident to responsibly and ethically deal sensitively with religious/spiritual issues in the patient; one about the task of the psychiatric educator when religious/spiritual issues intersect with the resident's role as a professional; and one about professionalism as a competence, and more specifically, the question of what professionalism implies with respect to how psychiatrists in general should deal with religious/spiritual issues. These three questions can each be divided into two sub-questions, one focusing on the object of attention and one on the subject who pays attention to religious/spiritual issues. Objects of attention may be religious/spiritual issues in the patient, the resident who has to learn certain skills, or the profession as it develops a view on these matters. Subjects of attention are, respectively, the resident, the educator, and the professional as a person. The psychiatric educator may focus on how residents try to find a proper (i.e., morally sensitive and responsible) stance with respect to religious/spiritual issues in either the patient or themselves. But educators may also reflect on their own role fulfillment as educators. They may deal with the general question of how to instruct residents to act morally sensitively and responsibly at the intersection between religious/spiritual issues and psychiatry. And they may struggle with their own doubts, concerns, and convictions with regard to religious/spiritual matters and how these interfere with their educational roles and duties. All of these questions are, finally, related to a set of more general questions about how values and virtues that are intrinsic to the profession are related to the management of religious/spiritual issues, either in the patient or in oneself as a professional. A summary of these six themes is presented in Table 22.1. Each topic corresponds to a section in this chapter. In the remainder of this chapter, this categorization of questions will be used as a framework to structure the discussion. The focus will be, first on the resident, then on the educator, and finally on the concept of professionalism.

THE RESIDENT 1: ETHICAL ASPECTS OF LEARNING TO DEAL WITH RELIGIOUS AND SPIRITUAL ISSUES IN THE PATIENT

Should residents learn to discuss religious/spiritual issues with their patients? In a systematic literature survey, Best, Butow, and Olver (2015) found that a majority of patients with somatic

TABLE 22.1 Actors, Roles and Topics; Self- and Other-Related

Who	Role	Topic
Resident	Being a trainee	1. Ethical aspects of learning to deal with religious/spiritual issues in the patient
		2. Ethical aspects of learning to deal with religious/spiritual issues in one's role fulfilment
Educator or Supervisor	Professionalism of the educator/supervisor	1. Finding a proper (moral) stance as educator with respect to how residents have to deal with religious/spiritual issues
		2. Responsibly dealing with the interference of one's own religious/spiritual issues with one's role as educator
Professional (including residents)	Professionalism as core competence; reflection on moral implications of one's professional role	1. Ethical implications of professionalism with respect to religious/spiritual issues in the patient
		2. Ethical implications of professionalism with respect to religious/spiritual issues in one's own role fulfillment

or psychiatric disorders want to be asked about religion/spirituality by their doctor. A significant minority do not desire this, however, and patients and doctors do not always agree on what such spiritual enquiry should entail. The authors concluded that, given this mismatch, doctors need to learn to identify patients' needs in this respect. In a systematic literature review among doctors, the same authors found that religion/spirituality issues are infrequently discussed and that many physicians prefer chaplain referral to discussing them (Best et al., 2016). The most often reported barriers for discussion were insufficient time and lack of training. Prior training and increased physician religiosity appeared to facilitate spiritual enquiry. In a study among 1144 US psychiatrists and non-psychiatrists, Curlin et al. (2007) found that a vast majority of psychiatrists (94%) and somewhat more than half of non-psychiatrists (53%) were open to address religious/spiritual issues with patients. Psychiatrists generally endorsed positive influences of religion and spirituality on health but were also more likely to report that religion and spirituality may lead to negative emotions and increased suffering.

These and similar earlier findings have resulted in a number of initiatives aimed at including the topic of religion and spirituality in psychiatric training programs (Josephson & Peteet, 2007; Josephson, Peteet, & Tasman, 2010; Larson, Lu, & Swyers, 1997; Lawrence & Duggal, 2001; Puchalski, Kheirbek, Doucette, Martin, & Yang, 2013; Puchalski, Larson, & Lu, 2000) and to the development of model curricula (Grabovac, Clark, & McKenna, 2008; Grabovac & Ganesan, 2003; Kozak, Boynton, Bentley, & Bezy, 2010; McCarthy & Peteet, 2003). These initiatives were stimulated by award programs inaugurated by the John Templeton Foundation between 1997 and 2002 and by the George Washington Institute for Spirituality and Health (GWISH) between 2001 and 2006. Since then, several professional organizations have issued standards, recommendations, guidelines, or position statements regarding religion and spirituality in relation to psychiatric training (Bowman, 2009; Cook, 2013; Verhagen & Cook, 2010; Verhagen & Cox, 2010; see also American Psychiatric Association [APA], 1990, 2006a). The model curricula typically aim at acquiring clinical skills and attitudes to address religious/spiritual issues. These skills and attitudes help the resident to assess spiritual needs in a respectful and nonjudgmental way; they enable the trainee to gather and interpret information about the religious/spiritual history of the patient; and they help the trainee identify resources of spiritual care. Ideally, teaching should also provide an introduction to empirical findings on spirituality and mental health and to techniques of addressing the topic in psychotherapy (Baetz & Toews, 2009; Huguelet & Koenig, 2009). An elaborate set of learning objectives and outcome goals for psychiatric residency training can be found on the Web site of GWISH and is represented in a slightly adapted form in Box 22.1.

Most recently, the Accreditation Council on Graduate Medical Education (ACGME), in collaboration with the American Board of Psychiatry and Neurology, has moved to evaluating psychiatric trainees through the use of milestones. The Milestones in the Psychiatry Milestone Project (2014) are "descriptors and targets for resident performance as a resident progresses from entry into residency through graduation." A Milestone typically describes knowledge, skills, attitudes, and other attributes for each of the ACGME roles. The six roles are divided into 22 subcompetencies, which in turn are subdivided in threads (66 in total). Milestones are defined at the level of these threads. Relevant in this context are the thread "Compassion, reflection, sensitivity to diversity," which belongs to the domain PROF1 (professionalism 1) and the subcompetence "Compassion, integrity, respect for others, sensitivity to diverse patient populations, adherence to ethical principles." At level 2, the thread "requires capacity for self-reflection, empathy, and curiosity about and openness to different beliefs and points of view, and respect for diversity" and

---

Box 22.1. Learning Objectives and Outcome Goals for Psychiatry Residency (George Washington Institute for Spirituality and Health)

LEARNING OBJECTIVES

The resident should demonstrate competence in the following:

Knowledge

- ☐ Defining spirituality, including these phenomenological aspects: experiences/attitudes/practices/beliefs (from here on these items are called simply "experiences").
- ☐ Understanding the unique impact of spiritual/cultural experiences on human development and health in infancy, childhood, adolescence, and adulthood.
- ☐ Understanding a differential diagnosis for spiritual/cultural phenomena at the individual and spiritual/cultural system levels.
- ☐ Understanding the impact of spiritual/cultural experiences on the relationship between the physician and patient, including transference and counter-transference.
- ☐ Understanding of spiritual/cultural issues and treatment preferences surrounding the end-of-life affect medical ethics as applied to family practice and internal medicine.
- ☐ Understanding of the variety of spiritual experiences and traditions, with unique perspectives on transpersonal issues.
- ☐ Understanding of the research data on the impact of patients' cultural identity, beliefs and practices on their health and access to and interaction with health care providers.
- ☐ Understanding that differences in cultural identity between physicians and patients can impact delivery of health care.
- ☐ Understanding of their own spirituality and how truly compassionate care giving can come from knowing and respecting the role spirituality has in their own life.
- ☐ Understanding of the role of culturally based healers and care providers.
- ☐ Understanding how physician's role encompasses patient care and the care of their family during the entire transition between life and death.
- ☐ Understanding the dimensions of palliative care (physical, emotional, social and spiritual) at the end-of-life of a patient.

Skills

- ☐ Interviewing patients with sensitivity to communication styles, vulnerabilities, and strengths as well as their cultural identity, beliefs and practices.
- ☐ Listening for, eliciting, and understanding accurate histories, including the importance of spiritual issues, cultural identity and beliefs/rituals and their impact on the patient's life.
- ☐ Identifying and eliciting patients' values, beliefs, and preferences for treatment during the course of illness.
- ☐ Identifying how, as influential caregivers, cultural identity, beliefs and practices might affect their relationship with patients, as well as their case formulation, diagnosis and management plans.
- ☐ Recognizing when a patients' spiritual views or cultural beliefs/rituals are harmful to the patient and making appropriate interventions and referrals (for example to chaplains, spiritual directors or culturally-based healers).

☐ Diagnosing, assessing and formulating treatment plans for patients, with an understanding of spiritual and cultural realm of experiences.

☐ Recognizing and using specific transference and countertransference reactions.

☐ Recognizing possible biases against the spiritual/cultural issues found in the medical literature and understanding their origins.

☐ Demonstrating the ability to deliver difficult news to patients and their families in a caring and compassionate manner.

☐ Learning to work with a multi-disciplinary team delivering end-of-life care and appreciate each member's contribution.

☐ Effectively listening to and responding to patients about their suffering.

Attitudes

☐ Awareness of their spiritual and cultural experiences and the impact of these experiences on their identity and world view.

☐ Avoidance of stereotyping and over-generalization and an appreciation for diversity of spiritual and cultural identities, belief, ritual and practices.

☐ Awareness of their own attitudes toward various spiritual and cultural experiences and the possible biases that could influence their treatment of patients.

☐ Respect for patients from a variety of spiritual and cultural backgrounds.

☐ Non-judgmental attitudes when eliciting a spiritual history and preferences for treatment during the course of illness.

☐ An appreciation for the systems and venues for health care delivery at the end-of-life (hospice, home nursing, institutional care).

OUTCOME GOALS

The overall goal for the program is to encourage the full integration of a more compassionate and holistic approach to healthcare. Spiritual care is the foundation of compassionate care. It speaks to the connection we form with our patients and colleagues with the altruistic goals of providing the best care for those we serve—our patients. By being attentive to all dimensions of our patients' lives—the physical, emotional, social, and spiritual—we can deliver the best healthcare possible for our patients.

From https://smhs.gwu.edu/gwish/education/residency-programs#psychiatry.

"examples of the importance of attention to diversity in psychiatric evaluation and treatment." Milestone at level 3 is the ability to demonstrate "eliciting beliefs, values and diverse practices of patients and their families," understanding of "their potential impact on patient care," and display of "sensitivity to diversity in psychiatric evaluation and treatment." At level 4, the resident should be able to develop a "mutually agreeable care plan in the context of conflicting physician and patient and/or family values and beliefs" and "to discuss own cultural background and beliefs and the ways in which these affect interaction with patients." This formulation is remarkable and important, given the traditional hesitance about bringing in one's own values and spiritual points of view as a doctor. Level 5 refers to a degree of performance beyond that of residents (i.e., a level that is typical for role models and teachers).

Defining these learning objectives and outcome goals is one issue, but effectively teaching them and having these skills and attitudes really integrated in clinical work is another. One way of approaching the issue is by making use of the Cultural Formulation Interview (CFI), which can be found in the appendixes of the *Diagnostic and Statistical Manual of Mental Disorders, Fifth Edition* (DSM-5), in both a patient and an informant version (APA, 2013, pp. 750–754, 755–757). The interview addresses in 16 questions the cultural identity of the patient (including religiosity/spirituality), cultural conceptualizations of distress (including spiritual reasons), cultural features of vulnerability and resilience (including religious ways of coping), cultural features of the relationship between the individual and the clinician; and overall cultural assessment.

THE RESIDENT 2: ETHICAL ASPECTS OF THE RESIDENT'S ROLE FULFILLMENT

In spite of all these recommendations and the availability of practical tools, there may arise all manner of difficulties in daily practice. Balboni et al. (2015) addressed this topic from the angle of what has been called the hidden curriculum. The term *hidden curriculum* is not new; it refers to the actual socialization in medical practice, as contrasted with the ideal socialization described in training curricula (Hafferty & Franks 1994; Levinson et al., 2014, Chapter 8). Balboni et al. (2015) defined it as "the process of formation, largely based in apprenticeship, which instills behaviors, attitudes, and values among trainees." This actual socialization is often in tension with the overt ideals of medical professionalism, which aim at fostering virtues like compassion, unselfishness, and humanitarianism. The hidden curriculum may be so strong and so discrepant from what young professionals rightfully expect that it has toxic effects on them, including erosion of empathy, cynicism, burnout, thoughts of leaving medicine, depression, and/or suicidal ideation. Similar byproducts of medical training have been discussed and investigated in the context of research on ethics education (for a brief overview, see Roberts & Dyer, 2004, pp. 249–253).

Balboni et al. (2015) admit that it is unclear whether medical education alone can reverse these toxic effects. This is because the hidden curriculum is generated by deep, internal and external social structures—internal structures such as poor role modeling and rigid, hierarchal relationships, and external structures such as market forces, bureaucratization, and the so-called technological imperative. Educational reformers, they suggest, should try to connect with other partners within and outside medicine, aiming at reform of these structures. It is in this context that they ask for special attention to spirituality in the medical curriculum and to grounding of professional ideals and virtues in practices outside medicine, including moral and religious communities. The general idea is that the hidden curriculum—conceived as a socialization process—is so pervasive that it requires counterforces in social structures outside medicine that are at least equally powerful in internalizing the virtuous habits and ideals doctors need to possess (Daaleman, Kingman, Newton, & Meador, 2011; Kinghorn, McEvoy, Michel, & Balboni, 2007; Peteet, 2014).

In their exploratory study (33 subjects), Balboni et al. (2015) investigated how religion and spirituality, understood as primary socialization, intersects with medical training and the experience of the hidden curriculum. Three domains emerged as important for trainee socialization: differences in perceived difficulties during medical training between religious/spiritual and non-religious/spiritual respondents; differences in coping strategies between the religious/spiritual and non-religious/spiritual groups; and fluctuations in level of religion and spirituality during medical training. Religious/spiritual students appeared to struggle more than non-religious/spiritual students with issues related to personal identity and self-confidence but less with relational discord on teams, work-life balance, and emotional stress in patient encounters. Religious/spiritual trainees tended to adopt religious coping styles such as prayer, faith, and compassion, whereas non-religious/spiritual subjects were inclined to use compartmentalization and emotional repression as coping mechanisms. Religious/spiritual students also showed an increase in level of religiosity/spirituality during medical training.

Having a sense of calling might be one of the ideals that is associated with one's sense of identity as a professional (Gustafson, 1982). Yoon, Shin, Nian, and Curlin (2015) found that physicians and psychiatrists who score higher on measures of religiosity are more likely to report a strong sense of calling. The authors interpreted calling as an intrinsic motivating factor that helps students and physicians to sustain meaning and purpose in their work. Calling has references to spheres of life which are, again, broader than medicine alone. The experience of being called connects one's sense of professional identity with the heart of medicine. Calling includes a vision of life itself; it nourishes a sense of self-fulfillment, and it connects one's sense of self with a sphere that extends beyond the individual. It is this connection ("personal fit") that is assumed to provide the experience of meaning and purpose that is at the center of the experience of being called (see also Dik & Duffy, 2009; Duffy, Allan, & Bott, 2012; Duffy, Manuel, Borges, & Bott, 2011).

THE EDUCATOR 1: ETHICALLY DEALING WITH RELIGIOUS AND SPIRITUAL ISSUES IN PSYCHIATRIC TRAINING

The *Resource Document on Religious/Spiritual Commitments and Psychiatric Practice* of the APA (2006b) encourages psychiatrists to "maintain respect for their patients' commitments (values, beliefs and worldviews)." These guidelines warn clinicians against imposing "their own religious/spiritual, antireligious/spiritual, or other values, beliefs and world views on their patients." And they state that psychiatrists "should foster recovery by making treatment decisions with patients in ways that respect and take into meaningful consideration their cultural, religious/spiritual and personal ideals."

Respect, not imposing one's own values, and taking into consideration patients' values are important and uncontested preconditions for safe encounters between patients and physicians. It may be difficult enough to act according to these standards. An even more complex issue, however, is to assess how the intrinsic values of "normal" practices interact with values that deviate from them, either in the patient or in the clinician. The very concept of professionalism depends on commitments that are value-laden (Peteet, 2014)—commitments that refer to proper behaviors such as honesty, confidentiality, and appropriate relations with patients; to virtues such as trustworthiness, striving for excellence, and stewardship; and to taking responsibility for quality of care, access to care, and just distribution of finite resources. Ideally, these ideals and virtues are embodied in one's professional attitude.

How are clinicians supposed to negotiate about patient values and ideals if the clinical practice of psychiatry and psychotherapy itself is not value-neutral? If professionals do not stand on neutral and unshakeable ground, then their ideals and values are no longer self-evident and may become topics of discussion. There will sometimes be a need to renegotiate about them. Even more complex are situations in which the value system of the individual professional markedly differs from the prevailing group norms and values within the profession. How should clinicians deal with their own values in such cases? And how should young clinicians be learning to navigate through the intricate patchwork of interests, expectations, power relations, and conflicting values?

There is no blueprint for this. The least one may expect is that professionals learn to identify the patient's orientation on core values and on religious/spiritual issues; that they are able to address the patient's values and religious/spiritual concerns; that they are aware of their own values and religious/spiritual concerns and the possible biases that may result from them; and that they are able to discuss their biases and concerns in a professional context (e.g., consultation, coaching). In the literature on medical specialist training, much emphasis is put on learning on the spot, and rightly so. Teaching should take place in the clinical setting, by role modeling, by case discussions, in clinical rounds, and via interdisciplinary exchanges (Marrero, Bell, Dunn, & Roberts, 2013). Teaching should preferably focus on process rather than content when it aims at a change of attitude. There is some evidence that a process-oriented, clinically focused approach results in positive change in perceived competency in residents (Awaad, Ali, Salvador, & Bandstra, 2015).

THE EDUCATOR 2: RESPONSIBLY DEALING WITH ONE'S RELIGIOUS AND SPIRITUAL ISSUES

Dealing with religious/spiritual issues by definition interferes with one's own value system. Value negotiation is at the heart of the encounter with the patient (Woodbridge & Fulford, 2004). Professionalism is the competence that is relevant in this context. There is a tendency in the medical educational literature to focus on professional behavior as a more or less measurable aspect of professionalism. This seems wise, given the fact that theoretical accounts of professionalism are easily perceived as just words—words that strongly contrast with lapses in professionalism which are inevitable and part of the hidden curriculum. However, it is precisely the intersection with religiosity/spirituality that may make clinicians aware of the presence of another dimension of professionalism: the ability to reflect on value-laden issues that interfere with the therapeutic relationship; the capacity to address relevant normative issues in a sensitive way; and, most of all, the ability to embody these competences in an attitude that is open-minded, respectful, sensitive, and interested. It is a competence that requires verbal skills and a sufficiently rich vocabulary.

Professionalism, conceived in this way, is a second-order capacity that helps clinicians to relate to their own role fulfilment and to integrate their (usually implicit) professional self-understanding with an understanding of what the patient needs and what psychiatry as a medical specialty may offer. Acquiring this competence is not easy and requires a safe space to explore one's personal engagement and to disclose possibly sensitive material (Campbell, Stuck, & Frinks, 2012; Willen, 2013). It is a learning process that runs parallel with the development of psychotherapeutic skills. One of the most important psychotherapeutic skills is the ability to assess and identify content and process synchronically. What the patient says should be compared with how she behaves, in relation to the therapist/psychiatrist and to herself. Early in their training, psychiatry residents often say that the synchronic monitoring of content and interaction is among the most difficult skills they have to acquire. Something similar holds for the process of value negotiation. This process requires a synchronic monitoring of the implicit and explicit values of the patient and of oneself (content) as well as the interaction between the patient and oneself (process). It presupposes a clear view of one's targets and an ability to adapt these targets pragmatically according to what patients allow and need in a given situation.

Interestingly, there has been some discussion in the literature about this issue from the perspective of religion and spirituality. Kuczewski (2007), who endorses the view of professionalism as a second-order (reflective) competence, discussed the role of religiosity/spirituality in the context of decision making and treatment planning. He suggested that there are two promising approaches for helping patients and their families to productively engage in the decision-making process. First, patient-centred interviewing techniques can be employed to explore the patient's religious/spiritual beliefs and successfully incorporate them into choices. This approach goes one step further than just trying to know more about the patient's worldview. Patient-centered interviewing is an attempt to contextualize diagnostic reasoning and shared decision making by engaging with the patient's world and by doing more than mere information gathering. This engagement begins by showing interest in how patients interpret what is going on. And it extends to attempts to make sense of treatment options by explaining their rationale in terms that fit with the patient's view of life.

A second, more radical approach to the decision process may be needed in some more recalcitrant conflicts regarding treatment plans. Such situations may require that clinicians become more involved and personally engaged in discussion and disclosure of religious/spiritual worldviews. Kuczewski (2007) referred in this context to what he called "rich models of informed consent," such as the transparency model. The transparency model, originally proposed by Brody (1989), sees as the goal of informed consent that patients and physicians, when needed, make their own thinking transparent to each other. Both parties, in other words, disclose relevant aspects of their attitude toward their roles, either as patient or as clinician. This self-disclosure may include information about one's worldview and/or perspective on life insofar as it is relevant for the purpose of the consultation.

Kuczewski (2007) discussed several examples in which such self-reflective disclosure diminishes the interpersonal gap between the clinician and patient (see also Lidz, Appelbaum, & Meisel, 1988). Treatment decisions are often intertwined with affectively highly loaded and existential issues. The discussion about treatment options can sometimes be better addressed at this affective and existential level. Traditional models of informed consent and shared decision making are based on exchange of information and on free and rational choice. These models leave little room for the exploration of affective and existential themes and how the affective-existential dynamic interferes with clinical decision making. The heat of the professional's own existential involvement may sometimes be needed to bring the client to a point at which he or she is able to give up self-destructive closure or acting out (see, for example, in Case 1 in this chapter).

THE PROFESSIONAL 1: ETHICAL IMPLICATIONS OF PROFESSIONALISM WITH RESPECT TO RELIGIOUS/ SPIRITUAL ISSUES IN THE PATIENT

How one thinks about the ethical implications of professionalism with respect to religious/ spiritual issues depends, finally, on one's appreciation of the role and relevance of values and worldviews for professionalism. There are different ways of conceptualizing this role and relevance. Balboni, Peteet, and Puchalski (2014) described three models of integration, each of which put emphasis on different aspects of the intersection between religiosity/spirituality and psychiatric practice, without excluding one another.

The whole-person model builds on the World Health Organization's definition of health and the interprofessional model of spiritual care (Puchalski et al., 2009). It opts for a biopsychosocial-spiritual model of care (Sulmasy, 2002) and sees it as an obligation of every professional to attend to the whole person. This approach considers religiosity/spirituality as a domain of care in its own right, one requiring expertise that is as specialized as the expertise that is needed for other domains. It implies teamwork, given the diversity in expertise between professions, and expects the chaplain, as spiritual care specialist, to be fully integrated in the team. It entails a view of medical care that puts emphasis on healing, which goes further than curing. The notion of healing aims at wholeness and meaningfulness and at the relation between physician and patient, which ideally should be characterized by authenticity, compassion, and awareness of the transformative potential of the clinical encounter.

Case 1

Sarah, a 23-year-old fashion student, was in psychotherapy because of an eating disorder and depressive complaints. Her early attachment relations were unsafe and unstable. She has had regular episodes with suicidality, automutilation, and different forms of manipulative behaviour. After 1½ years of psychotherapy and another suicidal episode, she finally told her therapist (Monica) about her sense of utter isolation and loneliness and her inability to give shape to her life. Sarah's sense of isolation resonated with the therapist's own feelings of loneliness, isolation, and powerlessness related to her recent, painful divorce. Tears came up and Monica could not help but cry briefly. Sarah was shocked, and Monica apologized. She explained that she was moved by what Sarah said, that it resonated with a recent episode in her own life about which she could go into detail, but that she could feel how deep Sarah's sense of isolation was. Later, in an intervision group, Monica described what had happened and how ashamed she felt about not being in control. The group supported her, one member discussed a similar situation, and the group suggested that she wait to see how the patient would react.

The therapy moved on, and after a few months Sarah said: "You know, Monica, the moment I saw you crying, . . . it was the first time I really felt a connection with you. You really saw my pain, and I felt that. It is strange, but from that moment on, my feeling of isolation lost its grip on me. Other things became more important, and I am now more in control."

The existential functioning model requires clinicians to attend to existential themes in the lives of their patients. Examples of these themes are hope, identity, meaning/purpose, morality, and autonomy/authority. These themes may become important because of underlying spiritual distress, or they may give rise to such distress. Balboni et al. (2014) construed a difference between emotional, existential, and spiritual distress and suggested that existential distress is about how the world is experienced, whereas spiritual distress is about how the world "is." This distinction might sound somewhat artificial, but it is tenable to say that existential distress concerns a broad range of themes that all refer to one's being-in-the-world, whereas spiritual distress is more about what gives direction to this being-in-the-world—one's hopes, one's faith, and one's deepest motivations.

A third model is marked by open pluralism. This model includes the larger cultural and institutional contexts in which mental health care is delivered, including the values and ideas that are inherent to these contexts. The idea is that these contexts and spheres have their own normative anchor points, each with their own "plausibility structure." The term *plausibility structure* is adopted from the work of sociologist Peter Berger (1967), who argued that as a result of the process of division of labor, there has emerged a plurality of social spheres, each having its own set of values and arguments to explain and justify its existence and its relation to other social structures and institutions. The process of division of labor consists of "repeating and overlapping patterns of bifurcations" which finally has resulted in the dichotomization between the spiritual and the non-spiritual. In other words, the current separation of spirituality and medicine is not so much the result of developments within the science and practice of medicine as it is rooted in a larger historical and social process that has led to a division of tasks and, finally, to noncommunication between professionals working in the fields of medicine and spiritual care. Adherents of the open plurality model argue that this might not be the end point and that other constructions of social reality are possible, especially in open and plural societies. Hospitals and other care facilities can be seen as realities which are rooted in cultures and communities that perceive spirituality as interwoven with every aspect of human life. A fully developed pluralist approach would welcome expression of spiritual traditions on a social and institutional level (i.e., in the practice of medicine itself) (see also Curlin & Hall, 2005). A case example is given in Case 2.

Case 2

Fatima was a first-year resident in psychiatry. She was Muslim and had asked the director of residency training whether she would be allowed to wear a head scarf when working with patients. She said that for her it would be the proper thing to do and that it would not negatively interfere with her work. "By wearing a head scarf, I am expressing my faith," she said. "I am aware that this has an impact on how patients will perceive me, but I can explain to them that my faith teaches me to be trustworthy as a doctor and to value human life." The director of residency training hesitated and consulted the team of supervisors. It was decided that Fatima would be allowed to wear a head scarf and that her interaction with patients would be closely monitored. One of the arguments was that other residents also wore symbols and clothed themselves in ways that referred to who they were and what they believed. Another was that we live in a pluralist society and that this pluralism should also be reflected in the composition of future professional groups. It also was brought up that the problem was not having a religion as such but how to develop a reflective attitude that enables residents to deal with their personal beliefs without violating the ethics of the profession.

One of the most important insights of the open plurality view is that it points to the limitations of therapeutic neutrality (i.e., the view that considers separation between the medical and the spiritual as the default position). The historical process leading to the separation between medicine and spirituality is neither self-evident nor neutral. And the very fact of the separation between these fields construes its own reality—one in which professionals view religiosity/spirituality as outside their scope of competence and interest and in which they are more inclined to ignore religious/spiritual issues in the lives of their patients and to abstain from personal engagement with these issues in the consulting room. The open pluralism approach helps to show that the neutrality option is one among many other views on professionalism.

THE PROFESSIONAL 2: ETHICAL IMPLICATIONS OF PROFESSIONALISM WITH RESPECT TO RELIGIOUS/ SPIRITUAL ISSUES IN ONE'S ROLE FULFILLMENT AS A PROFESSIONAL

Balboni et al. (2014) emphasized that the three models do not exclude one another; rather, they highlight different elements of a more integrative view. In the context of mental healthcare, with its current emphasis on competencies, emphasis should be put on the affective, reflexive, and moral aspects of the competence of professionalism. The model depicted in Box 22.2 may help structure our thinking about what is meant here. It gives a sketch of how affective, reflexive, and morally sensitive attuning to the needs of the patient might be conceived (i.e., as embedded in relations, both to the patient and to oneself). It is especially this latter element, the attunement of one's own basic commitments and concerns to one's role in specific contexts, that is easily overlooked in hectic daily clinical life. One could conceive of this attuning as a narrative describing one's personal history in the profession of psychiatry, a history that itself is determined by role models, contexts, one's own morality, and spirituality, implicit or explicit, all in the context of larger institutional and societal changes (economic, juridical, social) and scientific developments. Attuning to the needs of the patient implies always and at the same time attuning to one's own role in all these contexts and in relation to all these factors.

The diagram depicts how the patient relates to her own illness (2), sketches the influence of contextual factors on the formation and manifestation of illnesses at different levels (individual, institutional, and societal [3]), highlights how the condition of the patient may contribute to the patient's relation to the illness (4), and pays attention to the influence of a whole range of person-related factors on how the patient relates to the illness—factors like as character, personal values, biographically determined preoccupations and sensitivities, and ultimate concerns. It depicts the activity of the professional as (ideally) focused on all five of these themes (A) and as related to a multilayered context (C), which itself influences all other relations. Relation (B) indicates that the professional as person relates to his or her own role. This self-relating as a professional is in turn influenced by one's factual role fulfillment (D) and by person-related factors such as personality, biographically determined preoccupations, and sensitivities (E).

Moral sensitivity and the capacity to reflect on one's own biases and inclinations belong to the core competences that are required for ethically appropriate dealing with religious/spiritual issues in mental healthcare. Box 22.2 underscores that the professional does not coincide with his or her professional role and is more than just a bundle of competencies and skills. (For a broader perspective, see Radden & Sadler, 2010.) The neutrality thesis, which as we have

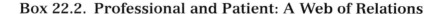

Box 22.2. Professional and Patient: A Web of Relations

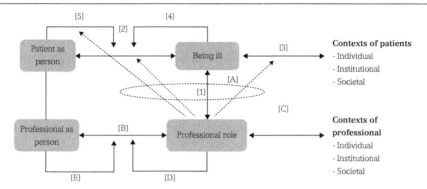

Attuning to the patient and to one's role as professional

In his or her professional role, the professional pays attention to different aspects of being ill [1–5]

1. Professional focuses on manifestations of illness
2. Interaction between patient and illness
3. Interaction between context and illness
4. Influence of being ill on the way the patient deals with the disorder
5. Influence of the person on the way the patient deals with being ill

In his or her professional role, the professional relates in different ways to his or her own professional role fulfilment [A–E]

A. Professional role in its fullest sense
B. Attitude toward and dealing with professional role
C. Interaction between professional role and context
D. Influence of professional role on attitude toward professional role
E. Influence of the person on attitude toward professional role

Source: Glas (in press).

seen leads to a separation between the fields of psychiatry and religiosity/spirituality, is not self-evident; nor is it the only tenable position in an era that puts emphasis on evidence and a solid scientific basis. The neutrality position is itself an expression of a particular stance toward professional role fulfilment, one that considers personal involvement to be relevant only insofar as it sustains the scientific integrity of professional work. The side effect of this stance is that something else is communicated as well, between the lines: The subjective reactions of the patient to his or her illness are relevant only insofar as they can be accounted for in terms that fit the science-based conceptual framework of the psychiatrist. Everything else will inevitably be seen as merely idiosyncratic and subjective, and this message will become part of religiosity/spirituality the hidden curriculum.

CONCLUSION

Our reflection on ethical considerations about religious/spiritual issues in psychiatric training has gone over into a discussion about the nature of professionalism and the identity of the psychiatrist. An important element of professionalism consists of morally sensitive reflection about, and dealing with, one's stance toward one's professional role. Being a psychiatrist is more than having a bundle of skills; relating, as a professional, to these skills is also an important element. Ethically sensitive dealing with religious/spiritual issues in psychiatry not only requires insight into the religious/spiritual needs of the patient. It also presupposes insight into the affective and moral and spiritual aspects of this intrapersonal dynamic of oneself as professional, given the impact of the contexts in which one's professional life evolves. This dynamic can be phrased in terms of a narrative—a story about oneself as professional. Sharing these narratives and probing for alternative routes may open up one's mind and provide fresh perspectives on how to deal with the tensions and brokenness that are inevitably part of our professional lives.

REFERENCES

American Psychiatric Association, Committee on Religion and Psychiatry. (1990). Guidelines regarding possible conflict between psychiatrists' religious commitments and psychiatric practice. *American Journal of Psychiatry, 147*(4), 542.

American Psychiatric Association. (2006a). *Practice guidelines for the psychiatric evaluation of adults* (2nd ed.). Washington, DC: American Psychiatric Publishing.

American Psychiatric Association. (2006b). *Resource document on religious/spiritual commitments and psychiatric practice.* Washington, DC: American Psychiatric Publishing.

American Psychiatric Association. (2013). *Diagnostic and Statistical Manual of Mental Disorders, 5th Edition.* Washington: American Psychiatric Publishing.

Awaad, R., Ali, S., Salvador, M., & Bandstra, B. (2015). A process-oriented approach to teaching religion and spirituality in psychiatry residency training. *Academic Psychiatry, 39,* 654–660.

Baetz, M., & Toews, J. (2009). Clinical implications of research on religion, spirituality, and mental health *Canadian Journal of Psychiatry, 54*(5), 292–301.

Balboni, M. J., Puchalski, C. M., & Peteet, J. R. (2014). The relationship between medicine, spirituality and religion: Three models of integration. *Journal of Religion and Health, 53,* 1586–1598.

Balboni, M. J., Bandini, J., Mitchel., C., Epstein-Peterson, Z. D., Amobi, A., Cahill, J, . . . Balboni, T. (2015). Religion, spirituality, and the hidden curriculum: Medical student and faculty reflections. *Journal of Pain and Symptom Management, 50*(4), 507–515.

Berger, P. L. (1967). *The sacred canopy: Elements of a sociological theory of religion* (1st ed.). Garden City, NY: Doubleday.

Best, M., Butow, P., & Olver, I. (2015). Do patients want doctors to talk about spirituality? A systematic literature review. *Patient Education and Counselling, 98,* 1320–1328.

Best, M., Butow, P., & Olver, I. (2016). Doctors discussing religion and spirituality: A systematic literature review. *Palliative Medicine, 30*(4), 327–337.

Bowman, E. S. (2009). Teaching religious and spiritual issues. In P. Huguelet & H. G. Koenig (Eds.), *Religion and spirituality in psychiatry* (pp. 332–353). Cambridge, England: Cambridge University Press.

Brody, H. (1989). Transparency: Informed consent in primary care. *Hastings Center Report, 19,* 5–9.

Campbell, N., Stuck, C., & Frinks, L. (2012). Spirituality training in residency: Changing the culture of a program. *Academic Psychiatry, 36*(1), 56–59.

Cook, C. C. H. (2013). Recommendations for psychiatrists on spirituality and religion: Position statement PS03/2013. Royal College of Psychiatrists. Retrieved from https://www.rcpsych.ac.uk/pdf/PS03_2013.pdf.

Curlin, F. A., & Hall, D. E. (2005). Strangers or friends? A proposal for a new spirituality-in-medicine ethic. *Journal of General Internal Medicine, 20*, 370–374.

Curlin, F. A., Lawrence, R. E., Odell, S., Chin, M. H., Lantos, J. D., Koenig, H. G., & Meador, K. G. (2007). Religion, spirituality, and medicine: Psychiatrists' and other physicians' differing observations, interpretations, and clinical approaches. *American Journal of Psychiatry, 164*, 1825–1831.

Daaleman, T. P., Kinghorn, W. A., Newton, W. P. & Meador, K. G. (2011). Rethinking professionalism in medical education through formation. *Family Medicine, 43*(5), 325–329.

Dik, B. J., & Duffy, R. D. (2009). Calling and vocation at work: Definitions and prospects for research and practice. *Counseling Psychology, 37*, 424–450.

Duffy, R. D., Allan, B. A., & Bott, E. M. (2012). Calling and life satisfaction among undergraduate students: Investigating mediators and moderators. *Journal of Happiness Studies, 13*, 469–479.

Duffy, R. D., Manuel, R. S., Borges, N. J., & Bott, E. (2011). Calling, vocational development, and well being: A longitudinal study of medical students. *Journal of Vocational Behavior, 79*, 361–366.

Gabbard, G., Roberts, L. W., Crisp-Hahn, H., Ball, V., Hobday, G., & Rachal, F. (2012). *Professionalism in psychiatry.* Washington, DC: American Psychiatric Publishing.

Glas, G. (in press). *Psychiatry as normative practice.* Philosophy, Psychiatry, Psychology.

Grabovac, A. D., Clark, N., & McKenna, M. (2008). Pilot study and evaluation of postgraduate course on "The Interface Between Spirituality, Religion and Psychiatry." *Academic Psychiatry, 32*, 332–337.

Grabovac, A. D., & Ganesan, S. (2003). Spirituality and religion in Canadian psychiatric residency training. *Canadian Journal of Psychiatry, 48*(3), 171–175.

Gustafson, J. M. (1982). Professions as "callings." *The Social Service Review, 56*, 501–515.

Hafferty, F. W., & Franks, R. (1994). The hidden curriculum, ethics teaching, and the structure of medical education. *Academic Medicine, 69*(11), 861–871.

Huguelet, P., & Koenig, H. G. (Eds.). (2009). *Religion and spirituality in psychiatry.* Cambridge, England: Cambridge University Press

Josephson, A. M., & Peteet, J. R. (2007). Talking with patients about spirituality and worldview: Practical interviewing techniques and strategies. *Psychiatric Clinics of North America, 30*, 181–197.

Josephson, A. M., Peteet, J. R., & Tasman, A. (2010). Religion and the training of psychotherapists. In P. J. Verhagen, H. M. Praag, J. J. López-Ibor, J. L. Cox, & D. Moussaoui (Eds.), *Religion and psychiatry: Beyond boundaries* (pp. 571–586). Oxford, England: Wiley-Blackwell.

Kinghorn, W. A., McEvoy, M. D., Michel, A., & Balboni, M. (2007). Professionalism in modern medicine: Does the emperor have any clothes?. *Academic Medicine, 82*, 40–45.

Kozak, L., Boynton, L., Bentley, J., & Bezy, E. (2010). Introducing spirituality, religion and culture curricula in the psychiatry residency programme. *Medical Humanities, 36*(1), 48–51.

Kuczewski, M. G. (2007). Talking about spirituality in the clinical setting: Can being professional require being personal? *American Journal of Bioethics, 7*(7), 4–11.

Larson, D. B., Lu, F. G., & Swyers, J. P. (1997). *Model curriculum for psychiatric residency training programs: Religion and spirituality in clinical practice.* Rockville, MD: National Institute for Healthcare Research.

Lawrence, R. M., & Duggal, A. (2001). Spirituality in psychiatric education and training. *Journal of the Royal Society of Medicine, 94*(6), 303–305.

Levinson, W., Ginsburg, S., Hafferty, F. W., & Lucey, C. R. (2014). *Understanding medical professionalism.* New York, NY: McGraw-Hill.

Lidz, C. W., Appelbaum, P. S., & Meisel, A. (1988). Two models of implementing informed consent. *Archives of Internal Medicine, 148*, 1385–1389.

Marrero, I., Bell, M., Dunn, L. B., & Roberts, L. W. (2013). Assessing professionalism and ethics knowledge and skills: Preferences of psychiatry residents. *Academic Psychiatry, 37*(6), 392–397.

McCarthy, M. K., & Peteet, J. R. (2003). Teaching residents about religion and spirituality. *Harvard Review of Psychiatry, 11*, 225–228.

Peteet, J. R. (2014). What is the place of clinicians' religious or spiritual commitments in psychotherapy? A virtues-based perspective. *Journal of Religion and Health, 53*(4), 1190–1198.

The Psychiatry Milestone Project. (2014). *Journal of Graduate Medical Education, 6*(1 Suppl 1), 284–304. http://doi.org/10.4300/JGME-06-01s1-11

Puchalski, C. M., Ferrell, B., Virani, R., Otis-Green, S., Baird, P., Bull, J., . . . Sulmasy, D (2009). Improving the quality of spiritual care as a dimension of palliative care. *Journal of Palliative Medicine, 12*(10), 885–904.

Puchalski, C. M., Kheirbek, R., Doucette, A., Martin, T., & Yang, Y. T. (2013). Spirituality as an essential element of person-centered compassionate care: A pilot training program for clinicians. *Journal of Medicine and the Person, 11*, 56–61.

Puchalski, C. M., Larson, D. B., & Lu, F. G. (2000). Spirituality courses in psychiatry residency programs. *Psychiatric Annals, 30*, 543–548.

Radden, J., & Sadler, J. Z. (2010). *The virtuous psychiatrist: Character ethics in psychiatric practice.* New York, NY: Oxford University Press

Roberts, L. W., & Dyer, A. R. (2004). *Concise guide to ethics in mental health care.* Washington, DC: American Psychiatric Publishing.

Sloan, R. P., Bagiella, E., VandeCreek, L., Hover, M., Casalone, C., Jinpu Hirsch, T., . . . Poulos, P. (2000). Should physicians prescribe religious activities? *New England Journal of Medicine, 342*(25), 1913–1916.

Sulmasy, D. P. (2002) A biopsychosocial-spiritual model for the care of patients at the end of life. *The Gerontologist, 42*(3), 24–33.

Verhagen, P. J., & Cook, C. C. H. (2010). Epilogue: Proposal for a World Psychiatric Association consensus or position statement on spirituality and religion in psychiatry. In P. J. Verhagen, H. M. Praag, J. J. López-Ibor, J. L. Cox, & D. Moussaoui (Eds.), *Religion and psychiatry: Beyond boundaries* (pp. 615–629). Oxford, England: Wiley-Blackwell.

Verhagen, P. J., & Cox, J. L. (2010). Multicultural education and training in religion and spirituality. In P. J. Verhagen, H. M. Praag., J. J. López-Ibor, J. L. Cox, & D. Moussaoui (Eds.), *Religion and psychiatry: Beyond boundaries* (pp. 587–613). Oxford, England: Wiley-Blackwell.

Willen, S. S. (2013). Confronting a "big huge gaping wound": Emotion and anxiety in a cultural sensitivity course for psychiatry residents. *Culture, Medicine and Psychiatry, 37*(2), 253–279.

Woodbridge, K., & Fulford, K. W. M. (2004). *Whose values? A workbook for values-based practice in mental health care.* London, England: Sainsbury Centre for Mental Health.

Yoon, J. D., Shin, J. H., Nian, A. L., & Curlin, F. A. (2015). Religion, sense of calling, and the practice of medicine: Findings from a national survey of primary care physicians and psychiatrists. *Southern Medical Journal 108*(3), 189–195.

Index

Page numbers followed by *f* indicate figures; page numbers followed by *t* indicate tables; page numbers followed by *b* indicate boxes

275